Critical Thinking, Clinical Reasoning, and Clinical Judgment

A Practical Approach

Critical Thinking, Clinical Reasoning, and Clinical Judgment

A Practical Approach

EDITION

Rosalinda Alfaro-LeFevre, MSN, RN, ANEF
President
Teaching Smart/Learning Easy
Stuart, Florida
http://www.AlfaroTeachSmart.com

ELSEVIER

Elsevier
3251 Riverport Lane
St. Louis, Missouri 63043

Notices

Practitioners and researchers must always rely on their own experience and knowledge in evaluating
and using any information, methods, compounds or experiments described herein. Because of rapid
advances in the medical sciences, in particular, independent verification of diagnoses and drug dosages
should be made. To the fullest extent of the law, no responsibility is assumed by Elsevier, authors, editors
or contributors for any injury and/or damage to persons or property as a matter of products liability,
negligence or otherwise, or from any use or operation of any methods, products, instructions, or ideas
contained in the material herein.

Previous editions copyrighted 2017, 2013, 2009, 2004, 1999, and 1995.

Library of Congress Control Number: 2019939196

Executive Content Strategist: Lee Henderson
Senior Content Development Manager: Ellen Wurm-Cutter
Content Development Specialist: Melissa Rawe
Publishing Services Manager: Shereen Jameel
Senior Project Manager: Umarani Natarajan
Design Direction: Patrick Ferguson

Printed in China

Last digit is the print number: 9 8 7 6 5 4 3 2 1

Working together
to grow libraries in
developing countries

www.elsevier.com • www.bookaid.org

ABOUT THE AUTHOR

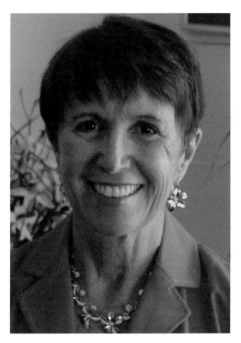

Known for making difficult content easy to understand, **Rosalinda Alfaro-LeFevre, MSN, RN, ANEF,** is a National League for Nursing Academy of Nursing Education Fellow. She has written about critical thinking and clinical reasoning since 1986 and has received a **Sigma Theta Tau Best Pick** and **AJN Book of the Year** award. Because her books bring clarity to difficult topics, they're used throughout the world.

Rosalinda has over 20 years of clinical experience—mostly in the ICU, CCU, and ED—and has taught in associate degree and baccalaureate nursing programs. She is the president of Teaching Smart/Learning Easy in Stuart, Florida, a company dedicated to helping people acquire the intellectual and interpersonal skills needed to deal with today's personal and workplace challenges.

Born in Buenos Aires, Argentina, to a British mother and an Argentine father, Rosalinda immigrated as a child to the United States from Argentina via Canada. Although Rosalinda says she's an American at heart, she points out that she is blessed with multicultural experiences, presenting nationally and internationally and enjoying close relationships with her family in Spain, Argentina, and the United Kingdom. You can learn more about Rosalinda at http://www.AlfaroTeachSmart.com.

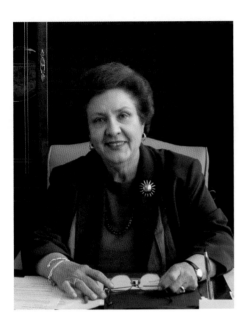

M. Louise Fitzpatrick, EdD, RN, FAAN, beloved Connelly Endowed Dean and Professor, led Villanova University's College of Nursing from 1978 until her death in 2017. During those years, she developed the college into a premier nursing program recognized repeatedly by the National League for Nursing as a Center of Excellence in Nursing Education. She is remembered as one of the most vibrant, transformative leaders in the history of Villanova University. To honor her legacy, the College of Nursing is now named the M. Louise Fitzpatrick College of Nursing. *Photo Courtesy of Villanova University.*

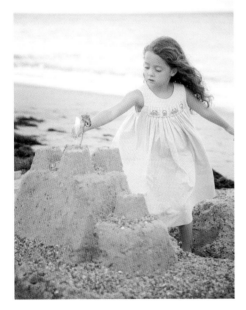

Lilly Roderick, a natural leader, lived in Kitty Hawk, North Carolina. Adopted, she and her mother, Tristan, were a match made in heaven. Lilly often called for group hugs with my twin grandsons, Reid and Grant. In 2016, Lilly died 3 weeks after her fifth birthday from a hemorrhage while recovering at home (9 days after a routine tonsillectomy). Later, I learned that there are three times when risk of post-tonsillectomy hemorrhage is high: 6 minutes, 6 hours, and 6 days after surgery (this is anecdotal evidence; most references say "around a week" rather than "6 days"). Lilly had an amazing life in the Outer Banks with her family and friends—the joy she brought will forever make us smile!
Photo courtesy of www.meganbeasleyphotography.com.

ADVISORS AND REVIEWERS

A note of thanks: Without the timely and insightful reviews and advice of the experts listed on these pages, this book would not have been possible. The author wishes to also acknowledge the diligent work of the translators of previous editions—you amaze me.

CONTENT REVIEWERS AND ADVISORS

Miriam de Abreu Almeida, PhD, RN
Professor, School of Nursing
Graduate Nursing Coordinator
Federal University of Rio Grande do Sul
Porto Alegre, Brazil

Ricardo Ernesto Blanco Alfaro
Murcia, Spain

Ledjie Ballard, MSN, CRNA, ARNP
Kalispell, Montana

Deanne A. Blach, MSN, RN, CNE
President, Nurse Educator
DB Productions of NWAR, Inc.
Green Forest, Arkansas

Judy Boychuk Duchscher, BScN, MN, PhD, RN
Associate Professor
Thomson Rivers University Nursing School
Kamloops, British Columbia, Canada
Executive Director, Nursing the Future (http://www.nursingthefuture.ca)

Susan A. Boyer, DNP, RN-BC
Executive Director, Vermont Nurses in Partnership
Ascutney, Vermont

Hilda H. Brito, MSN, RN, BC
Interim Director of Professional Development
University of Miami Hospital and Clinics
Miami, Florida

Ruth I. Hansten, MBA, PhD, RN, FACHE
Principal, Hansten Healthcare PLLC
Santa Rosa, California
www.Hansten.com, www.RROHC.com

Robert Hess, PhD, RN, FAAN
CEO and Founder
Forum for Shared Governance
Hobe Sound, Florida

Donna D. Ignatavicius, MS, RN, CNE, ANEF
President
DI Associates
Littleton, Colorado

Sharon E. Johnson, MSN, RNC, NE-BC
Former Director (Retired) of Home Health and
     Hospice
Main Line Health Home Care
Radnor, Pennsylvania

Nancy Konzelmann, MS, RN-BC, CPHQ
Quality Coordinator
Port St. Lucie Medical Center
Port St. Lucie, Florida

Corrine R. Kurzen, MEd, MSN, RN
Former Director (Retired), Practical Nursing
     Program
School District of Philadelphia
Philadelphia, Pennsylvania

Heidi Pape Laird
Systems Programmer
Partners HealthCare
Boston, Massachusetts

Holly B. Laird, DO
Resident Physician
Osteopathic Neuromusculoskeletal Medicine
SBH Health System
Bronx, New York

Nola Lanham, MSN, RN-BC
Manager, Clinical Education
Baptist Health
Jacksonville, Florida

Maria Teresa Luis, PhD, RN
Barcelona, Spain

Bette Mariani, PhD, RN, ANEF
Associate Professor of Nursing
M. Louise Fitzpatrick College of Nursing
Villanova University
Villanova, Pennsylvania
2018–2019 President, International Nursing
    Association for Clinical Simulation and
    Learning

Melani McGuire, MSN, CRNP
Malvern, Pennsylvania

Jeanne Liliane Marlene Michel, PhD, RN
Professor, Nursing Department
Federal University of São Carlos
São Carlos, São Paulo, Brazil

Judith C. Miller, MS, RN
Nursing Tutorial and Consulting Services
Henniker, New Hampshire

Charles L. Nola
Aerospace Engineer
Madison, Alabama

Marilyn H. Oermann, PhD, RN, ANEF, FAAN
Thelma M. Ingles Professor of Nursing
Duke University School of Nursing
Durham, North Carolina
Editor, *Nurse Educator* and *Journal of Nursing Care*
    Quality

Terri Sue Patterson, MSN, RN, CRRN,
    FIALCP
President, Nursing Consultation Services
Plymouth Meeting, Pennsylvania

William F. Perry, MA, RN
Informatics Consultant
Beavercreek, Ohio

Andrew Phillips, PhD, RN
Assistant Professor, School of Nursing
MGH Institute of Health Professions
Partners Healthcare
Boston, Massachusetts

Joanne Profetto-McGrath, PhD, RN
Professor, School of Nursing
University of Alberta
Edmonton, Alberta, Canada
Inaugural Fellow – Canadian Nurse Educator Institute

Cherie R. Rebar, PhD, MBA, RN, COI
Professor of Nursing
Wittenberg University
Springfield, Ohio

James Riley
Healthcare Executive
Richmond, Virginia

Matthew Riley, PsyD, BCBA
Executive Director
The Timothy School
Berwyn, Pennsylvania

Michael H. Riley, MBA, MSW, LPC, EMT
Account Manager
Praesidium, Inc.
Arlington, Texas

Laura Sherburn
Chief Executive Officer, Primary Care
Doncaster Ltd.
Doncaster
South Yorkshire, England

Rose O. Sherman, EdD, RN, NEA-BC, FAAN
Professor, Christine E. Lynn College of Nursing
Director, Nursing Leadership Institute
Florida Atlantic University
Boca Raton, Florida

Jean Shinners, PhD, RN-BC
Executive Director
Versant Center for the Advancement of Nursing
Las Vegas, Nevada

Kathleen R. Stevens, EdD, RN, ANEF, FAAN
Castella Endowed Distinguished Professor
Director, Improvement Science Research Network
University of Texas Health Science Center
San Antonio, Texas

Carol Taylor, PhD, RN
Senior Clinical Scholar
Kennedy Institute of Ethics
Washington, D.C.
Professor of Nursing and Medicine
Georgetown University, School of Nursing and
    Health Studies
Washington, D.C.

Brent W. Thompson, PhD, RN
President
HandheldCare LLC
Associate Professor (Retired) Department of Nursing
West Chester University of Pennsylvania
West Chester, Pennsylvania

Elizabeth M. Tsarnas, DNP, ARNP, FNP-BC
Nurse Practitioner
Santoriello Gynecology
Stuart, Florida
Adjunct Professor
Florida Atlantic University
Boca Raton, Florida

**Theresa M. Valiga, EdD, RN, CNE, ANEF,
    FAAN**
Professor Emerita
Duke University School of Nursing
Durham, North Carolina

Esperanza Zuriguel-Pérez, PhD
Head of Nursing Research Group
Knowledge Management Department
Hospital Vall d'Hebron
Barcelona, Spain

CRITICAL THINKING: AN INTERNATIONAL HEALTH CARE IMPERATIVE

Sweeping changes in health care and nursing education—many driven by information technology and research on best practices that improve quality, safety, and learning while decreasing costs—are revolutionizing how we think, learn, and give patient care.

Although the amount of change we deal with on a daily basis can sometimes feel overwhelming, revising this edition gave me "a front-row seat" to the significant progress we're making. This edition has been completely transformed to address what it takes to think critically and succeed in 21st-century practice and education.

Critical thinking, clinical reasoning, decision-making, and clinical judgment are challenging to teach and learn. Using plain language, practical examples, and easy-to-understand illustrations, this book brings the clarity needed to make profound changes in personal and professional reasoning. It encourages you to become self-aware and helps you chart a course to developing thinking habits that promote sound reasoning in clinical, teaching, and testing challenges.

Here's the big picture of how this book is organized:

- **Chapters 1 to 3 provide the foundation for developing critical thinking, clinical reasoning, decision-making, and clinical judgment skills.** They describe the relationship among these skills and explore how personal factors like personality, upbringing, and culture affect reasoning. You learn the importance of *safety and learning cultures*—in which everyone focuses on safety and everyone teaches and learns—and gain strategies for simulated, conceptual, and clinical learning, as well as taking high-stakes tests (e.g., the NCLEX® exam).
- **Chapters 4 to 6 focus on reasoning, decision-making, and judgment in the clinical setting,** detailing the knowledge and skills needed to give safe and effective nursing care. These chapters focus on applying clinical reasoning *principles*. Chapter 5 gives the foundation for moral and ethical reasoning, evidence-based practice, quality improvement, professionalism, and leadership. Chapter 6 gives opportunities to practice clinical reasoning and decision-making skills addressed in Chapter 4 by working with case scenarios that are based on real incidents. Example skills in this section include *assessing systematically, detecting signs and symptoms (cues), distinguishing relevant from irrelevant, drawing valid conclusions,* and *setting priorities.*
- **Chapter 7 helps you develop the communication, teamwork, and self-management skills** needed to lead and succeed in interprofessional practice (e.g., dealing with conflict and complaints, navigating change, giving and receiving feedback, and managing time).

WHAT'S NEW TO THIS EDITION

Although the main focus of this book is *practice readiness*—being able to think critically in the context of today's patient-centered, outcome-driven, interprofessional clinical setting—you'll find clear connections between *clinical* terms and terms used in the *Next-Generation NCLEX (NGN)* exam. For example, clinicians tend to use *signs and symptoms;* the NGN clinical judgment model uses *cues* to refer to *signs and symptoms.* Solid content that moves from simple to complex will help you gain virtually all the skills that are likely to be tested in NGN (e.g., recognizing and analyzing cues, evaluating outcomes, generating hypotheses, judging options, and taking action).[1]

Other new content includes:
- How to become a critical thinker
- A detailed discussion of Quality and Safety for Nursing Education (QSEN) and Nurse of the Future (NOF) competencies as addressed by key nursing and health care organizations and publications (see Chapter 1)
- How to apply conceptual learning principles to maximize learning
- The roles of preceptors and nurse residencies
- More on simulation and debriefing
- Strategies to evaluate clinical reasoning
- A completely rewritten Chapter 4 that now includes:
  - Nursing accountability and how to think like a nurse to ensure that "nursing thinking" is included in interprofessional clinical reasoning (you'll see that it's not so much *how* nurses think that makes their contributions unique as it is what they think *about*).
  - How ADPIE (assess, diagnose, plan, implement, and evaluate) and AAPIE (assess, analyze, plan, implement, and evaluate) relate to the nursing process, new clinical judgment models, practice standards, and interprofessional clinical reasoning
  - How to think *with* health information technology (HIT)
  - Detailed clinical reasoning principles that promote sound clinical judgments across health care professions
  - How to make scope-of-practice decisions, set priorities, and delegate care
- The importance of leadership and professionalism
- Virtually all new exercises to promote application and retention of content

WHAT'S THE SAME ABOUT THIS EDITION

The following content and features are retained:
- Making patient and caregiver safety and welfare top priorities in all thinking, including taking responsibility for being "a safety net" when helping co-workers, anticipating what they may need, and pitching in to prevent mistakes
- Using predictive models (*Predict, Prevent, Manage, Promote*)
- Maintaining surveillance (continually monitoring patients to detect signs and symptoms and keep them safe)
- The importance of developing inquisitiveness and self-efficacy
- The roles of logic, intuition, and creativity
- The importance of thinking ahead, thinking-in-action, and thinking back (reflecting on practice)
- How to use *critical thinking indicators* (CTIs) and the 4-Circle Model to facilitate critical thinking development (these models are now used throughout the world[2])
- *Think, Pair, Share* exercises throughout that promote deep learning through peer and expert collaboration
- A full-color design with elements that help you gain a sense of "salience" (what's most important)
- **Access to additional resources**—including the most up-to-date *Evidence-Based Critical Thinking Indicators* document and other tools—at http://www.AlfaroTeachSmart.com

WHO SHOULD READ THIS BOOK?

You should read this book if:
- You're an educator, leader, or preceptor in need of evidence-based strategies and tools to promote critical thinking in students and staff.

- You're a student or beginning nurse and want to be more confident and competent in making patient care decisions.
- You need to prepare for standard tests like the NCLEX exam and professional certification exams.

SUGGESTIONS FOR EDUCATORS

You can use this book to guide a specific course or as an adjunct to other courses. You get the best results if you start to use it in beginning courses and continue to refer to it as you progress through various learning stages. You may even consider making parts of the book required reading *before* starting nursing school. For example, prenursing students can generally benefit from reading Chapters 1 to 3.

Rather than spending endless hours developing PowerPoints and lectures, tell learners to *bring the book to class* and *interact with the content in the book* (a *lot* of time has been spent on presenting the content in logical, understandable ways). Spend your time thinking about *how you can stimulate discussion*. For example, using the *Think, Pair, Share* approach, say, "Take a few minutes to review Table 4.1, then give me your thoughts on novice versus expert thinking." Not only is this approach interactive, it keeps everyone grounded on where content can be found in the text. Developing sound reasoning requires learners to first become aware of content, then *revisit and apply it consistently* until they have developed new habits. All too often, content is inadvertently diluted or changed due to the time and brain power going to *PowerPoint development*. In turn, students say, "You don't have to read the book … it's all in the *PowerPoints*." (We all know how misleading this can be.)

You can download the *Think, Pair, Share* PowerPoint to discuss with students from the POWERPOINT section of www.AlfaroTeachSmart.com.

Box 1 addresses the best way to read this book. Box 2 addresses assumptions and promises that drive how this book has been written and designed.

BOX 1   The Best Way to Read This Book

The best way to read this book is however you choose to read it.

1. If you like the traditional approach, read it from beginning to end. You'll enjoy the narrative, logical approach and numerous scenarios and examples designed to help you understand and remember content.
2. If you like to use your own unique approach—for example, the back-to-front approach (read summaries before text), the "skip around to the stuff that looks interesting" approach, or the "read the stuff that will be on the test first approach"—here are some of the features that help you focus on what's most important.

Preceding Each Chapter
- **This Chapter at a Glance:** Allows you to scan major headings.
- **Learning Outcomes and Key Concepts List:** Help you focus on what's most important and decide where you stand in relation to what you need to learn.

Following Each Chapter
- **Critical Thinking and Clinical Reasoning Exercises:** Direct you to use content, helping you clarify understanding and move information into long-term memory.
- **Key Points/Summary:** Reminds you of the most important content.

Continued

BOX 1   The Best Way to Read This Book—cont'd

Other Features You Need to Know About

- **Response Key:** You can find example responses to all exercises, except *Think, Pair, Share* exercises, in Appendix I.
- **Critical Moments and Other Perspectives:** These sections give simple strategies that make a big difference in results and offer interesting (and sometimes amusing) points of view.

Reading Efficiently

Use an organized and efficient learning approach, for example:

- **Survey:** Scan the abstract, major headings, tables, and illustrations.
- **Question:** Turn major headings into questions.
- **Read:** Read, taking notes and answering your questions.
- **Review, Recite, and Reread:** Review the chapter (or your notes), reciting key content out loud, and then ask yourself, "What's still not clear here?" Read the sections you don't understand again, and raise questions to ask in class or discuss with your peers.

BOX 2   Assumptions and Promises

Before I began to write this book, I made some assumptions:

- You want to learn.
- Your time is valuable, and you don't want to waste it.
- You like to learn the most important things first.
- You learn better when you're motivated, know why information is relevant, and choose your own way of learning.
- You know yourself best, so it's inappropriate for *me* to tell *you* how to think.
- You feel a sense of accomplishment when you gain the knowledge and skills that help you be more independent.

  Because of these assumptions, I promise to:

- Let you know what's most important.
- Use lots of examples and present information in a usable way.
- Give the "reasons behind the rules."
- Encourage you to choose what works for you.
- Help you develop the skills required to be a better thinker, independent learner, and more effective nurse.

PATIENTS, CLIENTS, CONSUMERS, STAKEHOLDERS, AND "HE/SHE"

To reflect that patients and clients are health care consumers who are *individuals* with unique needs, values, perceptions, and motivations, often a fictitious name or "someone," "person," "consumer," or "individual" is used (instead of "patient" or "client"). The term *stakeholder* is now used when talking about all the individuals and groups who have a vested interest in how care is given (e.g., patients, significant others, caregivers, and insurance companies.) *He* and *she* are used interchangeably to avoid the awkwardness of using "he/she."

TELL US WHAT YOU THINK

We want to hear your struggles and concerns. If you have a problem with something, it's likely that others do too. Your problems are our opportunities to learn, improve, and help others with similar issues. Please let me know what you think.

Rosalinda Alfaro-LeFevre, MSN, RN, ANEF
President, Teaching Smart/Learning Easy
http://www.AlfaroTeachSmart.com

REFERENCES

1. NCSBN. *NGN News - Summer 2018*. Retrieved from, www.ncsbn.org; 2018.
2. Zuriguel-Pérez E, Falcó-Pegueroles A, Roldán-Merino J, et al. Development and psychometrics properties of the nursing critical thinking in clinical practice questionnaire. *Worldviews Evidence-Based Nursing*. 2017;14(4):257–264. https://doi.org/10.1111/wvn.12220.

ACKNOWLEDGMENTS

I want to thank my husband, Jim; my stepson, Alex; my daughter-in-law, Hillary; and my grandsons, Reid and Grant, for their love, support, and sense of humor and fun. I also want to thank the rest of my family and the following people for their ongoing support and contribution to my personal and professional growth: Heidi Laird, Ledjie Ballard, Terri Patterson, Grace and Frank Nola, Charlie Nola, Chuck and Pat Morgan, Dan Hankison, Ivonne Bullon, Virginia McFalls, Bill Perry, Brent Thompson, Carol Taylor, Sharon Johnson, Terry Valiga, Mary Ann Rizzolo, Annette Sophocles, Melani McGuire, Maria Sophocles, Barbara Cohen, Patti Cleary, Ruth Hansten, Nancy Konzelman, Hilda Hernandez-Piloto Brito, Esperanza Zuriguel-Pérez, Louise Fitzpatrick, the M. Louise Fitzpatrick College of Nursing Faculty, and the past and present staff nurses of Paoli Hospital, Paoli, Pennsylvania. I can't thank enough those of you who have been willing to advise and give so freely of your time and expertise.

My special thanks go to the following people at Elsevier: Lee Henderson, Executive Content Strategist; Ellen Wurm-Cutter, Senior Content Development Manager; Melissa Rawe, Content Development Specialist; Patrick Ferguson, Designer; Umarani Natarajan, Senior Project Manager; and the sales and marketing staff for their vital roles in making this book successful.

Rosalinda Alfaro-LeFevre, MSN, RN, ANEF
http://www.AlfaroTeachSmart.com

CONTENTS

What Are Critical Thinking, Clinical Reasoning, and Clinical Judgment?

THIS CHAPTER AT A GLANCE...

LEARNING OUTCOMES

After completing this chapter, you should be able to:

1. Compare and contrast *thinking* and *critical thinking*.
2. Explain (or map) how *communication, critical thinking, clinical reasoning, clinical judgment, decision-making, problem-solving*, and *nursing process* are related to one another.
3. Explain why ADPIE gives the foundation for clinical reasoning and passing the NCLEX® and other standard tests.
4. Address the importance of gaining 21st-century Nursing Skills and Quality and Safety for Nursing Education (QSEN) competences.
5. Describe how healthy workplaces, learning cultures, and safety cultures support critical thinking.
6. Describe the key elements of interprofessional practice.
7. Explain (or map) the reasoning phases represented by the acronym ADPIE or AAPIE.
8. Discuss how ADPIE relates to interprofessional clinical reasoning, the nursing process, National Council Licensure Examinations (NCLEX®), and certification exams.
9. Describe (or map) critical thinking as it relates to the scientific method and problem-solving method.
10. Compare and contrast *problem-focused thinking* and *outcome-focused thinking*.
11. Define the term *personal critical thinking indicator* (CTI).
12. Explain why interpersonal skills are as important as clinical skills.
13. Use CTIs, together with the 4-Circle CT model, to identify five critical thinking characteristics or skills you'd like to improve.
14. Compare and contrast *thinking ahead, thinking-in-action*, and *thinking back*.

CRITICAL THINKING: BEHIND EVERY HEALED PATIENT

A powerful quote from an online blog sets the stage for this chapter: "Behind every healed patient is a critical thinking nurse."[1] Critical thinking—your ability to focus your thinking to get the results you need—makes the difference between whether you succeed or fail. It makes the difference between keeping you and your patients safe and being in harm's way. Whether you're trying to set priorities, collaborate with a difficult person, or develop a plan of care, critical thinking— deliberate, informed thought—is the key.

Most students find that they're *well prepared* to do the critical thinking needed to pass the NCLEX® (National Council Licensure Examination). But when they start their first job, they'll realize that they're *underprepared* to function in today's complex clinical setting, where increased patient acuity and decreased length of stay are the norm.[2-4] They find that becoming competent critical thinking clinicians is intellectually, emotionally, and physically challenging, leaving many of them feeling overwhelmed. Because of these issues, retaining new nurses at a time when we really need them is increasingly difficult.

Throughout this book you'll find an interplay of how to develop your *own personal critical thinking abilities* (how to become a critical thinker) and how to gain *nursing critical thinking skills* (key 21st-century nurse skills[5-17]). In short, this book helps you:

- Connect with your talents and blind spots, giving you the clarity and strategies you need to make the most of your own unique way of thinking.
- Gain the insights and confidence you need to need to achieve your personal and professional goals. Many of you—like me when I was young—are unaware of your own amazing potential.
- Develop critical thinking skills that serve patients, families, communities, and yourself well.
- Be prepared to take your place as a valuable member of the health care team, making profound contributions that change the safety and quality of health care.

Developing critical thinking starts with having a good understanding of what it *is*. As a colleague of mine says, too many people think that critical thinking is like an "amorphous blob" that you can't describe—something that you're "just supposed to *do*." To improve thinking, you must be specific about exactly what's involved when thinking critically in various situations.

This chapter helps you start the journey to improving your ability to think critically in two steps: (1) First, you learn why health care organizations and nursing schools stress the need for critical thinking. (2) Second, you examine exactly what it is and how it relates to clinical reasoning, clinical judgment, the nursing process, decision-making, and problem-solving and prevention.

> **GUIDING PRINCIPLE**
>
> **The first step to developing critical thinking is to gain a deep understanding of what it entails in various circumstances.** The saying "one size *doesn't* fit all" applies—critical thinking changes depending on context; what works in one situation may be inappropriate in another.

CRITICAL THINKING: NOT SIMPLY BEING CRITICAL

Critical thinking (CT) doesn't mean simply being negative or full of criticism. It means not accepting information at face value without carefully evaluating it. When you think critically, you examine assumptions, evaluate evidence, and uncover underlying values and reasons before drawing conclusions and making decisions.

In *critical thinking*, the term *critical* may be replaced with *important*. In other words, CT is "important thinking" you need to do in various situations—for example, using evidence-based strategies to assess, prevent, and manage problems. For example, "We're implementing an evidence-based fall prevention protocol to help nurses predict when patients are at risk for falls."

REWARDS OF LEARNING TO THINK CRITICALLY

Learning what CT is—what it "looks like" and how you "do it" when circumstances change—helps you:

- **Gain confidence,** a trait that's crucial for success; lack of confidence is a "brain drain" that impedes thinking.
- **Be safe and autonomous;** it helps you decide when to take initiative and act independently and when to get help.
- **Keep patients safe and improve care quality and job satisfaction** (nothing's more rewarding than seeing patients and families thrive because you made a difference).

Consider how the following points relate to the importance of developing CT skills:

- CT is the key to preventing and solving problems. If you can't think critically, you become a part of the problem.
- CT is crucial to passing tests that demonstrate you're qualified to practice nursing—for example, the NCLEX® and other certification exams.
- In all settings, nurses are expected to take on new responsibilities, collaborate with diverse individuals, and make more independent decisions.
- Nurses' roles within the context of today's workforce, the nursing shortage, social issues, and technology continue to expand. As a nurse, you must be a key player in designing and implementing more effective and efficient health care.
- Today's care complexity requires knowledgeable professionals who are thought oriented rather than task oriented. For the public to value the need for nurses, we must change our image from being simply "a caring, helpful hand" to one that shows we have specific knowledge that's vital to keeping patients safe and helping them get and stay well.
- Patients and families must be active participants in making decisions; as the saying goes, "Nothing about me, without me." Knowing how to teach and empower patients and families to manage their own care requires excellent CT and interpersonal skills.
- CT skills are key to establishing the foundation for lifelong learning, a healthy workplace, and an organizational culture that's more concerned with reporting errors and promoting safety than "pointing fingers" and "blaming" (Box 1.1).

21ST-CENTURY NURSE SKILLS

To gain insight into the complexity of care today, consider the following qualities and skills that key publications and nursing organizations stress you must have to be able to function as a 21st-century nurse (next page).[5–17]

BOX 1.1   Healthy Workplace and Safety and Learning Cultures

Healthy Workplace Environment

Healthy workplace standards form the foundation for a climate that fosters critical thinking by providing an atmosphere that's respectful, healing, and humane. These standards stress the need for (1) effective communication, (2) true collaboration, (3) effective decision-making, (4) appropriate staffing, (5) meaningful recognition, and (6) authentic leadership. A safe and respectful environment requires each standard to be maintained, because studies show that you don't get effective outcomes when any one standard is considered optional.

Safety Culture

When a group has a culture of safety, everyone feels responsible for safety and pursues it on a regular basis. Patient safety is top priority. To identify the main causes of mistakes and build systems to prevent them, there's more concern about reporting errors than placing blame. Nurses, physicians, and technicians look out for one another and feel comfortable pointing out unsafe behaviors (e.g., when hand sanitation has been missed or when safety glasses should be worn). Safety takes precedence over egos or pressures to complete tasks with little help or time. The organization values and rewards such actions.

Learning Culture

In a learning culture, teaching and learning are key parts of daily activities. Everyone is encouraged to create learning opportunities and share information freely. Leaders, teachers, and staff are approachable and promote self-esteem and confidence by treating learners with kindness and showing genuine interest in them as people. Learners are encouraged to feel that they belong to the team. Teaching strategies are tailored to individuals, not tasks. Promoting research and improving care quality is "everyone's job."

References

American Association of Critical Care Nurses. Is Your Workplace Healthy? Retrieved from: https://www.aacn.org/nursing-excellence/healthy-work-environments

The Joint Commission. National Patient Safety Goals. Retrieved from: http://www.jointcommission.org/PatientSafety/NationalPatientSafetyGoals/

© 2018 Alfaro-LeFevre, R. http://www.AlfaroTeachSmart.com

Quality and Safety Education for Nurses (QSEN) Competencies[5]

- **Patient-centered care:** Recognize that patients and families (or their designees) must be the source of control. They must be full partners in the process of giving compassionate, coordinated care that's based on respect for individual preferences, values, and needs.
- **Teamwork and collaboration:** Function effectively within nursing and interprofessional teams, fostering open communication, mutual respect, and shared decision-making to achieve quality patient care.
- **Evidence-based practice:** Integrate the best current evidence with clinical expertise and patient/family preferences and values for delivery of optimal health care.
- **Quality improvement:** Use data to monitor the outcomes of care processes, and use improvement methods to design and test changes continually to improve the quality and safety of health care systems.
- **Safety:** Minimize the risk of harm to patients and providers through both system effectiveness and individual performance.
- **Informatics:** Use information and technology to communicate, manage knowledge, mitigate error, and support decision-making.

Additional Qualities and Skills[6–17]

- **Personal qualities:** Demonstrate independence, self-confidence, self-management, sociability, integrity, resilience, responsibility, and accountability.
- **Stress management:** Make stress reduction and self-renewal a habit; get enough rest and exercise; set priorities considering work (career/ambitions) and lifestyle (health needs, leisure, family).
- **Critical thinking, clinical reasoning, decision-making, and clinical judgment:** Know how to focus your thinking to achieve outcomes (results) and minimize risks and wasted time.
- **Ethical reasoning:** Maintain privacy and confidentiality; apply professional standards of what's right or wrong to act in patients' best interests.
- **Teaching/learning:** Commit to lifelong learning and self-improvement; assess health literacy; teach patients, families, caregivers, and co-workers; and foster a culture of learning.
- **Documentation:** Ensure health records demonstrate adherence to practice, care management, and documentation standards.
- **Maximizing resources:** Allocate time, money, materials, space, and human resources.
- **Building relationships:** Foster an atmosphere of mutual respect, trust, and support; work with diverse, multigenerational patients, families, and co-workers.
- **Leadership and professionalism:** Organize and prioritize care for a group of patients; guide patients, families, and co-workers toward common goals; advocate for patients, families, and nurses; and resolve conflicts professionally. Demonstrate behaviors in accordance to the standards of professional conduct.
- **Interprofessional collaboration:** Engage with professionals from various disciplines to promote learning and enable cooperation to improve patient outcomes.
- **Systems thinking:** Recognize connections, predict consequences of actions, and learn how clinical problems tend to unfold over time.
- **Function in systems-based practice:** Recognize all the processes in the health care system that interact to provide cost-effective care to individual patients and specific populations.
- **Spiritual, cultural, and population health competence:** Respond to needs related to spiritual beliefs, culture, race, gender, age, and various groups/populations (language, personality, sexual orientation, disability, and socioeconomic factors).
- **Navigate and facilitate change:** Chart a course to adapt to change and help others do the same.
- **Develop innovative approaches:** Think creatively, and generate and evaluate ideas.

As you work on developing CT and 21st-century nurse skills, there's one overarching principle that applies to everything you do:

GUIDING PRINCIPLE

All reasoning depends on the quality of communication. Has there been a *mutual exchange* of information, thoughts, and feelings? Has the most important information been shared? Has the information been exchanged in a timely, factual, complete, and respectful way? Faulty communication is a common critical thinking error.

HOW THIS BOOK HELPS YOU IMPROVE THINKING

To keep your interest and help you understand and remember what you read, this book is designed based on principles of brain-based learning.[18] Let's first look at what brain-based learning is and then how this book is organized to help you improve, regardless of your skill level.

Brain-Based Learning

Brain-based learning uses strategies that help your brain get "plugged into learning." For example:

1. **You learn best when there's a logical progression of content** and you're engaged by a conversational style that gives lots of examples, strategies, and exercises to help you apply content to the "real world."
2. **Gaining deep understanding requires intensive analysis,** which means thinking about the same topics in various ways.
3. **Understanding and retaining what you read requires that you make learning meaningful** by using your own unique way of processing how content relates to you personally, rather than trying to memorize a bunch of facts.
4. **Humor reduces stress, keeps your interest, and helps you learn.**
5. **Thinking is like any skill (e.g., music, art, and athletics).** We each have our own styles and innate or learned capabilities. We all can improve by gaining insight, acquiring instruction and feedback, and deliberately working on the skills in real and simulated situations.

Organized for Novices and Experts

Whether you're a novice or an expert, the following organization helps you connect with what you already know and move on to developing the complex skills you need to succeed today.

- Chapters 1 to 3 give the foundation for developing critical thinking, clinical reasoning, decision-making, and clinical judgment. You learn the "what and how" of critical thinking; how things like personality, upbringing, and culture affect thinking; and what strategies can help you overcome personal challenges. You explore the importance of learning cultures—in which "everyone teaches and everyone learns"—and get strategies for simulated, conceptual, and clinical learning, as well as passing high-stakes tests (e.g., NCLEX®).
- Chapters 4 to 6 address clinical reasoning, judgment, and decision-making. Here, you examine the knowledge and skills needed to develop sound clinical judgment and make safe and effective decisions. You learn key clinical reasoning principles and how to "think *with* health information technology." You gain a foundation for moral and ethical reasoning, evidence-based practice, quality improvement, professionalism, and leadership. In Chapter 6, you apply what you learned in Chapters 4 and 5 by working with case scenarios that are based on real incidents. You practice key skills such as assessing systematically, drawing valid conclusions, and setting priorities.
- Chapter 7 helps you develop the communication, teamwork, and self-management skills you need to lead and succeed in interprofessional practice (e.g., giving and taking feedback, navigating change, and managing your time). These are the skills you need to collaborate with other professionals and advocate for your patients, yourself, and your community.

DESCRIBING CRITICAL THINKING

When trying to get an in-depth understanding of something, we sometimes call this "peeling the onion." When you peel an onion, you go through many layers to get to the core. Let's "peel the critical thinking onion" by looking at various descriptions of what it entails.

Thinking Versus Critical Thinking

You may be wondering what the difference is between *thinking* and *critical thinking*. The main differences are *purpose* and *control*. Thinking refers to any mental activity. It can be "mindless," like when you're daydreaming or doing routine tasks like brushing your teeth. CT is controlled and purposeful, using well-reasoned strategies to get the results you need.

The Best Definition

CT is a complex process that changes depending on context (circumstances). For this reason, there is no one *right* definition. Depending on context, one or more definitions may apply. Many authors develop their own descriptions to complement and clarify someone else's (which is, by the way, a good example of thinking critically: CT requires you to "personalize" information—to analyze it and decide what it means to you, rather than simply memorizing someone else's words). In fact, the description that you put in your own words may be the best one because it's most likely to impact your reasoning abilities.

A Synonym: Reasoning

A good synonym for critical thinking is *reasoning* because it implies careful, deliberate thought. As early as kindergarten, students start to learn the "four *Rs*": reading, 'riting, 'rithmetic, and reasoning.

Common Critical Thinking Descriptions

Consider how the following CT descriptions complement and clarify one another:
- "Knowing how to learn, reason, think creatively, generate and evaluate ideas, see things in the mind's eye, make decisions, and solve problems"[10]
- "Reasonable, reflective thinking that focuses on what to believe or do"[19]
- "The ability to solve problems by making sense of information using creative, intuitive, logical, and analytical mental processes … and the process is continual"[20]
- "Knowing how to focus your thinking to get the results you need (includes applying logic, intuition, standards, and evidence-based practice)"[21]

Critical Thinking, Clinical Reasoning, Decision-Making, and Judgment

The terms *critical thinking, clinical reasoning, decision-making,* and *clinical judgment* are often used interchangeably. But there is a slight difference in how we use these terms:
- **Critical thinking**—a broad term—refers to reasoning *both* inside and outside of the clinical setting.
- **Clinical reasoning and decision-making**—specific terms—refer to the process you use to think about patient problems in the clinical setting—for example, deciding how to prevent and manage mobility issues. For reasoning about other clinical issues (e.g., teamwork, collaboration, and streamlining workflow), nurses usually use the term ***critical thinking.***
- **Clinical judgment** refers to the result (outcome) of critical thinking, clinical reasoning, and decision-making—the conclusion, decision, or opinion you make after analyzing information.

To clarify the relationships among critical thinking, clinical reasoning, decision-making, and clinical judgment, study Fig. 1.1. This figure, from previous editions, corresponds to with how the National Council of State Boards of Nursing defines *clinical judgment* ("the observed outcome of critical thinking and decision making"[22]).

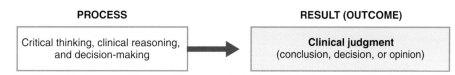

FIG. 1.1 Clinical judgment—the result of critical thinking, clinical reasoning, and decision-making.

Critical Thinking Versus Nursing Process

American Nurses Association (ANA) standards state that the nursing process—*assessment, diagnosis, planning, implementation,* and *evaluation* (ADPIE)*—serves as a CT model that promotes a competent level of care.[23] To maintain ANA standards, think your way through licensing and certification exams, and give competent care, you must know how to apply nursing process principles as described in this book. For example, always assess before you act and monitor patient responses (outcomes) closely as you act.

Applied Definition: Thinking in the Clinical Setting

To understand important points about thinking in the clinical setting—a setting that's challenging, complex, and regulated by laws and standards—study the following applied definition.

Critical thinking in nursing—which includes clinical reasoning, decision-making, and clinical judgment—is purposeful, informed, outcome-focused thinking that:[24]

- **Is guided by standards**, policies, ethics codes, and laws (individual state practice acts and state boards of nursing regulations).
- **Is driven by patient, family, and community needs**, as well as nurses' needs to give competent and efficient care (e.g., streamlining charting to free up nurses for patient care).
- **Is based on principles of the nursing process, problem-solving, and the scientific method** (requires forming opinions and making decisions based on evidence).
- **Focuses on safety and quality**, constantly re-evaluating, self-correcting, and striving to improve personal, professional, and system practices.
- **Carefully identifies the key problems**, issues, and risks involved and includes patients, families, and key stakeholders in decision-making early in the process. Stakeholders are the people who will be most affected (patients and families) or from whom requirements will be drawn (e.g., caregivers, insurance companies, third-party payers, and health care organizations).
- **Uses logic, intuition, and creativity** and is grounded in specific knowledge, skills, and experience.
- **Calls for strategies that make the most of human potential** and compensate for problems created by human nature (e.g., preventing errors by using technology).

Study Fig. 1.2, which shows the relationships of many aspects of CT.

GUIDING PRINCIPLE

Critical thinking, clinical reasoning, decision-making, and clinical judgment are guided by professional standards, policies, ethics codes, and laws (individual state practice acts and state boards of nursing regulations). You aren't expected to know everything, but you are expected to ask for help when you're unsure about how to proceed in clinical situations that are new to you. Being unfamiliar with standards, policies, and laws isn't an excuse for inappropriate actions.[14]

---

* ANA standards add *outcome identification,* which is a part of *planning.*

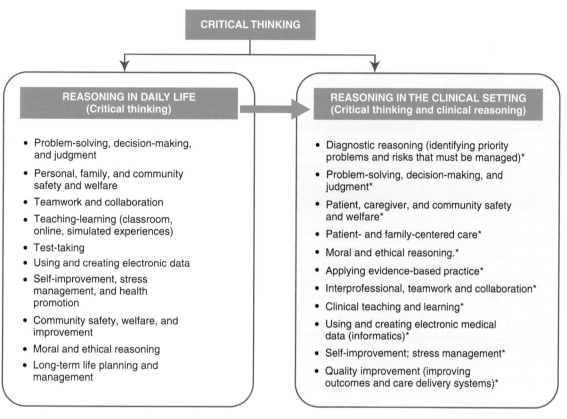

*Relates to ANA practice standards, The Joint Commission Standards, Quality and Safety Education for Nurses competencies, and Institute of Medicine competencies

FIG. 1.2 *Critical thinking* **is an "umbrella term" that includes reasoning both inside and outside of the clinical setting.** The terms *clinical reasoning, critical thinking, clinical judgment, problem-solving,* and *decision-making* are closely related and often used interchangeably. Your ability to reason well in your daily life affects your ability to reason in the clinical setting. (Copyright 2018 by R. Alfaro-LeFevre. http://www. AlfaroTeachSmart.com.)

INTERPROFESSIONAL CLINICAL PRACTICE AND REASONING

The most common clinical reasoning framework that's used among health care professionals is **ADPIE** (*assess, diagnose, plan, implement, evaluate*). The focus of ADPIE changes depending on the health care professional's role. **Examples:**

- **Physicians focus on medical problems** (promoting body system functioning, curing diseases, and alleviating symptoms).
- **Respiratory therapists** focus on promoting lung function.
- **Nurses focus on nursing concerns** (e.g., monitoring health status and patient responses to health problems; managing treatment regimens; preventing complications; and promoting comfort, mobility, well-being, and independence, as detailed in Chapters 4 and 6).

ADPIE guides clinicians to document in a way that clearly communicates care to the interprofessional team, meets legal standards, and provides the data researchers need to develop evidence-based practices. Some nurses use **AAPIE** instead of **ADPIE**, naming the second phase, *Analysis*. Calling the second phase *Diagnosis* focuses on the end result of analysis: drawing conclusions (diagnosing problems and risks).

Review the following summary of ADPIE phases—keep in mind that these phases happen in the context of unfolding (evolving) human situations and that the terms *diagnosis* and *problem identification* are often used interchangeably.

CLINICAL REASONING PHASES*

- A̲ssessing: Detecting/**noticing** cues (signs, symptoms, risks)
- D̲iagnosing: Analyzing, synthesizing, and **interpreting** data; differential diagnosis (creating a list of problems; weighing the probability of one problem against that of another that's closely related); NCLEX considers this phase *generating hypotheses*
- P̲lanning: **Responding**; predicting complications; anticipating consequences; considering actions; setting priorities; decision-making; ensuring safety
- I̲mplementing: **Responding**; taking actions; monitoring responses; **reflecting**; making adjustments
- E̲valuating: **Reflecting**; repeating ADPIE as indicated

* Bold terms indicate Tanner's clinical judgment model (noticing, interpreting, responding, reflecting)[25]

Rather than being linear and step-by-step, ADPIE is a dynamic cycle of interrelated thinking processes. Fig. 1.3 summarizes you do during each of the phases.

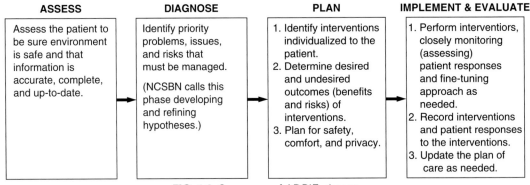

ASSESS	DIAGNOSE	PLAN	IMPLEMENT & EVALUATE
Assess the patient to be sure environment is safe and that information is accurate, complete, and up-to-date.	Identify priority problems, issues, and risks that must be managed. (NCSBN calls this phase developing and refining hypotheses.)	1. Identify interventions individualized to the patient. 2. Determine desired and undesired outcomes (benefits and risks) of interventions. 3. Plan for safety, comfort, and privacy.	1. Perform interventiors, closely monitoring (assessing) patient responses and fine-tuning approach as needed. 2. Record interventions and patient responses to the interventions. 3. Update the plan of care as needed.

FIG. 1.3 Summary of ADPIE phases.

As health care evolves, you're likely to learn other models to guide thinking. ADPIE should be the *first* tool you learn to think critically in nursing because it underpins virtually all care management approaches. When there are issues with reasoning when using other models, clinicians often revert to ADPIE, asking, "Did we assess, diagnose, plan, implement, and evaluate well enough?" No matter what model you use, keep the following in mind.

GUIDING PRINCIPLE

Engaging patients, families, and caregivers and ensuring their safety and welfare must be given top priority in all reasoning and decision-making.

PROBLEM-FOCUSED VERSUS OUTCOME-FOCUSED THINKING

Problem-focused thinking and outcome-focused thinking are closely related. You need excellent problem-solving skills to achieve desired outcomes (results) and minimize risks. But consider the following:

- **There are many ways to solve problems.** There are quick fixes, as well as long-term and temporary solutions. Outcome-focused (results-oriented) thinking aims to fix problems in ways that get you *the best results over time.*
- **Sometimes there are so many problems that the best approach may be to focus on** *outcomes* **rather than** *problems*. For example, if you work on a team with many interpersonal problems, your manager might say, "I want us all to work as a team. I ask you to put the problems aside and get agreement on roles, responsibilities, and behavior so that our patients get good care and we enjoy coming to work." If you focus only on the problems, you may miss easy solutions (Fig. 1.4).

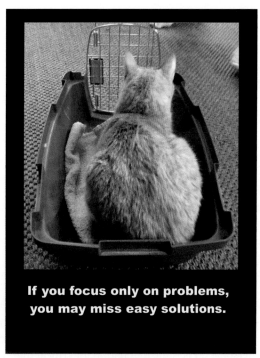

**If you focus only on problems,
you may miss easy solutions.**

FIG. 1.4

WHAT ABOUT COMMON SENSE?

Is CT simply common sense, something that can't be taught? The answer is "no." Some people are born with the gift of common sense, but a lot of it is *learned from experience*. You can put someone with great common sense in a new or stressful situation, and you're likely to see behaviors that don't seem at all sensible. Think about the following scenario, a true story.

SCENARIO CRITICAL THINKING: SIMPLY COMMON SENSE?

As an evening supervisor, I stopped to check on a new graduate who was in charge for the first time. She appeared to be "in over her head," nervous, and running around. Calmly, I asked how things were going. She replied, "Fine, except for the man in Room 203. His temperature was 104° F an hour ago. We drew blood cultures, gave aspirin, and started him on antibiotics." I asked, "What's the temperature now?" She replied, "He's not due until 8 PM" (3 hours later). It seemed common sense to me that you would check the temperature more frequently when it was that high. Wanting to set a collaborative tone, I stressed the need to check it more frequently and asked her to keep me informed. I also made sure I came back frequently to see how things were going. At the time, I believed this nurse had no common sense, but she went on to be an excellent clinician with a track record of success. She was simply inexperienced, nervous, and overwhelmed in a new situation. She may even have been subconsciously defending an oversight.

Common sense may be innate, but it also comes from knowledge and experience. What may be common sense to you, based on your upbringing, schooling, or experience, may not be so to someone else. If you encounter someone who seems to have no common sense, don't jump to conclusions. Dig a little deeper to determine the real issues: Are there knowledge, confidence, communication, or organizational skills problems? Is the person simply inexperienced or stressed by a new environment? Has the person become complacent? Could a learning disability be contributing to the problem? Like CT, common sense often can be taught if you determine the underlying problems and do something about them.

WHAT DO CRITICAL THINKERS LOOK LIKE?

Research shows that most critical thinkers have high foreheads and furrowed brows, probably because of all the thinking they do. If you're not questioning this statement, then you're not thinking critically about what you're reading. When I ask, "What do critical thinkers look like?" I mean, "What characteristics do we see in someone who thinks critically?" To answer this question, consider the next section on *critical thinking indicators*, which were developed after an extensive review of the literature and surveys of nurse experts.[24] Keep in mind that *indicators* suggest that something is happening—for example, a green light on an appliance is an indicator that the power is on.

CRITICAL THINKING INDICATORS (CTIs)

An *indicator* is something observable that serves to define a concept in a practical way (e.g., an intelligence test is an indicator of intelligence). Studying critical thinking indicators (CTIs)—observable behaviors that indicate CT—gives you insight into what critical thinkers "look like." Review Box 1.2, which lists personal CTIs—the behaviors and characteristics of critical thinkers. Developing personal CTIs is the foundation for critical thinking. Decide where you stand in relation to each indicator, using the following 0–10 scale:

0 = I need to work on this indicator
10 = This indicator is habit for me

As you evaluate yourself, keep in mind that some of you—because of your nature—will be harder on yourself than others will be. If you have some trusted friends, peers, or family members, ask them how they see your behavior. Ask them to focus on *usual patterns of behaviors* (not single incidents) and to give you specific examples. The results of this exercise may reaffirm or surprise you.

BOX 1.2 Personal Critical Thinking Indicators

SELF-AWARE: Identifies own learning, personality, and communication style preferences; clarifies biases, strengths, and limitations; acknowledges when thinking may be influenced by emotions or self-interest.

GENUINE/AUTHENTIC: Shows true self; demonstrates behaviors that indicate stated values.

EFFECTIVE COMMUNICATOR: Listens well (shows deep understanding of others' thoughts, feelings, and circumstances); speaks and writes with clarity (gets key points across to others).

CURIOUS AND INQUISITIVE: Asks questions; looks for reasons, explanations, and meaning; seeks new information to broaden understanding.

ALERT TO CONTEXT: Looks for changes in circumstances that warrant a need to modify approaches; investigates thoroughly when situations warrant precise, in-depth thinking.

REFLECTIVE AND SELF-CORRECTIVE: Carefully considers meaning of data and interpersonal interactions; asks for feedback; corrects own thinking; is alert to potential errors by self and others; finds ways to avoid future mistakes.

ANALYTICAL AND INSIGHTFUL: Identifies relationships; expresses deep understanding.

LOGICAL AND INTUITIVE: Draws reasonable conclusions (if this is so, then it follows that because …); uses intuition as a guide; acts on intuition only with knowledge of risks involved.

CONFIDENT AND RESILIENT: Expresses faith in ability to reason and learn; overcomes problems and disappointments.

HONEST AND UPRIGHT: Looks for the truth, even if it sheds unwanted light; demonstrates integrity (adheres to moral and ethical standards; admits flaws in thinking).

AUTONOMOUS/RESPONSIBLE: Self-directed, self-disciplined, and accepts accountability.

CAREFUL AND PRUDENT: Seeks help as needed; suspends or revises judgment as indicated by new or incomplete data.

OPEN AND FAIR-MINDED: Shows tolerance for different viewpoints; questions how own viewpoints are influencing thinking.

SENSITIVE TO DIVERSITY: Expresses appreciation of human differences related to values, culture, personality, or learning style preferences; adapts to preferences when feasible.

CREATIVE: Offers alternative solutions and approaches; comes up with useful ideas.

REALISTIC AND PRACTICAL: Admits when things aren't feasible; looks for useful solutions.

PROACTIVE: Anticipates consequences; plans ahead; acts on opportunities.

COURAGEOUS: Stands up for beliefs; advocates for others; doesn't hide from challenges.

PATIENT AND PERSISTENT: Waits for right moment; perseveres to achieve the best results.

FLEXIBLE: Changes approaches as needed to get the best results.

HEALTH-ORIENTED: Promotes a healthy lifestyle; uses healthy behaviors to manage stress.

IMPROVEMENT-ORIENTED (SELF, PATIENTS, SYSTEMS): Self—Identifies learning needs; finds ways to overcome limitations; seeks out new knowledge. **Patients**—Promotes health; maximizes function, comfort, and convenience. **Systems**—Identifies risks and problems with health care systems; promotes safety, quality, satisfaction, and cost containment.

From Alfaro-LeFevre, R. (2019). *Evidence-based critical thinking indicators*. All rights reserved. Available at http://www. AlfaroTeachSmart.com

NOTE: This list is the ideal—no one is perfect.

GUIDING PRINCIPLE

There are no ideal critical thinkers—no one's perfect. Even the best thinkers' abilities vary, depending on circumstances such as confidence level and previous experience. What matters are *patterns* over time (does the person demonstrate critical thinking characteristics most of the time?).

Box 1.3 shows how other authors describe CT traits. These traits were incorporated into the CTIs using simple terms. Table 1.1 gives examples of what CT is and what it's not.

BOX 1.3 How Other Authors Describe Critical Thinking Traits

Scheffer and Rubenfeld's Habits of the Mind[1]
- **CONFIDENCE:** Assurance of one's reasoning abilities.
- **CONTEXTUAL PERSPECTIVE:** Consideration of the whole situation, including relationships, background, and environment relevant to some happening.
- **CREATIVITY:** Intellectual inventiveness used to generate, discover, or restructure ideas. Imagining alternatives.
- **FLEXIBILITY:** Capacity to adapt, accommodate, modify, or change thoughts, ideas, and behaviors.
- **INQUISITIVENESS:** An eagerness to know, demonstrated by seeking knowledge and understanding through observation and thoughtful questioning to explore possibilities and alternatives.
- **INTELLECTUAL INTEGRITY:** Seeking the truth through sincere, honest processes, even if the results are contrary to one's assumptions and beliefs.
- **INTUITION:** Insightful sense of knowing without conscious use of reason.
- **OPEN-MINDEDNESS:** A viewpoint characterized by being receptive to divergent views and sensitive to one's biases.
- **PERSEVERANCE:** Pursuit of a course with determination to overcome obstacles.
- **REFLECTION:** Contemplation on a subject, especially on one's assumptions and thinking for the purposes of deeper understanding and self-evaluation.

Facione's Critical Thinking Dispositions[2]
- **TRUTH SEEKING:** A courageous desire for the best knowledge, even if such knowledge fails to support or undermines one's preconceptions, beliefs, or self-interest.
- **OPEN-MINDEDNESS:** Tolerance of divergent views; self-monitoring for possible bias.
- **ANALYTICITY:** Demanding the application of reason and evidence; alert to problematic situations; inclined to anticipate consequences.
- **SYSTEMATICITY:** Valuing organization; focusing; being diligent about problems at all levels of complexity.
- **CRITICAL THINKING SELF-CONFIDENCE:** Trusting one's own reasoning skills; seeing oneself as a good thinker.
- **INQUISITIVENESS:** Curious and eager to acquire knowledge and learn explanations, even when the applications of the knowledge are not immediately apparent.
- **MATURITY:** Prudence in making, suspending, or revising judgment; awareness that multiple solutions can be acceptable; appreciation of the need to reach closure even in the absence of complete knowledge.

Paul and Elder's Intellectual Traits[3]
- **INTELLECTUAL HUMILITY:** Consciousness of limits of your knowledge; willingness to admit what you don't know.
- **INTELLECTUAL COURAGE:** Awareness of the need to face and fairly address ideas, beliefs, or viewpoints to which you haven't given serious listening.
- **INTELLECTUAL EMPATHY:** Consciousness of the need to imaginatively put yourself in the place of others to genuinely understand them.
- **INTELLECTUAL AUTONOMY:** Having control over your beliefs, values, and inferences; being an independent thinker.
- **INTELLECTUAL INTEGRITY:** Being true to your own thinking; applying intellectual standards to thinking; holding yourself to the same standards to which you hold others; willingness to admit when your thinking may be flawed.
- **CONFIDENCE IN REASON:** Confidence that, in the long run, using your own thinking and encouraging others to do the same gets the best results.
- **FAIR-MINDEDNESS:** Awareness of the need to treat all viewpoints alike, with awareness of vested interest.

TABLE 1.1 Critical Thinking: What It Is and What It Is Not		
Critical Thinking	**Not Critical Thinking**	**Critical Thinking Example**
Critical for the sake of improvement and doing things in the best interest of the key players involved	Being critical without being able to identify improvements; critical for the sake of having it your way	Figuring out ways to achieve the same (or better) outcomes more efficiently
Inquisitive about intent, facts, and reasons behind ideas or actions; thought and knowledge oriented	Unaware of motives, facts, and reasons behind ideas or actions; task oriented, rather than thought oriented	Seeking to fully understanding situations and procedures before giving care; modifying approaches as needed.
Sensitive to the powerful influence of emotions, but focused on making decisions based on what's morally and ethically the right thing to do	Emotion driven; unclear about what these emotions are or how they influence thinking	Finding out how someone feels about something, then moving on to discuss what's morally and ethically right

WHAT'S FAMILIAR AND WHAT'S NEW?

We understand something best by comparing it with things we already know: How is it the same, and how is it different? Let's examine what's familiar and what's new about CT.

What's Familiar
Problem-Solving

Knowing specific problem-solving and prevention strategies is a key part of CT (and the NCLEX exam). For example, if you're caring for someone after heart surgery, you must know what strategies are used to prevent and manage complications. Be aware, however, that using *problem-solving* interchangeably with *critical thinking* can be a "sore subject." Problem-solving is missing the important concepts of prevention, creativity, improvement, and aiming for the best results. Even if there are no problems, you should be thinking creatively, asking, "What could we do better?" and "Are there risks we need to address to prevent problems before they happen?"

Analyzing

Although being analytical is important, CT requires more than analyzing. It requires coming up with new ideas (right-brain thinking) and judging the worth of those ideas (left-brain thinking). Some overly analytical people suffer from "analysis paralysis," overthinking problems when they should be taking action.

Decision-Making

Decision-making and *critical thinking* are sometimes used interchangeably. Making decisions is an important part of critical thinking and clinical judgment.

Scientific Method

The scientific method is an excellent CT tool. It has been well studied and applies the following principles of scientific investigation (all applied in NCLEX)[22]:

- **Observing:** Continuously collecting data to gain understanding and check for changes in circumstances.
- **Classifying data:** Grouping related information so that patterns and relationships emerge.
- **Drawing conclusions** that follow logically: "If this is so, then it's likely that …."
- **Generating hypotheses (hunches, assumptions, or suspicions).** Creating a list of suspected problems and solutions.

- **Conducting experiments/analyzing data:** Performing studies to examine and analyze data.
- **Testing hypotheses:** Determining whether there's factual evidence to support hunches, assumptions, or suspicions.
- **Drawing conclusions and making judgments** that follow logically based on the previous steps: "If our analysis and studies give us evidence that this is so, then it's likely that …."

What's New
Emotional Intelligence(EI)/Emotional Quotient (EQ)

Emotional intelligence (EI), also called *emotional quotient (EQ)* and *emotional intelligence quotient (EIQ)*—the ability to recognize and manage your own emotions and help others do the same—is as important to CT as the intelligence quotient (IQ).

So-Called "Soft Skills" Aren't Soft

For years, we called communication and interpersonal skills the "soft skills" of nursing, implying that clinical skills such as managing intravenous lines are the most important skills. We now know that communication and interpersonal skills such as engaging patients, dealing with difficult people, and resolving conflicts are crucial to CT.

Right-Brain and Left-Brain Thinking

CT requires right-brain thinking (creative and intuitive—generating new ideas) and left-brain thinking (logical and analytical—judging the worth of those ideas). You probably have a tendency toward either right- or left-brain thinking, but you should work to use both sides of your brain.

Maximizing Human Potential

We're only just beginning to identify ways to maximize the human potential to think critically. For example, new brain imaging techniques show us what parts of the brain are being used in various thinking and tasks, helping us learn how we use our brains. People survive brain injuries that used to be fatal, and we continue to learn from their rehabilitation. For example, some people who have had strokes can't speak, but they can sing words.

Mapping as a Strategy to Teach and Learn

Maps and decision trees created by experts guide seasoned and new nurses alike. Maps created by learners promote deep personal understanding. They help learners make connections between concepts and information in their own unique way. You can find the "how-to's" of concept mapping in Appendix A.

Changing How We View Mistakes

Experts agree that "to err is human" and that most errors happen because of multiple factors and system problems (e.g., look-alike drugs or inadequate staffing or staff preparation). Humans are vulnerable to making mistakes because of "human factors" (e.g., stress, fatigue, and information overload).[26] Reducing errors related to human factors (e.g., using computers and decision support systems) is now a priority. We also know that being allowed to make mistakes in safe situations (e.g., simulations) is a powerful way to learn.

Preparing for "What-If" Scenarios

In today's world we emphasize the need to develop policies and procedures to be prepared for "what-if" scenarios (e.g., terrorist attacks, including bioterrorism).

Evidence-Based Thinking

Clinicians are expected to provide evidence that supports opinions, solutions, and courses of action. We must be confident when we're asked questions like, "What evidence do you have that this will work?" or "What data are you using to support that this is the problem or that this is a good solution?"

Measuring Outcomes (Results)

Rather than measuring results subjectively (e.g., *"the patient seems to be managing his pain well"*), CT requires focusing on outcomes—very specific, objective ways of measuring results (e.g., *"2 hours after medication, the patient rates his pain at 2 on a scale of 0 to 10, with 0 meaning pain-free and 10 meaning the worst possible pain"*).

Collaborative Thinking

Collaborative approaches are the norm today. The workforce is diverse, and we need to facilitate "meetings of the minds" to achieve the best outcomes. We continue to develop ways to promote interprofessional care and ensure that patients are engaged in problem identification and care management processes.

Relating on a "Human Level" Matters

Maintaining professionalism, understanding patients' personal interests and passions, and showing your "human side" help build the relationships needed for CT (Fig. 1.5).

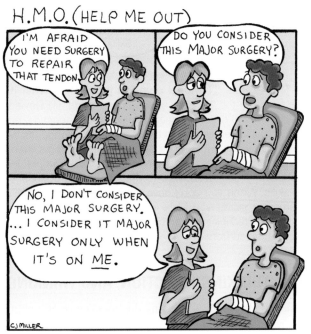

FIG. 1.5 Showing your "human side" helps build the relationships needed for critical thinking.

4-CIRCLE CT MODEL: GET THE PICTURE?

Whereas CTIs describe behaviors that promote CT, the 4-Circle CT Model (Fig. 1.6) gives you "a picture" of what CT involves. This model—used in many regions, from South America, to Europe, to Africa—is the basis for a clinical practice CT questionnaire, as addressed in an article in *Worldviews on Evidence-Based Nursing.*[27] Study the four circles below. Note that CT requires a blend of CT characteristics, theoretical and experiential knowledge, interpersonal skills, and technical skills. Realize that the top circle—CT characteristics—corresponds with the personal CTIs listed in Box 1.2. In the next chapters, we'll discuss the other circles in more depth. For now, remember that if you develop the CT characteristics and attitudes in the *top* circle (e.g., confidence, resilience, and being proactive), developing the skills in the *other* three circles of the model will be easier.

4-CIRCLE CRITICAL THINKING (CT) MODEL

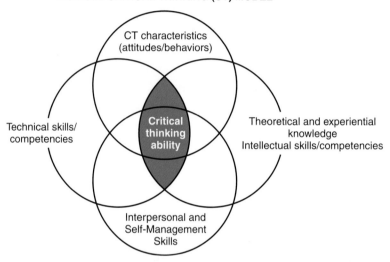

4-CIRCLE CT Model © 2015 R. Alfaro-LeFevre www.AlfaroTeachSmart.com

FIG. 1.6 The 4-Circle CT Model gives "a picture" of what it takes to think critically. Going clockwise from the top, here's what you need to do: (1) Develop critical thinking characteristics and behaviors. If you develop critical thinking characteristics, the skills in the other circles come readily. (2) Acquire theoretical and experiential knowledge, as well as intellectual skills related to problem-solving and the nursing process (e.g., assessing systematically and setting priorities). (3) Gain interpersonal and self-management skills. For example, learn how to resolve conflicts and engage patients in care; learn how to manage your emotions, stress, and time. (4) Expand your technical skills. When you don't have the related technical skills—for example, IVs, nasogastric tubes, computer skills—you have less brain power for critical thinking (because of the "brain drain" of learning technical skills). (From Alfaro-LeFevre R. Evidence-based critical thinking indicators. 2019. Retrieved from http://www.AlfaroTeachSmart.com. No use without permission.)

THINKING AHEAD, THINKING-IN-ACTION, AND THINKING BACK (REFLECTING)

Let's finish this chapter by addressing the importance of looking at CT from three perspectives: *thinking ahead, thinking-in-action*, and *thinking back (reflective thinking).*

Consider the following descriptions and think about the differences in each circumstance.

1. **Thinking Ahead:** Anticipating what might happen and being proactive by identifying what you can do to be prepared. For novices, thinking ahead is difficult and sometimes restricted to reading

procedure manuals and textbooks. An important part of being proactive is asking questions like, "What can I bring with me to help jog my memory and stay focused and organized?"

2. **Thinking-in-Action:** Often, this is called "thinking on your feet." It's rapid, dynamic reasoning that considers several things at once, making it difficult to describe. For example, suppose you find your stove on fire. As you spring into action, your mind races, thinking about many things at once ("How can I put this out?" "Where's the fire extinguisher?" "Should I call the fire department?"). Thinking-in-action is highly influenced by previous knowledge and hands-on experience. To keep safety first in all important situations, keep experts nearby who have extensive experiential knowledge stored in their brains. If you encountered a fire, wouldn't you like to have a fireman standing at your side? Thinking-in-action is prone to "knee-jerk" responses and decisions. To use the fire example again, an untrained person may throw water on a grease fire, which can make it worse.

3. **Thinking Back (Reflecting on Thinking):** Analyzing and deconstructing your reasoning to look for flaws, gain more understanding, and make corrections. Experienced nurses double-check their thinking in dynamic ways during thinking-in-action. However, this doesn't replace reflective thinking that *happens after the fact* (using debriefing to examine clinical experiences and identify lessons learned).

Considering all three of these phases of thinking helps you examine thinking in a holistic way. If you look only at *one phase*, you'll miss important parts of thinking.

PUTTING IT ALL TOGETHER

By now, you should have an initial idea of what critical thinking, clinical reasoning, decision-making, and clinical judgment entail. To increase your understanding of this chapter, first review the following shaded section on how to make the most of the exercises throughout this book. Then go on to complete the critical thinking exercises and review end-of-chapter key points.

Making the Most Out of the Exercises in This Book

- **Apply strategies that use your own learning style preferences.** For example, consider drawing pictures, diagrams, and maps to make connections between concepts. If you need help with mapping, see *Concept Mapping: Getting in the "Right" State of Mind* (Appendix A).
- **When writing responses, at first be more concerned with substance than grammar** (as you would if you were writing a diary). However, as you progress, apply grammar rules and make your responses clear to others. Making your responses clear to others helps you clarify your thoughts. Following grammar rules improves clarity and gives you practice for writing other important papers and communications.
- **Don't be afraid to paraphrase.** Paraphrasing helps you gain understanding because you explain what you read using familiar language (your own). To avoid concerns of plagiarism, cite the page numbers you're paraphrasing.
- **Consider how the exercises can be improved.** Give suggestions to your instructor or send them to us by clicking on "Contact Us" at http://www.AlfaroTeachSmart.com. If your suggestion is unique, we'll post it on our web page and cite you as the contributor.
- **You can find example responses for all exercises, except for the ones labeled *Think, Pair, Share*** in Appendix I.

Think, Pair, Share Exercises

This strategy promotes efficient, cooperative learning and has three main steps:

1. Think about a question or issue independently, jotting down three thoughts or questions that seem important to you.
2. Pair off with a partner. Discuss what you each jotted down; write down things your partner listed that you did not; together with your partner, choose one to three of the most important points you want to share with the group.
3. Share these in a group discussion. You can find a template for completing *Think, Pair, Share* exercises at http://www.AlfaroTeachSmart.com.

❓ CRITICAL THINKING EXERCISES

Find example responses in Appendix I (page 215).

1. **Fill in the following blanks, choosing from the following words:** ADPIE; assessment; clinical judgment; CTIs; cycle; laws; welfare; priority; process; critical; safety; context, ethics codes; dynamic
   A. Patient and caregiver (a) _____ and (b) _____ must be given top (c) _____ in all critical thinking in health care.
   B. While thinking refers to any mental activity (whether focused or not), _____ thinking implies reasoning that's purposeful, deliberate, and focused.
   C. Critical thinking and clinical reasoning describe the (a) _____ you use to come to a (b) _____ (conclusion, opinion, or decision).
   D. Critical thinking often changes, depending on _____.
   E. Developing personal critical thinking characteristics and behaviors, as described by _____, is the foundation for critical thinking.
   F. _____ is the most common reasoning model used among health care professionals.
   G. Reasoning is a (a) _____ of thinking processes that are fluid and (b) _____, rather than linear and step-by-step.
   H. Critical thinking, clinical reasoning, and clinical judgment are guided by professional standards, policies, (a) _____, and (b) _____ (individual state practice acts and state boards of nursing regulations).
2. When you form an opinion, you draw a conclusion from facts (evidence).
   A. What's the difference between facts and opinions?
   B. How can you determine if an opinion is valid?
3. What is the relationship between critical thinking indicators (see Box 1.2) and behavior?
4. What is the relationship between achieving outcomes (desired results) and identifying problems, issues, and risks involved?
5. If you are in a new or uncomfortable situation, what is likely to happen to your ability to demonstrate critical thinking indicators?
6. What do the following "five Cs" (context, confident, courage, curious, committed) have to do with critical thinking?
7. Why is it important to consider thinking from three perspectives: thinking ahead, thinking-in-action, and thinking back (reflecting)?

👥 THINK, PAIR, SHARE

With a partner, in a group, or in a journal entry:

1. Complete the following sentences and then compare your responses with those of others:
   a. If I were to explain to someone else what critical thinking is, I would say that …
   b. I do my best thinking when …
   c. I do my worst thinking when …

2. Discuss how the focus of ADPIE changes depending on whether you're a physician, a respiratory therapist, a dietician, or a nurse.

3. Draw a map that shows the fluid, cyclic nature of ADPIE.

4. Discuss times when you've experienced some of the descriptions listed under "Not Critical Thinking" in Table 1.1. How did it affect your thinking?

5. Discuss how having a healthy workplace, learning culture, and safety culture affects critical thinking skill development.

6. Identify five personal CTIs (see Box 1.2, page 13) that are especially challenging for beginning nurses. Share your thoughts on why they are challenging.

7. Discuss where you stand in relationship to gaining the skills addressed in the 4-Circle CT Model.

8. Share where you stand in relation to understanding the key concepts and achieving the learning outcomes mentioned at the beginning of this chapter.

9. Discuss your thoughts on the following *Critical Moments and Other Perspectives*.

CRITICAL MOMENTS AND OTHER PERSPECTIVES

Good Question!

Socrates learned more from questioning others than he did from reading books. Learn to be confident asking questions. Seek other opinions, and question deeply to gain understanding. Don't think you have to know all the answers. Simply saying "Good question!" often sparks great critical thinking.

Aha!

We say "Aha!" when we suddenly realize something or have our suspicions confirmed. We say "Aha!" when we connect with something that was in the back of our minds but never put into words. As you read this book, share your "Aha's." These moments of "light bulbs going off in your head" are energizing. They bring new ideas and stimulate you to learn more.

What Matters More—Knowing or Caring?

People won't care how much you know until they know how much you care.

Teddy Roosevelt

Effects of Nurses' Quality of Life

"We know [that] if health care providers are healthy themselves, they are more likely to talk [to patients about health] and be credible when they talk to clients about health." Registered nurses, who account for 1% of the U.S. population, are responsible for the well-being of their patients, yet they are a largely unhealthy population. They know what they need to do to improve their health, yet they fall below the rest of the population in every health metric besides smoking.[28]

Marla Weston, ANA Enterprise CEO

Healthy Versus Unhealthy Work Environments

"I worked on a unit where no one got along, you never heard thank you, and I hated coming to work. Now I work on a unit where the work I do is appreciated. Not once have I heard my boss talk badly about other colleagues. I'm not someone who comes to work to look for friends, but I want us to work together and get the job done. What a difference it feels to work in an environment where you're appreciated!" (Adapted from an American Nurses Association LinkedIn posting.[19])

KEY POINTS/SUMMARY

- This chapter focuses on describing what critical thinking entails in various situations (the next focuses on how to become a critical thinker).
- Critical thinking doesn't mean simply being critical. It means not accepting information at face value without evaluating whether it is factual and reliable.
- Critical thinking is a broad term that includes clinical reasoning, judgment, and decision-making.
- There's no *one* right definition of CT—there are several that complement and clarify one another, and one definition may apply to one situation but not another.
- The term *critical thinking* is often used interchangeably with *clinical reasoning, clinical judgment, problem-solving,* and *decision-making.*
- Critical thinking, clinical reasoning, and judgment are guided by professional standards, policies, ethics codes, and laws (individual state practice acts and state boards of nursing regulations)—you must know what you're legally allowed to do and how you should do it.
- Like the nursing process, the most common clinical reasoning framework used among health care professionals is ADPIE (*assess, diagnose, plan, implement, evaluate*); the focus of ADPIE changes depending on the health care professional's role.
- Clinical reasoning happens in a context of unfolding (evolving) human situations; it's fluid, dynamic, and cyclic, rather than linear and step-by-step.
- Communication and interpersonal skills such as engaging patients, collaborating with others, and resolving conflicts are essential for critical thinking.
- Personal CTIs (see Box 1.2) are behaviors that demonstrate characteristics that promote critical thinking. Ability to demonstrate CTIs varies depending on circumstances such as familiarity with the people and situations at hand.
- The 4-Circle CT model (see Fig. 1.6) gives you a picture of what it takes to think critically.
- Critical thinking is like any skill (e.g., music, art, athletics). We each have our own styles and innate or learned capabilities. We can improve by becoming self-aware, obtaining instruction, practicing, and seeking feedback from others.
- It's important to consider critical thinking from three different perspectives: thinking ahead, thinking-in-action, and thinking back (reflective thinking).
- Scan this chapter to review the illustrations and Guiding Principles.

REFERENCES

1. Behind every healed patient is a critical thinking nurse. (Website). Retrieved from http://www.hcpro.com/NRS-257219-868/Blog-spotlight-Behind-every-healed-patient-is-a-critically- thinking-nurse.html.
2. Kavanagh J, Szweda C. A Crisis in competency: the strategic and ethical imperative to assessing new graduate nurses' clinical reasoning. *Nursing Education Perspectives.* 2017;38(2):57–62. https://doi.org/10.1097/01.NEP.0000000000000112.
3. Boyer S, Valdez-Delgado K, Huss J, et al. Impact of a nurse residency program on transition to specialty practice. *Journal of Nurses in Professional Development.* 2017;33(5):220–227. https://doi.org/10.1097/NND.0000000000000384.
4. Buttaccio J. *3 Reasons Many Nurses are Leaving the Profession.* Retrieved from http://dailynurse.com/3-reasons-many-nurses-leaving-profession/; 2017.
5. Quality and Safety for Nursing Education (QSEN) Competencies. (Website) Retrieved from http://qsen.org/competencies
6. Beauvais A, Kazer M, Aronson B, et al. After the gap analysis: education and practice changes to prepare nurses of the future. *Nursing Education Perspectives.* 2017;8(5):250–254. https://doi.org/10.1097/01.NEP.0000000000000196.
7. Institute of Medicine. *Assessing Progress on the IOM Report: The Future of Nursing.* Washington, DC: National Academies Press; 2015. Retrieved from http://www.nationalacademies.org/hmd/Reports/2015/Assessing-Progress-on-the-IOM-Report-The-Future-of-Nursing.aspx.
8. Sroczynski M, Conlin G, Costello E, et al. Continuing the creativity and connections: the Massachusetts initiative to update the nurse of the future nursing core competencies. *Nursing Education Perspectives.* 2017;38(5):233–236. https://doi.org/10.1097/01.NEP.0000000000000200.

9. Benner P. Educating nurses: A call for radical transformation five years later. In: *Northeast Ohio Deans' Roundtable 10th Anniversary Conference, Cleveland, Ohio.* 2015.

10. Secretary's Commission on Achieving Necessary Skills (SCANS). Learning a living: A blueprint for high performance. U.S. Department of Labor. Retrieved from http://wdr.doleta.gov/SCANS/lal/

11. American Association of Colleges of Nursing (Website). Retrieved from www.aacn.nche.edu

12. American Nurses Association (Website). Retrieved from http://nursingworld.org/

13. National Association for Associate Degree Nursing (Website). Retrieved from https://www.oadn.org/

14. National Council of State Boards of Nursing (Website). Retrieved from https://www.ncsbn.org

15. National League For Nursing (Website). Retrieved from http://nln.org/

16. The Joint Commission (Website). Retrieved from https://www.jointcommission.org/

17. The National Center for Interprofessional Practice and Learning (Website). Retrieved from https://nexusipe.org/

18. Tang Y. *Brain-based leaning and education: Principles and practice.* San Diego, CA: Academic Press-Elsevier, Inc; 2017.

19. Ennis R. *What is critical thinking?* Retrieved from http://criticalthinking.net/definition.html; 2017.

20. Snyder M. Critical thinking: A foundation for consumer-focused care. *The Journal of Continuing Education in Nursing.* 1993;24:206–210.

21. Alfaro-LeFevre R. *Improving critical thinking, clinical reasoning, and clinical judgment.* Retrieved from https://www.nurse.com/; 2018.

22. NCSBN. *NGN News—Summer 2018.* Retrieved from www.ncsbn.org; 2018.

23. American Nurses Association. *Nursing scope and standards of performance and standards of clinical practice.* Washington, DC: American Nurses Publishing; 2015.

24. Alfaro-LeFevre R. *Evidence-based critical thinking indicators.* Retrieved from www.AlfaroTeachSmart.com; 2019.

25. Tanner CA. Thinking like a nurse: a research-based model of clinical judgment in nursing. *Journal of Nursing Education.* 2006;45(6):204–211.

26. Institute of Medicine. *To err is human: building a safer health system.* Washington, DC: National Academies Press; 2000. Retrieved from http://www.nap.edu/openbook.php?record_id=9728&page=1.

27. Zuriguel-Pérez E, Falcó-Pegueroles A, Roldán-Merino J, et al. Development and psychometrics properties of the nursing critical thinking in clinical practice questionnaire. *Worldviews on Evidence-Based Nursing.* 2017;14(4):257–264. https://doi.org/10.1111/wvn.12220.

28. Leins C. *Health Care Professionals' Quality of Life is Critical to Hospital Performance, Industry Leaders Say.* Retrieved from https://health.usnews.com/health-news/hospital-of-tomorrow/articles/2017-11-02/health-care-professionals-quality-of-life-is-critical-to-hospital-performance-industry-leaders-say; 2017.

2

Becoming a Critical Thinker

LEARNING OUTCOMES

After completing this chapter, you should be able to:

1. Summarize five key strategies to becoming a critical thinker.
2. Explain why having self-efficacy is central to developing critical thinking.
3. Address how personality, learning style, upbringing, culture, and generational differences affect thinking.
4. Identify strategies to make the most of emotional intelligence.
5. Explain why building trust in relationships and following a code of conduct are key to promoting critical thinking.
6. Summarize personal and situational factors that affect reasoning.
7. Name at least three habits that promote critical thinking and three that impede critical thinking.
8. Explain the relationship between goals and outcomes.
9. Describe how critical thinking relates to logic, intuition, and trial and error.
10. Evaluate your progress toward knowledge and intellectual critical thinking indicators (CTIs)

KEY CONCEPTS

Bias; prejudice; code of conduct; emotional intelligence; goals; intuition; logic self-efficacy; systems thinking; *See also previous chapter*

LEARNING TO READ YOUR OWN MIND

A first-grade teacher I know tells this great story: "One of my kids came into class looking pleased with himself. Pointing to the middle of his forehead, he announced, 'I just realized that I can read my *own mind*!'" Another of my friends talks to herself a lot. When asked, "Why are you talking to yourself?" she replies, "Because I'm the only one who makes any sense around here."

Many people have little understanding of their own thinking and even *less* understanding of how *others* think. While I can't promise that reading this chapter will stop you from talking to yourself, it *will* help you gain insight into how and why you think the way you do, how and why *others* think the way *they* do, and what you can do to become a critical thinker. When critical thinking is so much a part of you that your mind makes it a habit, it becomes the foundation for success in virtually all aspects of life—from managing personal and professional challenges to achieving your goals.

In this chapter, you'll examine factors that affect thinking and learn strategies you can use to make the most of your critical thinking potential.

FIVE KEY STRATEGIES

The following five strategies for becoming a critical thinker provide the organization for this chapter:

1. **Gain insight and self-awareness:** How do experts describe critical thinking? How do you personally describe it? How aware are you of how your personality, learning style, and upbringing affect your thinking? Are you aware of how others view your thinking and behavior (e.g., you may think you're being helpful, yet others may think you're controlling)? What factors influence thinking? What thinking habits should you develop? (Chapter 1 addressed the first two questions; this chapter helps you answer the rest.)
2. **Build trust in relationships by adopting a code of conduct that promotes respectful communication in all interactions** (Box 2.1). Skilled communication and open, honest *exchange* of facts, thoughts, ideas, and feelings are key.
3. **Be committed to developing the knowledge, attitudes, and skills needed for critical thinking.** These form the foundation for thinking habits that serve you well in personal, professional, and learning situations.
4. **Use an evidence-based reference** to ensure that everyone in your group has a common understanding of what critical thinking entails. These references serve as "talking points" to discuss what's going well and what needs to be improved. Everyone must be "on the same page."
5. **Reflect on your reasoning processes and ask for feedback.** You need to know what you're doing well and what you can do to improve. Formal and informal evaluation related to your thinking and performance is crucial to improve.

Let's start by examining the first strategy above Gaining insight and self-awareness.

HOW YOUR PERSONALITY AFFECTS THINKING

Your personality plays a major role in how you think and learn. It determines what information you notice, the way you make decisions, and how much structure and control you like. Connecting with your own particular personality's needs helps you understand how and why you think and act the way you do. It helps you get in touch with your talents and blind spots and find ways to improve. Understanding personality types different from your own helps you realize how and why *others* think the way they do. Armed with this information, you can facilitate "meetings of the minds."

To better understand your personality and thinking style, think about where you and others you know "fit" into the various styles described in Boxes 2.2 and 2.3.

BOX 2.1   Health Team Code of Conduct

As a member of this group/team, I agree to work to make the following a part of my daily routine.

1. **To keep patient and caregiver safety and welfare as the primary concern in all interactions, including:**
   - Always introducing myself to patients, family, and staff who are new to me.
   - Being vigilant and monitoring for care practices that increase risks for errors.
   - Remembering that no one is perfect and that all humans are vulnerable to making mistakes.
   - Taking responsibility for being "a safety net" when helping co-workers, anticipating what they may need, and pitching in to prevent mistakes (e.g., "I think that glove is contaminated; let me get you a new one." or "Here's a new needle.").
   - Making it a team principle that "If we witness unethical or unsafe practices, it's our responsibility to address them." (First directly with the person, then through policies and procedures if needed.)

2. **To promote empowered partnerships by**:
   - Valuing your time and the contribution you make to the team/group.
   - Accepting the diversity in our styles—recognizing that you know yourself best and should be allowed to choose your own approaches.
   - Promising to be honest, and treating you with respect and courtesy.
   - Promoting independence and mutual growth by applying the Platinum Rule[1] (Treat others as *they* want to be treated, not assuming they have the same needs *you* do).
   - Listening openly to new ideas and other perspectives.
   - Trying to "walk a mile in the other person's shoes."
   - Committing to resolving conflict without resorting to using power.
   - Taking responsibility for my own emotional well-being (if I feel bad about something, it's my responsibility to do something about it).
   - Ensuring that we both:
     - Stay focused on our joint purpose and responsibilities for achieving it.
     - Make decisions together as much as possible.
     - Realize that we're accountable for the outcomes (consequences) of our actions.
     - Have the right to say no, so long as it doesn't mean neglecting responsibilities.

3. **To foster open communication and a positive work environment by:**
   - Addressing specific issues and behaviors.
   - Acknowledging/apologizing if I've caused inconvenience or made a mistake.
   - Doing my "homework" before drawing conclusions; validating any rumors I hear.
   - Maintaining confidentiality when I'm used as a sounding board.
   - Using only ONE person as my sounding board before I decide to either give feedback or drop the issue.
   - Verifying any rumors I hear.
   - Redirecting co-workers who are talking about someone to speak directly to the person.
   - Addressing unsafe or unethical behavior directly and according to policies.
   - Offering feedback as indicated:
     - Within 72 hours, using "I" statements ("I feel … ." rather than "You make me feel … .").
     - Describing behaviors and giving specific examples.
     - Limiting discussion to the event at hand and not discussing history and telling you honestly and openly the impact of the behavior.

4. **To be approachable and open to feedback by:**
   - Taking responsibility for my actions and words.
   - Reflecting objectively, rather than blaming, defending, or rejecting criticism.
   - Asking for clarification of the perceived behaviors.
   - Remembering that there's always a little bit of truth in every criticism.
   - Staying focused on what I can learn from the situation.

© 2019 R. Alfaro-LeFevre. Retrieved from http://www.AlfaroTeachSmart.com.

BOX 2.2 Do You Know What to Do When Someone Turns Blue?

Here's a theory that gives new meaning to turning blue, red, white, or yellow (no, it doesn't mean becoming cyanotic, inflamed, shocky, or jaundiced). Psychologist Taylor Hartman uses colors to represent personality types.* (By the way, he says you can't really *turn* one color or another—you are what you are *born*.) Hartman thinks that each of us from birth is blessed with a core motive—a drive to approach life from a certain perspective. Using colors as labels, here's how he describes four distinct personality types.

REDS have a drive for power. They know how to take charge and make things happen. Reds' strengths are that they are confident, determined, logical, productive, and visionary. However, they can be bossy, impatient, arrogant, argumentative, and self-focused.

BLUES are driven to achieve intimacy. They love getting to know people well, have strong feelings, and like talking about the daily details of life. Blues are creative, caring, reliable, loyal, sincere, and committed to serving others. On the flip side, they can be judgmental, worry-prone, doubtful, and moody and often have unrealistic expectations.

WHITES strive for peace. They're independent, contented people who ask little of those around them. Whites are insightful, flexible, tolerant, easygoing, patient, and kind. But Whites tend to avoid conflict at all costs, are indecisive, are silently stubborn, and may "explode" because they hold things in until there are so many things bothering them that just one more problem pushes them over the edge.

YELLOWS are driven to have fun and enjoy the moment. They wake up happy, know how to enjoy life in the present moment, and are simply fun to be around. Yellows are outgoing, enthusiastic, optimistic, popular, and trusting. However, they tend to avoid facing facts and can be impulsive, undisciplined, disorganized, and uncommitted.

Applying the *Color Code* principles helps you connect with inner drives that often lie dormant, waiting to be harnessed in positive ways. Armed with this knowledge, you can make better "people decisions," like how to nurture a team or get along with difficult people. Imagine how you could apply this theory to help a group come together to give a presentation. You might get a productive, visionary Red to coordinate and lead the project; a caring, detail-oriented Blue to do the handouts; a peace-loving, insightful White to be a "human suggestion box" (no one's afraid to approach a White); and a fun-loving Yellow to make sure that the class is more than serious stuff (a little fun, humor, and refreshment make it an enjoyable, memorable, learning experience).

Think about what could happen in this situation if you switched some of those personalities and tasks around! The *Color Code* facilitates a crucial first step to improving thinking—understanding how and why we think the way we do (and how and why others think the way they do). These are challenging times that require us to think and work in teams. Applying these principles helps us spend less time spinning wheels and more time "in gear," fully engaged in progress. To take the Color Code test or order the book, go to http://www.ColorCode.com.

*Summarized from Hartman, T. (2013). *The color code; the people code for dealing effectively with different personalities.* Sandy, UT: Author

Source: Adapted from Alfaro-LeFevre R. *Do You Know What to Do When Someone Turns Blue?* 1998. Retrieved from http://www.nurse.com.

BOX 2.3 What's Your Thinking Style? (Myers-Briggs Type)

Extrovert	Introvert
Thinks out loud	Thinks inside
Draws energy from being with people	Draws energy from being quiet
Sensate	**Intuitive**
Perceives the world discretely through the five senses	Perceives the world overall
Looks for facts	Looks for meaning
Thinking	**Feeling**
Uses objective data	Uses subjective data
Seeks just decisions	Seeks fair decisions
Judging	**Perceiving**
Orders the environment	Keeps things flexible and open
Likes to plan	Likes to be spontaneous

Data from http://www.humanmetrics.com.

Keep in mind that one personality style isn't *better* than another. What matters is that you understand that there are distinct style differences and that you (1) connect with your own style, celebrating your strengths and working to overcome limitations, and (2) learn to connect with people with styles that are different from your own, respecting their need to approach things in their *own* way. Box 2.4 lists the benefits of being sensitive to personality types.

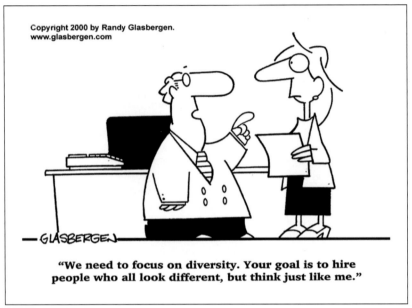

Copyright 2000 by Randy Glasbergen.
www.glasbergen.com

— GLASBERGEN

"We need to focus on diversity. Your goal is to hire people who all look different, but think just like me."

Reprinted with special permission from http://www.glasbergen.com.

BOX 2.4 Benefits of Being Sensitive to Personality Types

Partnering and Team Building
- Help diverse personalities come together with understanding and respect, promoting solid relationships
- Keep the focus on common goals, improving quality and efficiency
- Help identify strategies to reduce and resolve conflicts
- Facilitate collaboration and make the most of individual and team talents

Performance and Retention
- Promote critical thinking (people think better when they understand and trust one another)
- Reduce stress, allowing more brainpower for finding solutions
- Increase self-confidence by providing style-specific strategies
- Promote an environment that nurtures professional and personal growth

Consumer and Patient Satisfaction
- Facilitate communication with "difficult" patients and families
- Improve outcomes by helping you tailor approaches to consider different personalities' wants and needs
- Patients and families feel understood, empowered, and motivated by receiving care that's "in sync" with their own specific styles

CONNECTING WITH YOUR LEARNING STYLE

Connecting with your preferred learning style can make the difference between struggling to learn—feeling frustrated and like a failure—and learning efficiently.

Many people believe they are poor learners. However, the reality is that they're simply unaware of their own learning preferences. For example, a friend once said, "What I like best about computers is that I never was a good learner … but with computers, it doesn't matter because I just have to figure things out for myself … and I'm good at that." Learning is *figuring things out for yourself*. When you figure things out for yourself, you "own the material and make it yours." You understand deeply, and you retain more. If you're unsure about your learning style preferences and strategies to use, study Table 2.1.

TABLE 2.1 Strategies for Learning Style Preferences	
Learning Preference	**Strategies to Promote Learning**
Observers (Visual Learners) Learn best by watching. For example, you'd rather watch someone give an injection before reading the procedure.	**Sit in the front of the room, so you stay focused on the teacher, not on what's going on around you.** Visualize procedures in your mind's eye, rather than trying to follow individual steps. In skills labs, don't go first. Rather, watch your classmates and take a later turn. Ask for observational experiences. Take lots of notes, draw maps, and use a highlighter. Recopy your notes when you're studying. When learning new terms or concepts or trying to remember something, write them on sticky notes and put them where you'll see them frequently (e.g., the bathroom mirror, the computer). Preview chapters by scanning headings and illustrations.
Doers (Kinesthetic Learners) Learn best by moving, doing, experiencing, or experimenting. For example, you'd rather play with a syringe and inject a dummy before reading the procedure.	**Start by doing (e.g., play with equipment before reading about how to use it)** because it will make observing, reading, and listening more meaningful. Be sure you know the risks of doing without much knowledge, and find ways to minimize them (e.g., if you're playing on the computer, make sure you can't inadvertently erase a file). When taking notes, use arrows to show relationships. Draw boxes and circles around key concepts; use arrows when you make diagrams and maps. Pace up and down while reciting information to yourself; ride a bicycle while listening to an audio educational program. Record the information you're trying to learn, and listen to what you recorded while exercising (e.g., riding a bike). Write key words in the air; use your fingers to help you remember (bend the forefinger as you memorize a concept, and then bend the next for the next concept, and so on). Change positions frequently while studying; take frequent short breaks involving activity. Study in a rocking chair; play background music. Ask if you can do assignments in an active way (e.g., create a poster, be part of a discussion group).

Continued

TABLE 2.1 **Strategies for Learning Style Preferences—cont'd**	
Learning Preference	**Strategies to Promote Learning**
Listeners (Auditory Learners) Learn best by hearing. For example, you learn best when you can listen without worrying about taking notes.	**Whisper as you read, listening to your words (especially important when reading test questions).** Listen in class without taking notes, focusing on understanding what the teacher says, and then copy someone else's notes. Record classes and listen to what you recorded two or three times before exams. Ask if you can give an oral report or hand in an audio report for extra credit. Memorize by making up songs or rhymes. Study with a friend so you talk about the information. Record yourself as you read key information out loud.

GUIDING PRINCIPLE

There are no right or wrong ways to think or learn—there are only *differences*. Connecting with your preferred style helps you identify strategies to learn efficiently in your own way. When you figure things out *in your own way*, you're thinking critically.

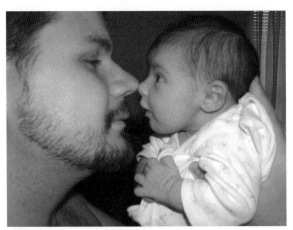

You are born with unique and inherited personality traits. Your birth order, gender, upbringing, and culture also affect your personality and learning preferences.

SELF-EFFICACY: BELIEVE IN YOURSELF

Self-efficacy—having confidence in your ability to accomplish all that you need to do to achieve your goals—is crucial to developing critical thinking. Today, independent learning in a complex world is the norm. We must all be self-sufficient. People with a strong sense of self-efficacy tend to challenge themselves, recover better from setbacks, and put forth a high degree of effort to meet commitments.[2] On the other hand, people with a poor sense of efficacy think they can't be successful. They're less likely to make a serious, extended effort and may see difficult tasks as threats to avoid. These people often have low aspirations, which may result in disappointing academic and clinical performances and become a self-fulfilling prophecy.[2]

With so much competition in the world today, it's easy to have dips in confidence levels, thinking things like, *Do I really have what it takes to do this?* Developing self-efficacy takes considerable self-coaching, as noted in the following quote:

> *"You must be your own coach. If you don't talk to yourself and give yourself pep talks, start now. Time was, only crazies talked to themselves; now, you miss the boat if you don't. Our minds are tricky things. We can't give in to self doubt or negativity. We must focus on the positives, as learning and performance depend on it."*
>
> *—Jean T. Penny, PhD, ARNP[3]*

If you have a low sense of self-efficacy, don't feel bad about it. Many of the challenges you face are common. It's not just you! You can overcome problems with self-efficacy through formal and informal coaching. A sensible mentor, teacher, or coach can help you put things in perspective and identify underlying feelings. They can help you get in touch with your strengths and develop ways to help you succeed.

EFFECTS OF BIRTH ORDER, UPBRINGING, AND CULTURE

Your birth order—whether you were the first born, who was expected to lead, or the "baby," who had few responsibilities—affects how you think, as does your parents' parenting style. If you were raised by strict, authoritarian parents who insisted that you "do as you are told, without asking questions," it's likely that you'll find it difficult to approach teachers or leaders to discuss problems, ask for feedback, or offer suggestions. Many of us need to muster courage to overcome deep-seated insecurities that come from hard lessons learned as a child.

Where you grew up and the culture you embrace also affect thinking. For example, in some countries, questioning teachers is considered rude. Yet when students ask questions, everyone learns. Think about the courage it took for the following nurse to come forward in one of my workshops and tell me her struggle with asking questions:

> *"In my culture, asking questions is discouraged and a sign of weakness and embarrassment. What I'm working on and want to know is how to become more confident and capable [of] asking questions. I realize it's essential to critical thinking."*
>
> *—Workshop Participant*

GENERATIONAL DIFFERENCES

Each generation has collective life experiences that shape their values, communication style, and what's expected in relationships. Whether you're dealing with personal, work, or patient relationships, understanding generational differences can make the difference between misunderstandings and making connections that make the most of individual talents. Study Table 2.2, which shows values and characteristics of various generations.

TABLE 2.2   Generational Values and Characteristics

Generation	Values and Characteristics
Veterans/Silent Generation (Born 1922 to 1946)	Respect for authority; hard work; stoicism; minimal or no technology use.
Baby Boomers (Born 1946 to 1964)	Social consciousness; teamwork; competition; optimism; long work hours expected; love–hate relationship with authority; lifelong learning; many are technologically challenged.
Gen X (Born 1964 to 1980)	Life/work balance; self-reliance; technological literacy: irreverent humor; informality; risk taking; lifelong learning; want feedback; pessimism and skepticism; acceptance of diversity; varying degrees of technology savvy.
Gen Y / Millenials (Born 1980 to 2000)	Life/work balance; empowerment; authentic leadership; security; privacy; preparedness; healthy workplaces; safety and learning cultures; diversity; confidence; optimism; teamwork; authority figures not held in awe; like change, multitasking, and need positive feedback; casual dress; fun; skeptical and less trusting of others; readily use technology.
Gen Z (Born 2000 to 2012)	Similar to Gen Y, plus: Life/work flexibility: work online at a rapid pace; share observations on various issues, media, and products; digital technology is second nature.

APPLYING PRINCIPLES OF EMOTIONAL INTELLIGENCE

Emotions affect reasoning in deep and intense ways. Since 1995—when science journalist Daniel Goleman wrote the ground breaking book, *Emotional Intelligence: Why It Can Matter More Than IQ*—many experts have studied how emotional intelligence affects thinking and performance.[4]

While the terms *emotional intelligence (EI)*, *emotional quotient (EQ)*, and *emotional intelligence quotient (EIQ)* are used interchangeably, we'll use EQ to keep it simple. Goleman describes EQ as the ability to:

- **Recognize your own emotions and those of others** (e.g., "I'm getting upset because I feel like all I'm hearing is that I'm *wrong*" or "This person seems to be getting upset and I need to find out why").
- **Discriminate between different feelings and label them appropriately** (e.g., "Are the main feelings here anger or insecurity?").
- **Use emotional information to guide thinking and behavior** (e.g., "If you feel insecure here, let's talk about this first").
- **Manage or adjust your emotions and behavior to reach your goals** (e.g., "I need to remain calm, even though I feel like I'm being attacked" or "I need to change how I approach people because it seems like they feel like I'm attacking them").

Being sensitive to others' emotions and learning how to work through difficult communications profoundly affects your ability to think critically. If you can't apply EQ principles, your great ideas and intentions will be lost in emotional issues. Many people aren't aware of their own deep, strong feelings. Pay attention to facial expressions, one of the best indicators of emotions (Fig. 2.1). Clarify what you think and feel and what others think and feel—then adjust your behavior to get the best results. Box 2.5 gives strategies for developing your EQ.

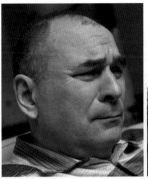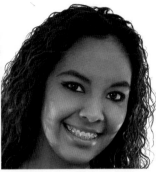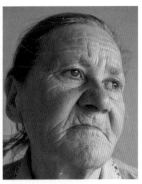

FIG. 2.1 Facial expressions are the best indicators of emotions. What emotions do you read in these photos?

BOX 2.5 Developing Emotional Intelligence

Definition: Knowing how to recognize and manage emotions to get positive results.
1. **Connect with emotions.** Put your feelings into words and, through dialogue, help others do the same ("I feel ... because ... ." If you're trying to connect with others' emotions, ask, "What are your thoughts and feelings on this?"). Never assume you know what someone else is feeling. Never expect others to know what you're feeling.
2. **Accept true feelings** for what they are. No one's to blame for what he or she feels.
3. **Learn mood management.** Recognize the importance of connecting with how emotions are affecting thinking. Learn to manage feelings like anger, anxiety, fear, and discouragement.
4. **Don't be too concerned with isolated events.** Patterns of behavior are what matter. Don't sweat the small stuff.
5. **Keep in mind that emotions are "catching."** If you're depressed, you may trigger depression in someone else. If you're enthusiastic, you may trigger enthusiasm.
6. **Pay attention to stress levels.** When the going gets rough, take time out, focus on the positives, find a sense of humor, play a game, or take a walk.
  Recommended: Consortium for Research on Emotional Intelligence in Organizations (http://www.eiconsortium.org/); Daniel Goleman website (http://www.danielgoleman.info/)

COMMUNICATING EFFECTIVELY

If you said, "Name one habit we should all work on to improve reasoning," I'd reply, "Communicating effectively." Becoming a critical thinker requires developing three main communication skills:
1. Listening deeply to understand other people's point of view.
2. Probing to gain the most important information in a nonjudgmental way.
3. Getting your point across clearly and succinctly.

Paying attention to both verbal and nonverbal messages is crucial to effective communication. Communication is usually based on more than one interaction and is highly influenced by messages sent by *behavior over time*. For example, you may be committed to giving good patient care, but if you constantly arrive late for work, you send a different message.

Communicating with patients, families, and health care team members is an ongoing challenge. For example, you must choose the best communication channel to use to get the best results (e.g., face to face, phone, or electronic messages). Adapting your style to meet others' communication preferences promotes timely exchange of information. For example, many of us use text messages because it's the only way we can get our families, patients, and clients to respond.

In all important communications, ask, "What's the best way to communicate with this person in this situation?" Often, this means using more than one communication channel (e.g., sending a follow-up e-mail after a verbal discussion). With communication problems ask (1) "What, from the other person's perspective, am I doing that contributes to this issue?" and (2) "What can I change to do better?" Also consider where you stand in relation to your CT potential (Fig. 2.2)

Throughout this book, you have many opportunities to practice specific communication skills in the context of various challenges (e.g., giving change-of-shift hand-off reports, dealing with conflict, and dealing with complaints). For now, study the communications in the following scenario. What went wrong? What went *right?* How might it have been handled differently?

SCENARIO COMMUNICATION SKILLS AFFECT OUTCOMES

Parents bring a young boy to the emergency department with a painful broken arm. They're greeted by Jane, the nurse, who decides which patients will be seen first. As Jane puts a splint on the child, she announces, "It will be at least 4 hours before he'll be seen." The parents ask, "Should we go somewhere else?" Jane replies, "Well, there will be a fee for this." Upset by her son's injury, the mother angrily shouts, "Four hours is unacceptable!" Jane calls security, who stands by on call. The mother announces, "This is humiliating! We're leaving!" As the parents go out the door, Bob, another nurse, pulls them aside and says, "Write a letter to Risk Management about this … this was BADLY handled."

The parents write a letter describing their bad experience. They also point out how much it meant to have Bob's kindness and concern. They wonder if Jane was just having a bad day. A few weeks later, they receive a call from the hospital explaining that due to privacy issues, not much could be said. But the caller did say one thing: "Jane will not be having any more bad days at our hospital."

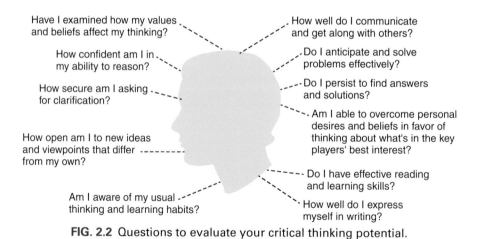

FIG. 2.2 Questions to evaluate your critical thinking potential.

COMMUNICATION STRATEGIES

Here are communication strategies that significantly affect your ability to gain the information you need to think critically.

- **Overcome innate needs to be right or to know everything** by practicing saying things like, "You're right" and "That's a good question!" (Yes, sometimes it takes practice saying the words ☺.)
- **Aim for mindful communication.** This means clearing your mind of "clutter" and paying attention to where you are in the present moment. Work to gain a keen awareness of the

situation, the information you gain, and the interaction of those engaged in the communication. To be mindful, pause before engaging in a communication and from time to time during the communication to allow yourself to get centered.

- **Sit down.** Sitting with someone gives the message that you'll take the time needed to exchange thoughts, feelings, and ideas. It also helps you be present "in the moment."
- **Think ahead—examine your "personal story" about the communication you're about to have.** What are your thoughts and feelings? Do you have preconceptions? What assumptions and judgments have you made? What's your confidence level? What can you do to be more objective and positive about the communication? Staying objective, overcoming bad feelings, focusing on the present, and expressing the desire for positive outcomes improve the quality of communication.
- **Consider how the other person may perceive both you and the situation.** Think about cultural differences and communication preferences. What can you do to make the other person more comfortable? Use clear, concise, simple language.
- **Evaluate your stress level and that of the other person.** Choose the right time and place.
- **Explain that your intent is not to judge, but to understand** (e.g., "I'm not here to judge. I just want to understand what's going on.").
- **Listen first.** Work to understand the thoughts and feelings that others are expressing before trying to get them to understand *you*.
- **Use strategies that help you see other points of view.**
  - Ask for clarification (e.g., "Can you clarify further?" or "Help me understand …").
  - Use phrases like, "From your way of looking at it " or "From your perspective."
  - Repeat back what you hear (e.g., "You're saying … is that correct?").
- **Listen empathetically.** Work to understand the other person's struggles and concerns. This is called "trying to walk a mile in someone else's shoes" and can be done by taking the following steps[5]:
  1. Clear your mind of thoughts about how you view the situation or concerns about how you're going to respond.
  2. Focus on listening to the person's feelings and perceptions.
  3. Rephrase the feelings and perceptions as you understand them to be (e.g., "I realize that you're frustrated and angry.").
  4. Detach and come back to your own frame of reference.
- Use strategies that help you get accurate and comprehensive information. For example, use open-ended questions (those requiring more than a one-word answer, such as, "How do you feel about leaving tomorrow?").
- Use strategies that help you get your point across:
  - Wait until the person is ready to listen.
  - When voicing an opinion, use phrases that convey that you're giving an opinion, rather than dictating what is so (e.g., "From my way of looking at it … " or "From my perspective …").
  - Ask the person to paraphrase what you said (e.g., "I need to know you understand. Can you tell me in your own words what I just said?").
- Demonstrate behaviors that send messages like *I'm responsible, I can be trusted,* and *I want to do a good job* (keep promises, be punctual, accept responsibility, and respect others' time).
- When you may have caused an inconvenience, made a mistake, or offended someone, offer a sincere apology, taking accountability (e.g., "I should have been more aware and I'm sorry this happened.").
- Be courteous and respect others' territory. Ask permission (e.g., "May I listen to your chest?" rather than "Sit up and let me listen to your chest.").

> ### BOX 2.6   The Importance of Listening
>
> **Listening: A Lost Art?**
> Not listening to each other separates us from family, friends, and co-workers. We haven't learned to listen and truly hear with empathy. We listen to prepare our responses, whether to tell our own story or to offer advice. Most of us are preoccupied with the rush of our own lives and give little thought to the needs of others to be heard. We listen as though we are expected to respond. When we want to be there for someone, we listen for where we can help. When we are spoken to heatedly, we become defensive and either talk back heatedly or withdraw. — Michael Nichols, Author of *The Lost Art of Listening: How Learning to Listen Can Improve Relationships*
>
> **Receptive Listening: Promoting Self-Awareness and Professional Growth**
> As part of a year-long nurse residency program at Dartmouth-Hitchcock Medical Center in New Hampshire, facilitators trained in receptive listening (listening without valuing, judging, helping, or changing) meet monthly in 90-minute sessions with small groups of new nurses. Nurses report that this type of listening creates a safe environment that contributes to their self-awareness, renewal, learning, problem-solving, and sense of belonging and connectedness to the organization. Receptive listening also has shown direct benefits to patients in an unpublished doctoral study. For more information, contact Ellen Ceppetelli at http://www.eliotgroupinstitute.com/.

- Keep an open mind, and practice listening skills (Box 2.6).
- For specific communication strategies in challenging situations, study the following skills in Chapter 7: *Communicating Bad News* (Skill 7.1), *Dealing With Complaints Constructively* (Skill 7.2), *Giving and Taking Constructive Criticism* (Skill 7.4), and *Managing Conflict Constructively* (Skill 7.5).

BUILDING RELATIONSHIPS

Whether you're dealing with patients or co-workers, building trust in relationships is crucial to getting the results you need. Without trust, you're likely to have superficial—rather than meaningful—discussions, because people are afraid to speak their minds. Open, honest dialogue happens only when there's trust between and among individuals. *Developing Empowered Partnerships* (Skill 7.3 in Chapter 7) gives strategies for building trust in relationships.

> ### GUIDING PRINCIPLE
>
> **People think best when they like and trust one another.** The first step to building trust is agreeing to a code of conduct and making roles and responsibilities clear. Be sensitive to style differences and follow the *Platinum Rule* ("Treat others as they want to be treated") rather than the *Golden Rule* ("Do unto others as you would have them do unto you").[1] This changes your thinking from "This is what I would want in this situation, so that's what I'll do" to "Let me first understand what others want so I can give it to them."

FACTORS INFLUENCING CRITICAL THINKING ABILITY

Have you ever found yourself saying, "I just wasn't thinking" or "This really got me thinking—I came up with some great ideas"? We all feel this way at one time or another. Our ability to think well varies, depending on personal factors and the current circumstances. This section addresses personal and situational factors that influence thinking.

Personal Factors Affecting Thinking

In addition to personality, learning styles, birth order, culture, upbringing, and generational tendencies described earlier, consider how the following personal factors affect thinking.

- **Health and Happiness.** If you're not feeling well, struggling with fatigue, stress, or other symptoms, you have little energy left for critical thinking. Studies show that unhappy people are prone to illness.[6,7] For this reason, leaders, organizations, and communities are studying what makes people happy and what can be done to improve happiness and sense of well-being. Some interesting facts from the *World Happiness Report*—an annual study published by the United Nations—include: (1) It's your human connections, not how much money you have, that makes you happy; and (2) Many people report being happier as they age.[7,8] Learning how to manage your moods and be optimistic can boost your ability to be a critical thinker—so much energy is lost on worry and negativity.

- **Mindfulness and Work–Life Balance.** Mindfulness (paying attention to your feelings, thoughts, and body sensations "in the moment") and work–life balance affect health and happiness. Life, school, and work stress can create "vicious cycles"—stressful days often mean sleepless nights. Make time to take care of yourself so you can take care of others. The saying goes, "People who worry about the glass being half-empty or half-full are missing the point: It's refillable." Make time to "refill your glass" (e.g., exercise, drink lots of water, eat well, and do things that bring peace and joy).

- **Fair-Mindedness and Moral Development.** People who are fair-minded and have a mature level of moral development are more likely to be critical thinkers.[8,9] It makes sense that those who are keenly aware of their own values, have a good sense of right and wrong, and approach situations with an attitude of "I must consider all viewpoints and make decisions in the key players' best interests" already are critical thinkers.

- **Age and Maturity.**[8-11] The older you get, the better thinker you become. There are two logical reasons for this: (1) Moral development usually comes with maturity; and (2) Most older people have had more opportunities to practice reasoning in various situations. Realize, however, that sometimes older people are rigid and set in their ways—in this case, age impedes critical thinking.

- **Personal Dislikes, Prejudices, and Biases.**[9] These are subtle but powerful factors that hinder critical thinking. Realize that bias differs from prejudice in that it includes things you are in favor of, as well as things you're against. Recognizing these factors and overcoming them to be objective helps you think more fairly and logically.

- **Self-Confidence.** Many authors address the need for self-confidence in reasoning. If you aren't confident, you spend much of your brain power worrying about failure, reducing the energy available for productive thinking. *Occasionally* self-confidence hinders critical thinking; some people become overly confident and believe they can't be wrong or have little to learn from others.

- **Past Experience.** Experience is usually considered an *enhancing* factor. You remember best what you learn from experience. If, however, your past experience is a bad one, it may be an inhibiting factor. For example, if a mother had a bad experience breast-feeding her firstborn child, she may be unwilling to consider breast-feeding subsequent children.

- **Knowledge of Problem-Solving, Decision-Making, the Nursing Process, and the Scientific Method.** Familiarity with these models enhances critical thinking because they form the foundation for sound reasoning.

- **Early Evaluation and Reflection.** When you make it a habit to evaluate early—reflecting on your thinking and checking whether your information is accurate, complete, and up-to-date—you can make corrections early. You avoid making decisions based on outdated, inaccurate, or incomplete information.

- **Effective Writing Skills.** When you learn how to make yourself clear in writing, you apply critical thinking principles like identifying an organized approach, deciding what's relevant, and focusing on others' perspectives.
- **Effective Reading and Learning Skills.** Because critical thinking often requires that you use resources independently, you must know how to read and learn well. Having effective reading skills doesn't mean knowing how to read rapidly. It means knowing how to read efficiently, identifying what's important, and drawing conclusions about what the material implies.

Situational Factors Affecting Thinking

Here are some situational factors that affect thinking.

- **Awareness of Risks.** Usually this is an enhancing factor. When you know the risks, you think more carefully (you "think before acting"). Sometimes awareness of the risks can increase anxiety to a level that impedes critical thinking. Most of us remember how hard it was to think critically when we gave our first injection.
- **Knowledge of Related Factors.** Knowing about factors that relate to creating solutions is central to clinical reasoning. For example, you might know about diabetes, but if you don't *know the person* you're going to teach about diabetes—the person's lifestyle, desires, and motivations—you'll be unlikely to design a plan that the person will follow.
- **Awareness of Resources.** Awareness of resources is essential for critical thinking. No one knows everything. You must know where to get reliable help (from human and other information resources).
- **Positive Reinforcement.** Positive reinforcement promotes critical thinking by building confidence and focusing on what's being done *right*.
- **Negative "Talk."** Focusing too much on what could go wrong impedes thinking because it drains your confidence and takes your attention away from what you need to do *right*.
- **Evaluative (Judgmental) Styles.** These impede critical thinking. When you think someone is judging you, you spend more brain power worrying about what the *other person* is thinking than what *you're* thinking.
- **Presence of Motivating Factors.** Having motivating factors (things that make you want to think critically) entices you to get your brain "in gear." For example, think how motivated you are to learn something when a teacher says, "You must know this because it will be on the test, and you'll run into it a lot in the clinical setting."
- **Time Limitations.** These can be enhancing or impeding factors. Time limitations can be motivating factors—deadlines stimulate us to get things done. If there's too little time, however, you may make decisions more quickly than you'd like and come up with less-than-satisfactory answers. It's interesting to note that the courts give more leeway to decisions that were made in emergency situations than to those made with plenty of time for thinking.
- **Distractions and Interruptions.** These impede thinking for obvious reasons—the more distractions, the more difficult it is to stay focused. Because distractions and interruptions cause mistakes, many organizations are working on how to minimize them.

Habits Causing Barriers to Critical Thinking

As humans, we all have deeply ingrained habits that may create barriers to critical thinking. Keeping in mind that the following habits are simply human nature, consider how they impede reasoning:

- **Self-Focusing.** Focusing on ourselves is a carryover from primitive survival instincts. In the early days of humans, people had to be keenly centered on their own needs to survive. We still have this instinct. Critical thinking requires you to overcome this natural tendency and work to understand needs, perspectives, and challenges that are *different* from your own.

- **Mine Is Better.** We tend to regard our ideas, values, religions, cultures, and points of view as being superior to those of others. To think critically, recognize when you are biased and have strong personal "pro" or "con" views that may influence your opinions.

- **Face-Saving.** We have a strong instinct to protect our image—we try to save face. Critical thinking requires us to learn and grow. As we learn and grow, we'll make mistakes or realize that our old ways of thinking or doing things can be improved. To be a critical thinker, we must be comfortable saying things like "I'm not sure," "I was wrong," or "I have to think about that."

- **Self-Deception.** This is the subconscious forgetting of things about ourselves we don't particularly feel good about. An example of this is experienced nurses who believe that they never made learning errors or were shy, nervous, or insecure when they were beginning nurses.

- **Resistance to Change.** We all tend to resist change. Too often change is considered "guilty until proved innocent." Overcoming this barrier doesn't mean embracing every new change uncritically. It means being willing to suspend judgment long enough to make an informed decision on whether the change is worthwhile (see *Navigating and Facilitating Change*, Skill 7.7, Chapter 7).

- **Conformity.** Although some conformity—like following policies and procedures—is good, there's also harmful conformity. Harmful conformity is when we conform to group thinking just to avoid being viewed as "different." Conforming without thought stifles the ability to be creative and improve. An example of harmful conformity is following policies blindly, even if there are circumstances that clearly indicate that the policy doesn't apply in *this* particular situation.

- **Stereotyping.** We stereotype when we have fixed, unbending overgeneralizations about others (e.g., *homeless people aren't very bright*). When our minds are fixed and unbending, we're unlikely to see the reality. By recognizing our tendency to stereotype, we can make a conscious effort to overcome this habit.

- **Needing to be right.** We all have a need to be right, often closing our minds to other possibilities. Feeling like you're being told you're wrong brings up subconscious feelings of insecurity. You have to be willing to rise above this instinct and ask yourself: Is it more important to be right than to gain the insights I need to improve and meet common goals?

- **Making assumptions (when our minds accept something as fact even though we haven't examined it closely).** We can all remember saying something like, "I was wrong when I assumed…" Stephen Covey, author of *The 7 Habits of Highly Effective People*, tells this touching story about making assumptions[5]: A man is sitting on a subway when another man gets on with three young children. The children are unruly, shouting and climbing all over the seats. The first man assumes the children lack discipline. Annoyed, he says to the father, "Don't you think you should talk to them and get them to behave?" The father, looking somewhat dazed, responds, "We're on the way home from the hospital—their mother just died and I don't know what to say to them."

- **Focusing on the first hypothesis we think of (jumping to conclusions).** Some clinicians use *hunches* instead of hypotheses (e.g., I have a hunch this person has mental issues). Unlike assumptions, which are often subconscious, hypotheses are *deliberate* (you decide something is true based on limited evidence). Hypotheses are important starting points for investigation or problem-solving. Yet our minds tend to anchor themselves on the *first* hypothesis we identify, before all the evidence is in. If the first hypothesis we think of is *incorrect*, we *start* with the wrong idea, causing the rest of our thinking to be flawed. Focusing on the wrong hypotheses is also what happens in the next habits listed here.

- **Tunnel Vision.** Our minds tend to focus exclusively on a limited point of view. A classic example of tunnel vision is when a psychiatric nurse fails to consider whether someone's confusion is related to a *medical problem*, and vice versa (a medical-surgical nurse fails to consider whether someone's confusion is related to a *psychiatric problem*).

- **One Size Fits All.** When we have strategies that have worked well in the past, it's natural for us to apply them to new situations. But if you're not getting the results you expected, overcome this tendency by asking questions like: "What have I assumed?" "What am I missing?" and "What should I do differently based on this particular person and situation?"
- **Choosing Only One.** When faced with more than one choice, we tend to choose only one. We forget to think about things like, "Are there other, better choices?" "Can we do *both*?" "Do we have to do *either*?" Beginners are most vulnerable to the *choosing-only-one* habit. They tend to blindly accept that if they've chosen at least one option, they've made a good decision. They also tend to make the assumption that there must be *one best way* to do something, instead of thinking that there probably are several good ways of getting things done and that each has advantages and disadvantages, depending on circumstances. You can overcome this tendency by remembering to ask, "Must I choose only one?" or "Is this the only way?" or "What approaches can we combine?"

Habits Promoting Critical Thinking

Developing habits that promote critical thinking is a constant "work in progress." Becoming a critical thinker requires ongoing self-reflection, self-correction, and practice. We gain insight and experience *over time*. Here are some thinking habits that can significantly affect your critical thinking ability:

- **Be proactive and responsible for your own life.** Anticipate responses, and act before things happen.
- **Affirm your path.** Your work is important, and it's a privilege to have it. Stay focused—fully present in everything you do—and give complete attention to each action, interaction, and task.
- **Communicate effectively.** Work to understand other points of view before presenting your own.
- **Become a systems thinker,** as described in the following shaded section.

Systems Thinking[12,13]

- **Look for *relationships among key pieces* of the whole** (e.g., How is my sense of well-being affected by what's going on in my personal life, at work [or school], and in my community?).
- **Think about the consequences of actions** (e.g., If I decide to move to another community, what are the consequences for my family?).
- **Learn how things tend to unfold over time** (e.g., According to what I read about moving, if I decide to move, there are likely to be feelings of stress and loss at the beginning, followed by better feelings of new beginnings and friendships after we settle in).

- **Begin with an end in mind.** Identify clear expected outcomes. What exactly do you want to accomplish? Make your goals and expectations explicit.
- **Know your priorities—put first things first.** Decide what's important, and stick to priorities moment by moment, day by day.
- **Stay grounded in who you are—"sharpen the saw"** (look after yourself physically, emotionally, and spiritually).[6] Covey explains "sharpening the saw" like this: *A man is sawing a tree trunk for hours. The saw is dull, and the man is exhausted. Someone suggests that he might do better if he sharpens the saw. The man responds, "I don't have time" and continues to work ineffectively.*
- **Show goodwill.** Your positive thoughts and actions help you and the people around you. Don't judge others or take part in gossip or negativity.
- **Think win-win.** Aim for *mutual benefit* in all human interactions.
- **Develop good learning habits and be committed to lifelong learning.** Learn something new every day and help others do the same.

FOCUSING ON OUTCOMES (RESULTS)

Critical thinkers are outcomes-focused (results-oriented). What exactly are you trying to accomplish? This section clarifies the relationship between goals and outcomes and explains why making it a habit to *focus on outcomes* is crucial for critical thinking.

Goal (Intent) Versus Outcome (Result)

The terms *goal, objective,* and *outcome* have similar meanings and are often used interchangeably. There is, however, a significant difference among these terms:

- **Goal (objective)** indicates general **intent,** what you **aim to do.** *Example:* My goal (or objective) is to teach Steve about diabetes.
- **Outcome** indicates specific, **measurable results.** *Example:* After I finish teaching Steve, he will be able to demonstrate insulin injection and explain how he will keep his blood sugar within normal range through diet, exercise, and medication.

Goals are often vague and can be idealistic. Outcomes center on *clearly observable benefits and desired ultimate results,* forcing you to be realistic and think things through. Use the following memory jog to help you remember these two terms.

G = G	**G**oals = **G**eneral intent (what you plan to accomplish)
O = O	**O**utcomes = **O**bservable results (what you will observe to determine how well you accomplished your goal or objective)

Think about the following scenario, which shows the importance and challenges of clarifying outcomes.

SCENARIO CLARIFYING OUTCOMES (END RESULTS): NOT THAT SIMPLE

A group gathers to discuss building a bridge in a small town. Someone says, "Let's first be sure that we all agree on the end result." Several members consider this a dumb statement. Isn't the end result simply that the town will have a bridge? A bridge is a clear and observable outcome, right? How about if I tell you this is very limited thinking? The real end result you need to focus on is that *whoever wants to get across that bridge is able to do so.* You must pay attention to the end users—the people who will use the bridge. This means starting by asking questions like, "Who will use this bridge?" "How much room will they need to get their vehicles across?" "When will there be the most traffic, and how much will that traffic weigh?" "Where is the best place for this bridge?" If these questions aren't raised in the beginning, it's likely that you'll end up with a costly, useless, inconvenient, or even dangerous bridge.

GUIDING PRINCIPLE

Determining outcomes requires you to stay centered on the key people who will demonstrate that the desired results are achieved. In the previous scenario, the key people are those who travel the bridge. In health care, it's the patients, families, clients, communities, and consumers.

You'll have opportunities to practice determining patient-centered (client-centered) outcomes in Chapter 6 (Skill 6.14). For now, just remember that if you haven't given enough thought to exactly what *end results* you need, you aren't thinking critically.

⚡ CRITICAL THINKING STRATEGIES

This section first summarizes 10 questions that are central to critical thinking, and then it addresses using logic, intuition, and trial and error.

Ten Main Questions

Here are 10 main questions you need to ask to promote critical thinking in various situations:

1. What major outcomes (observable beneficial results) do you and key stakeholders (e.g., patient, family, and care providers) expect to observe in the patient after care is complete? Be as specific as possible. For example, compare the vague outcome in the first situation here with the more specific outcome in the second situation.
   Situation 1: Jody will be discharged home in 2 days.
   Situation 2: Jody will be discharged home in 2 days in the care of her mother, who will be able to demonstrate sterile dressing change by then.

2. **What priority problems and risks must be managed to achieve the major outcomes?** Asking this question helps you prioritize. You have only so much time—assign top priority to addressing problems, issues, or risks that may impede progress toward getting results. Using the previous example, Jody's mother tells you that she knows nothing about changing sterile dressings and also wants to know how she can improve her parenting skills. If time is short, give top priority to teaching her about dressing changes and handle the issue of how to be a better parent by giving her information on reference materials and support groups.

3. **What are the circumstances (context) in this particular patient situation?** The approach to critical thinking changes, depending on the circumstances. For example, imagine that you're in class and you're asked how to manage a patient in shock. You aren't sure, but you think you know, so it's appropriate for you to answer. If you're in the clinical setting, however, trying to manage shock based on uncertain knowledge is dangerous.

4. **What knowledge and skills are required to care for this patient?** Having discipline-specific knowledge and skills is crucial to critical thinking. For example, how can you think critically about managing cardiac pain if you don't know the causes and common treatments of cardiac pain? If you don't know what knowledge and skills are required, you probably don't know enough to get involved—get help.

5. **How much room is there for error?** When there's less room for error, we must carefully assess the situation, examine all possible solutions, and make every effort to make prudent decisions. For example, which of the following situations has less room for error, and how might your approach to decision-making change in each situation?
   Situation 1: You need to decide whether to give an over-the-counter antihistamine to someone who is usually in good health.
   Situation 2: You need to decide whether to give an over-the-counter antihistamine to someone with multiple chronic health problems.
   The first situation has more room for error because the person is less likely to have preexisting conditions or be taking medications that might interact with the antihistamine. The second situation requires consultation with a physician.

6. **How much time do you have?** If you have plenty of time, you can take time to think independently, using resources such as textbooks. If you don't have much time, you should report the problem to your supervisor to ensure timely attention. **Patient safety and welfare is number one.**

7. **What human and information resources can help?** Identifying resources (e.g., textbooks, computers, or experts) is essential to getting the information you need to think critically. For

example, you don't have to know every side effect of every drug in a drug manual. Rather, know when you need detailed information. Look up the drug in a manual, or check with a pharmacist to carefully review *all* side effects.

8. **Whose perspectives must be considered?** Critical thinking requires you to consider the perspectives of all of the key players involved; otherwise you risk having conflicting purposes. For example, to develop an effective plan for home care, you must consider the perspectives of the patient, other household members, and other health care team members. Imagine what could happen if you sent a grandmother home with many brightly colored medications and everyone forgot to consider the perspective of a toddler in the home!

9. **What's influencing thinking?** Recognizing influencing factors such as personal biases helps us identify vested interests, an important step in making fair-minded choices. For example, a nurse who is strongly against abortion may avoid working in the field of gynecology, in which women's decisions might make it difficult to give objective nursing care.

10. **What must be done to monitor, prevent, manage, or eliminate the problems, issues, and risks identified in question 2 (and who's accountable for doing it)?** For example, if you have a bedridden patient who has surgery, preventing skin breakdown is a problem that must be managed to prevent dangerous pressure ulcers and ensure timely discharge. Deciding *who* is accountable for *what* is essential to ensure that nothing "falls through the cracks."

> ### GUIDING PRINCIPLE
> **Becoming a critical thinker means developing excellent problem-solving and prevention skills.** This includes always assessing situations thoroughly, being proactive, and determining (1) what outcomes (results) are most important and (2) what priority problems and risks must be addressed to achieve the outcomes.

Using Logic, Intuition, and Trial and Error

Let's consider how knowing principles of logic, intuition, and trial and error relate to critical thinking.

Logic—sound reasoning that's based on facts (evidence)—is the foundation for critical thinking. It's the safest, most reliable approach. For all important decisions and opinions, make sure you can explain the logic of your thinking.

Intuition—a valuable part of thinking—is best described as "knowing something without evidence." For experts, intuitive hunches speed up problem-solving, because they have a lot of experiential knowledge in their heads. For them, thinking-in-action is rapid, dynamic, and intuitive. Novices must rely more on step-by-step logic. Keep in mind that sometimes things are counterintuitive—the *opposite* of what your intuition tells you. In important situations, bring logic to your thinking and look for evidence to support gut feelings. If you have no evidence to support your intuition, consider the risks of acting on intuition alone. For example, can you remember a time when you did something on your computer based on intuition and ended up with a disaster? This also can happen with patients.

Trial and error—trying several solutions until you find one that works—is risky but sometimes necessary. Use trial and error only when there's plenty of room for mistakes, when the problem can be monitored closely, and when the solutions have been logically thought through. A common example of useful trial and error is trying to determine the best way for a dressing to be applied to an awkward wound—it may take several tries before the best way is determined.

Focusing on the Big Picture and the Details

Whether you see yourself as a "big picture" person or a "details" person, it's important to realize that critical thinking requires focusing on *both* the big picture *and* the details—the whole and the parts. Think about the following examples:

- **Mr. Martin has cardiac problems.** He tells you he has chest pain and is afraid he might die. Treating both "the whole" (Mr. Martin's pain and anxiety) and "the parts" (Mr. Martin's oxygen-deprived heart) is essential to resolving the chest pain (and, perhaps, to saving his life).
- **You're trying to teach Tonya how to care for her newborn.** You're well prepared with lots of nice pamphlcts. She seems interested, but she keeps yawning and doesn't seem to retain information very long. Finally you say, "Is there a better time we could do this?" She admits that she hasn't slept all night and is too tired. You come back later after Tonya's had a good rest. She learns readily. In this case, paying attention to an important detail (fatigue) helped you be a more effective teacher.

Remember to ask questions like, "What's the big picture here?" "Am I considering both the parts and the whole?" and "Am I paying attention to the most important details?"

Drawing Maps, Diagrams, and Decision Trees

When you draw maps, diagrams, and decision trees, you enhance your critical thinking ability by helping your brain grasp complex relationships. You apply *systems thinking* principles because with maps and diagrams, you make connections between one thing and another; when you draw decision trees, you illustrate consequences of actions and focus on how things are likely to unfold over time.

When you draw your own map, diagram, or decision tree, it helps you "personalize" information and "make it your own." When you study well-designed maps, diagrams, or decision trees, you learn more quickly, because your brain does better with "pictures" than words. Your brain handles information differently, depending on how it's presented. For example, which of the following ways of displaying percentages is easiest for you to grasp?

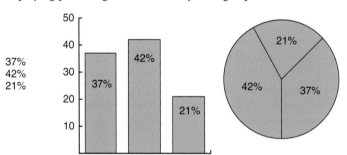

When trying to learn or teach someone something, consider questions like, "How can we look at this differently?" "What is the best way to represent this information?" "Is there a table, map, diagram, or decision tree that can add to understanding?"

Other Useful Strategies

Here are some more useful strategies that you can use to develop critical thinking habits:

- **Pay attention to how your communication style and behavior affect communication.** How are people responding to you? Do they seem confident, or are they unsure of themselves when communicating with you? Do you need to make some changes?
- **Develop good habits of inquiry.** Develop habits that aid in the search for the truth, such as keeping an open mind, verifying information, and taking enough time.

- **Anticipate questions others might ask.** These may include: "What will my instructor want to know?" "What do patients need to know?" "What will the doctor want to know?" This helps identify a wider scope of questions that have to be answered to gain relevant information.
- **Ask, "What else?"** Change "Have we done everything?" to "What else do we need to do?" Asking "What else?" pushes you to look further and be more complete.
- **Ask, "What if?"** For example, "What if the worst happens?" or "What if we try another way?" This helps you be proactive instead of reactive. It enhances your creativity and helps you put things in perspective.
- **Ask, "Why?"** To fully understand something, you must know what it is and *why it's so*. There's a saying: "She who knows what and how is likely to get a good job. She who knows why is likely to be her boss."
- **Think out loud or write your thoughts down.** When you put your thinking into words, you make your ideas, reasons, and logic explicit, making it easier to assess and correct yourself.
- **Ask an expert to think out loud** (e.g., Can you tell me how you usually deal with situations like this?"). When you ask experts to think out loud, you often learn systematic approaches to solving problems and making decisions.
- **Look for flaws in your thinking.** Ask questions like, "What's missing?" and "How could this be made better?" If you don't go looking for flaws, you'll be unlikely to find them. Once you've found them, you can make corrections early.
- **Ask someone else to look for flaws in your thinking** (e.g., Here's what I'm thinking ... am I missing anything?). This offers a "fresh eye" for evaluation and may bring new ideas and perspectives.
- **Paraphrase in your own words.** Paraphrasing helps you understand information using a familiar language (your own).
- **Compare and contrast (what's the same and what's different?).** This forces you to look closely at the *parts* of something as well as the *whole*, helping you become more familiar with both things you're looking at. For example, if I ask you to compare and contrast two kinds of apples, you have to look closely at both of them and get a taste of each one. As a result, you're more likely to remember each type of apple better.
- **Organize and reorganize information.** Organizing information helps you see certain patterns, but it may make you *miss* others. Reorganizing it helps you see some of those other patterns. For example, compare the following groups of numbers (each group contains the same numbers organized differently). What patterns do you see and which is easiest to remember?

36345643   34343656   33344566

- **Revisit information.** When you give something "a second pass"—coming back and studying it afresh—you see it differently.
- **Replace the phrases "I don't know" or "I'm not sure" with "I need to find out."** This shows you have the confidence and ability to find answers and mobilizes you to locate resources.
- **Don't take yourself too seriously—turn mistakes into learning opportunities.** You're not the only one who makes mistakes. Mistakes are often stepping-stones to improvement. If you aren't making mistakes, maybe you aren't trying new things. Create safety nets (things that help you avoid mistakes). Learn to laugh at your sensitive areas. For example, I tend to lose things, an embarrassing characteristic that I've tried to change. Since someone called me an "absent-minded professor," I just laugh and find ways to deal with this characteristic (like carrying keys on a lanyard around my neck). Humor reduces stress; "beating yourself up" increases it.

KNOWLEDGE AND INTELLECTUAL SKILLS CTIS

Being a critical thinker means recognizing that you need to gain discipline-specific knowledge and skills to reason well in various professions (e.g., engineering versus health care). This section addresses critical thinking indicators (CTIs) related to the knowledge and intellectual skills you need to have to give safe, effective care (Boxes 2.7 and 2.8). Understanding these *knowledge CTIs* and *intellectual skill CTIs* helps you answer the questions, "What do I have to know?" and "What do I have to be able to do?"

Keep in mind that developing *intellectual skill* CTIs (see Box 2.8) requires you to be able to apply *knowledge* CTIs (see Box 2.7). For example, to *distinguish normal from abnormal* (listed in Box 2.8), you have to apply *knowledge of normal and abnormal function* (listed in Box 2.7).

Determine where you stand in relation to having *knowledge* and *intellectual skills CTIs*; rate your ability to demonstrate each of the indicators using the 0–10 scaleat the bottom of the next page.

BOX 2.7 Critical Thinking Indicators Demonstrating Knowledge

(Requirements vary, depending on specialty practice [e.g., pediatrics versus adult health care].)

Clarifies Nursing Knowledge
- Nursing and medical terminology
- Nursing versus medical and other models, roles, and responsibilities
- Scope of nursing practice (qualifications; applicable standards, laws, and rules and regulations)
- Related anatomy, physiology, and pathophysiology
- Spiritual, social, and cultural concepts
- Normal and abnormal growth and development (pediatric, adult, and gerontological implications)
- Normal and abnormal function (bio-psycho-social-cultural-spiritual)
- Factors affecting normal function (bio-psycho-social-cultural-spiritual)
- Nutrition and pharmacology principles
- Behavioral health and disease management
- Signs and symptoms of common problems and complications
- Nursing process, nursing theories, research, and evidence-based practice
- Reasons behind policies, procedures, and interventions; diagnostic studies implications
- Ethical and legal principles
- Risk management and infection control
- Safety standards, healthy workplace standards, and principles of learning and safety cultures
- Interrelationship of health care disciplines and systems
- Reliable information resources

Clarifies Knowledge of Self
- Personal biases, values, beliefs, needs
- How own culture, thinking, personality, and learning style preferences differ from those of others
- Level of commitment to organizational mission and values

Demonstrates
- Focused nursing assessment skills (e.g., breath sounds or IV site assessment)
- Mathematical problem-solving for drug calculations
- Related technical skills (e.g., nasogastric tube or other equipment management)

BOX 2.8 Intellectual Skills Critical Thinking Indicators

Nursing Process and Decision-Making Skills
- Communicates effectively orally and in writing
- Applies standards, principles, laws, and ethics codes
- Makes safety and infection control a priority; prevents and deals with mistakes constructively
- Includes patient, family, and key stakeholders in decision-making; teaches patient, self, and others
- Identifies purpose and focus of assessment
- Assesses systematically and comprehensively as indicated
- Distinguishes normal from abnormal; identifies risks for abnormal
- Distinguishes relevant from irrelevant; clusters relevant data together
- Identifies assumptions and inconsistencies; checks accuracy and reliability (validates data)
- Recognizes missing information; gains more data as needed
- Concludes what's known and unknown; draws reasonable conclusions and gives evidence to support them
- Identifies both problems and their underlying cause(s) and related factors; includes patient and family perspectives
- Recognizes changes in patient status; takes appropriate action
- Considers multiple ideas, explanations, and solutions
- Determines individualized outcomes and uses them to plan and give care
- Manages risks and predicts complications
- Weighs risks and benefits; anticipates consequences and implications—individualizes interventions accordingly
- Sets priorities and makes decisions in a timely way
- Reassesses to monitor outcomes (responses)
- Promotes health, function, comfort, and well-being
- Identifies ethical issues and takes appropriate action
- Uses human and information resources; detects bias

Additional Related Skills
- Advocates for patients, self, and others
- Establishes empowered partnerships with patients, families, peers, and co-workers
- Fosters positive interpersonal relationships; addresses conflicts fairly; promotes healthy workplace and learning cultures
- Promotes learning and teamwork (focuses on common goals, respects diversity; encourages others to learn and contribute in their own way)
- Facilitates and navigates change
- Organizes and manages time and environment
- Gives and takes constructive criticism
- Delegates appropriately (matches patient needs with worker competencies; determines worker learning needs; supervises and teaches as indicated; monitors results personally)
- Leads, inspires, and helps others move toward mutually defined common goals.
- Demonstrates systems thinking (shows awareness of relationships existing within and across health care systems

Source: Alfaro-LeFevre R. *Evidence-Based Critical Thinking Indicators.* 2019. Retrieved from http://www.AlfaroTeachSmart. com. All rights reserved. No use without permission.

0 = I am unable to demonstrate this indicator at this time.
10 = This indicator is pretty much a habit for me.

If you're a beginner, don't be concerned about low scores when comparing yourself to the CTIs. These skills are developed on the job through practice and experience. You also get practice developing these skills as you complete the exercises throughout the book.

REFLECTING ON THINKING—ASKING FOR FEEDBACK

Let's end this chapter by briefly addressing the fifth key step to becoming a critical thinker: Making time to reflect on your reasoning, talking with others about reasoning strategies, and asking for feedback on how others view your thinking are crucial to improvement. What you learn from asking for feedback may surprise you—or it may confirm that you just need to keep doing what you're doing. Using evidence-based tools such as the CTIs helps give a reference point during discussions about critical thinking abilities. Fig. 2.2 (p. 34) gives you another way to reflect on where you stand in relation to achieving your critical thinking potential.

Because feedback is often associated with performance evaluation, we'll go into the complexity of evaluating reasoning in the next chapter, when we discuss best practices for evaluating thinking.

❓ CRITICAL THINKING EXERCISES

Find example responses in Appendix I (page 215).

1. **Fill in the following blanks, choosing from the following words:** hypothesis, self-efficacy, communication, conclusions, intent, developing, assumptions, starting, changing, personality, affect, results.
   A. Major steps to developing critical thinking potential include becoming aware of (a) _____ and learning preferences and identifying factors that (b)_____reasoning.
   B. Becoming a critical thinker requires (a) _____habits that promote critical thinking and (b)_____habits that deter critical thinking.
   C. If you had to choose only *one* skill to develop to become a critical thinker, it should be _____.
   D. Hypotheses are similar to _____ except that you make them deliberately, rather than subconsciously.
   E. Generating hypotheses is an important _____point for investigation
   F. Anchoring your mind on the first (a)_____you think of is a common reasoning error because you fail to consider alternative ideas and (b)_____.
   G. Your confidence level related to being able to learn specific skills is called_____.
   H. Goals and objectives usually focus on general (a)_____; outcomes focus on specific, measurable (b)_____.
2. Emotive thinking is thinking that's driven by feelings: How does this relate to critical thinking?
3. Compare and contrast the *Golden Rule* and the *Platinum Rule*.
4. There are some things that are almost impossible to grasp without mapping—yet they're easy to understand if you draw a map. For example, answer the following question.
   Margaret and Joyce are first cousins. Margaret has a daughter, Heidi, who has a son, Eric. Joyce has a daughter, Paula, who has a daughter, Laura. *How are Laura and Eric related?*
   a. First cousins
   b. Second cousins
   c. Third cousins
5. To get in touch with the human tendency to make assumptions, answer the following riddle.
   Riddle: Jack and Jill were found dead on the floor, surrounded by water and pieces of broken glass. There was no blood. What happened?
6. Using your own words and giving an example, explain the relationship between goals and outcomes.
7. What is the relationship between *knowledge* CTIs (see Box 2.7) and *intellectual* CTIs (see Box 2.8)?

THINK, PAIR, SHARE

With a partner, in a group, or in a journal entry:

1. Share how the behaviors in the *Health Team Code of Conduct* in Box 2.1 promote trusting relationships; address what could happen if the behaviors aren't a part of the code.

2. Discuss the following in relation to Do You Know What to Do When Someone Turns Blue? (see Box 2.3) and What's Your Thinking Style? (see Box 2.4).

   a. What's your thinking style and main motive according to Hartman's *Color Code* and Myers-Briggs Type Indicator?

   b. What personalities and thinking styles are difficult for you to work with, and how can you improve your ability to work with people who have these styles?

   c. How has your birth order, culture, and upbringing affected your thinking style?

3. Share where you stand in relation to Table 2.1; try going "out of your learning style box" and using some of the other style strategies.

4. Persistent negative thoughts may lead to—or be a sign of—*depression*, a major health care concern. Yet many people aren't even aware that most of their thinking is negative. Discuss what you can do if you or someone you know seems to have constant negative thoughts. Think of one thing you can do each day to feel happy; think of one thing you can do to help patients feel happy.

5. Share how you did when you assessed your ability to demonstrate the CTIs related to *knowledge* and *intellectual* skills (see Boxes 2.7 and 2.8).

6. Take the stress scale test at http://www.teachhealth.com. Share the stressful things in your life. How are you handling them? What healthy behaviors might help?

7. Study *Key Brain Parts Involved in Thinking* in Appendix F. Decide how thinking ability would be affected by brain damage in the frontal lobe or hippocampus.

8. Choose one of the following articles to discuss:

   - Train your mind to be stronger than your emotions or else you'll lose yourself every time. https://themindsjournal.com/gotta-train-mind-stronger/.
   - Bohem L. *Seven Elements of Effective Clinical Communication* (blog). Retrieved from https://www.vocera.com/blog/seven-elements-effective-clinical-communication.
   - Helliwell J, Layard R, Sachs J. World Happiness Report, 2018. Retrieved from http://world-happiness.report/.
   - Yoshikawa Y, Ohmaki E, Kawahata H et al. Beneficial effect of laughter therapy on physiological and psychological function in elders. *Nursing Open*. 2018. Retrieved from https://onlinelibrary.wiley.com/doi/full/10.1002/nop2.190https://doi.org/10.1002/nop2.190.
   - Alfaro-LeFevre R. Happiness: The evidence behind the emotion. 2018. Retrieved from https://www.nurse.com (fee may apply).

9. Share where you stand in relation to understanding the key concepts and achieving the learning outcomes at the beginning of this chapter.

10. Discuss your thoughts on the following *Critical Moments and Other Perspectives*.

CRITICAL MOMENTS AND OTHER PERSPECTIVES

Be Yourself, Change Yourself, Keep an Open Mind

- *Be yourself. Everyone else is taken.* —Oscar Wilde
- *Improving thinking helps you develop the most important tool you have: yourself. I have a very weird brain. But I like it—it's the only one I have.* —Ruth Hansten, RN, PhD[14]

- *Not being genuine and authentic—betraying your true feelings and beliefs—just to be agreeable and accepted creates an emotional toll that drains your brain and your soul.*
- *To change the world, you have to first change yourself.* —Unknown
- *Minds are like parachutes. They work best when open.* —Unknown

How to Think Like Einstein

- *It's not that I'm smart, it's just that I stick with problems longer.* —Albert Einstein
- *You don't inspire others by being perfect. You inspire them by how you deal with your imperfections.* —Unknown
- *Being a critical thinker means having the confidence to admit your flaws and what you don't know.* —Melani McGuire, ARNP[15]

Biggest Communication Problem

- *The biggest problem in communication is the illusion that it has taken place.* —George Bernard Shaw
- *Repeating back what you hear in communications (or asking others to do the same) helps ensure that communication has indeed taken place.*

Worried About Analysis Paralysis?

For every person paralyzed with excessive doubt, there are 100 who have too little doubt and charge off to take action without enough reflection. —Philip Hansten, Author of *Premature Fraculation: The Ignorance of Certainty and the Ghost of Montaigne*[16]

Considering Alternatives Promotes Critical Thinking

People aren't successful because they come up with one right answer or explanation. Rather, it's because they come up with many answers or explanations. To get the best results, make it a habit to look for alternative explanations, problems, or solutions.

Boundaries and Priorities—Not Guilt

Reducing stress and managing your time can help you find the time you need to focus on developing critical thinking. Many nurses feel guilty when they say no to requests for help. Yet there are only so many hours in the day. Don't feel guilty about setting boundaries for what you will and will not do. You can't do it all. When going through busy or stressful periods, avoid being distracted from the major priorities in your life. Set boundaries.

KEY POINTS/SUMMARY

- Five strategies for becoming a critical thinker are: (1) Gain insight and self-awareness. (2) Build trust in relationships by adopting a code of conduct that promotes respectful communication in all interactions. (3) Be committed to developing the knowledge, attitudes, and skills needed to think critically. (4) Use an evidence-based reference to ensure that everyone in your group has a common understanding of what critical thinking entails. (5) Reflect on your reasoning processes and ask for feedback.

- Formal and informal evaluation related to your thinking and performance is crucial to improve.
- Understanding your personal style—how and why you think and learn the way you do—is a key starting point for improving thinking.
- Understanding personality types and learning styles different from your own helps you realize how and why others think the way they do.
- Birth order, upbringing, and the culture you embrace have an impact on your thinking.

- Self-efficacy—having a strong sense that you're capable of accomplishing all that you need to do to achieve your goals—greatly affects your ability to gain the knowledge and skills needed for critical thinking.
- Developing your EQ—your ability to recognize emotions and make them work in positive ways—is as important as developing your IQ.
- Human habits can either promote or impede critical thinking; habits that impede critical thinking are often a *result of human nature*; those that promote critical thinking are often *learned*.
- Drawing maps, diagrams, and decision trees are all useful strategies to promote critical thinking.

- Goals, because they focus on intent, may be vague and unrealistic. Identifying observable, measurable outcomes (results) that focus on *who* must be able to accomplish *what* helps you be realistic and focused from the start.
- Logic—sound reasoning based on evidence—provides the foundation for critical thinking. Using intuition as a guide to look for evidence is an effective strategy that should be nurtured; before acting on intuition alone, be sure you consider the possible risks of harm.
- Trial and error (trying several solutions until you find one that works) is a risky but sometimes necessary approach to problem-solving.
- Scan this chapter to review the illustrations and Guiding Principles throughout.

REFERENCES

1. Alessandra, T. The platinum rule. Retrieved from http://www.alessandra.com/abouttony/aboutpr.asp.
2. Kirk. K. Self-efficacy: Helping students believe in themselves. Retrieved from http://serc.carleton.edu/NAGTWorkshops/affective/efficacy.html.
3. Penny, J. Personal communication.
4. Goleman Daniel. *Emotional Intelligence: Why It Can Matter More Than IQ*. New York: Bantam Books; 1995.
5. Covey S. *The 7 habits of highly effective people*®. New York: Simon & Schuster; 1989.
6. Helliwell J, Layard R, Sachs J. *World Happiness Report*. retrieved from http://worldhappiness.report/; 2018.
7. Alfaro-LeFevre R. *Happiness: The evidence behind the emotion*. Retrieved from https://www.nurse.com; 2018.
8. Paul R, Elder L. *Valuable intellectual traits* (Website). http://www.criticalthinking.org.
9. Alfaro-LeFevre R. *Evidence-based critical thinking indicators* (Website). http://www.AlfaroTeachSmart.com; 2019.
10. Facione P. *Critical thinking: What it is and why it counts* (Website). http://www.insightassessment.com; 2015 update.
11. Scheffer B, Rubenfeld M. A consensus statement on critical thinking in nursing. *Journal of Nursing Education*. 2000;39:353–359.
12. Dolansky M, Moore S. Quality and Safety Education for Nurses (QSEN): The Key is Systems Thinking OJIN: The Online Journal of Issues in Nursing Vol. 18, No. 3. *Manuscript*. 2013;1. https://doi.org/10.3912/OJIN.Vol18No03Man01.
13. Senge P, Fritz R, Wheattly M. *Learning organizations: The promise and the possibilities*. Retrieved from https://thesystemsthinker.com/learning-organizations-the-promise-and-the-possibilities/; 2018.
14. Hansten, R. Personal communication
15. McGuire, M. Personal communication
16. Hansten, P. Personal communication

3

Critical Thinking and Learning Cultures: Teaching, Learning, and Taking Tests

THIS CHAPTER AT A GLANCE...

Learning Cultures: Everyone Teaches, Everyone Learns

Conceptual Learning: Focusing on Big Ideas

Competency-Based Learning

Learning, Unlearning, and Relearning

Simulation and Debriefing

Preceptors and Nurse Residencies

Helping Others Learn: Promoting Independence

Assessing and Evaluating Thinking: Best Practices

Improving Grades and Passing Tests the First Time

NCLEX® Facts and Strategies

Critical Thinking Exercises

Key Points/Summary

LEARNING OUTCOMES

After completing this chapter, you should be able to:

1. Summarize key strategies for developing and sustaining learning cultures.
2. Describe or map the relationships among learning cultures, critical thinking, and safety.
3. Explain how concept-based and competency-based learning promotes efficient learning.
4. Detail your responsibilities related to educating patients and caregivers you supervise.
5. Identify three strategies you'll use to make the most of simulation and debriefing.
6. Explain why practicing what to do when things go wrong promotes critical thinking.
7. Explain the relationships among clinical learning, preceptors, nurse residencies, safety, and nurse retention.
8. Reflect on your clinical learning progress and ask for feedback appropriately.
9. Describe three best practices for assessing and evaluating nurses' critical thinking skills.
10. Identify strategies to help you study efficiently.
11. Explain why you need test-taking skills, as well as knowledge, to succeed in school and at work.
12. Use strategies that help you improve your test scores and pass the NCLEX® on the first try.

KEY CONCEPTS

Debriefing; competency-based education; conceptual learning; formative and summative evaluation; health literacy; mentor; preceptor; remediation; simulation; high-stakes testing; educated guess; *See also previous chapters*

LEARNING CULTURES: EVERYONE TEACHES, EVERYONE LEARNS

Building learning cultures that embrace the motto that "Everyone teaches, everyone learns" is central to promoting critical thinking in both schools and health care organizations. Engaging in critical thinking in today's rapidly changing world requires continuous learning and testing of that learning. Whether you're 18 years old or 80, embracing lifelong learning is the key to personal and professional success. This chapter helps you develop the teaching and learning skills you need to survive and thrive in today's fast-paced, ever-changing world. It also gives you strategies you can use to make it easier to succeed in testing situations (both routine and standard tests such as NCLEX®).

> **GUIDING PRINCIPLE**
>
> Building learning cultures—school and work environments that encourage all learners and staff at all levels to ask questions, share information freely, and create teaching and learning opportunities—is the foundation for developing critical thinking, improving outcomes, and keeping patients safe.

Building Learning Cultures

Here are five strategies to building and sustaining learning cultures:

1. **Start by changing single attitudes and behaviors—these then lead to becoming a culture.** Stress that being vigilant for safety issues and fostering research, quality improvement, and evidence-based practice are everyone's job. Create a safe, supportive environment in which peer-to-peer observations and feedback are encouraged in the spirit of enhancing organizational and personal performance. For example, if you see someone doing something that's unsafe, it's appropriate to say, "This looks risky (or unsafe); can I make a suggestion?"

2. **Make teaching and learning a key part of daily activities** of your workplace or school (address this in organizational values and performance evaluations). Don't assume that experts know it all or that learners have little to offer. Don't assume you know more than your patients. They may be your best teachers. Few things are more frustrating to patients with chronic problems than nurses who try standard approaches before asking something like, "Can you tell me how you've been managing this?"

3. **Promote self-esteem and confidence; be approachable and show that you care about learners' experiences.** Pay attention to context (what's happening in the moment that may be affect learning).[1]

4. **Uphold a good team spirit in which everyone works together toward common goals in a climate of trust and respect.** Help learners feel they belong to the team.

5. **Tailor teaching strategies to individuals, not tasks.** Encourage each person to learn in his or her own way. Promote independent learning in a safe environment; a lot of learning happens with trial and error and self-correction.

6. **Ensure that learners know how to evaluate the validity of information resources** (see shaded section below).

ABCDs of Evaluating Websites and Other Works

AUTHORITY: How well known is the author?

- Is the author a well-regarded name you recognize? What are the author's qualifications?
- Does the document give contact information (e.g., an e-mail address)?
- Did you access this document using a link from a site you trust?
- Are there statements about the review process for publication? Peer-reviewed publications—those published only after they've been reviewed by peer experts—are most reliable.

BIAS: Does the site or document try to persuade, rather than inform?
- What organization sponsors the site or document? Is the organization reliable?
- Is the page actually an advertisement disguised as information?

CITATIONS:
- Are full citations given to support the work?
- Does the author's content match the content in the citation?
- For web citations, is there a seal of approval posted? For example, the Health on the Net Foundation (http://www.hon.ch/) gives a seal of approval to websites that meet high standards.

DATES:
- How recent are the dates that are listed?
- Does the information you need demand more current data than are given in the documents you have?

CONCEPTUAL LEARNING: FOCUSING ON BIG IDEAS

Simply put, conceptual learning is a way to deal with information overload—instead of trying to learn everything all at once, you prioritize what you study by focusing on *big ideas* (major principles, concepts, and examples) before *details*. Let me give you an example of how conceptual learning works by applying it to this section. First, study the *big ideas* of conceptual learning in Fig. 3.1. After you've done that, go on to read the rest of this section, which gives you the *details* of conceptual learning.

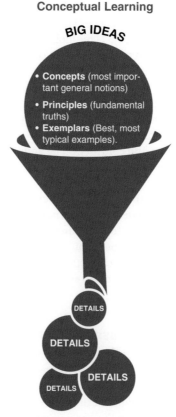

Conceptual Learning

BIG IDEAS

- **Concepts** (most important general notions)
- **Principles** (fundamental truths)
- **Exemplars** (Best, most typical examples).

DETAILS

DETAILS

DETAILS

DETAILS

FIG. 3.1 Concept-based curriculum. (From https://evolve.elsevier.com/education/concept-based-curriculum/conceptual-learning-definition/.)

Here's an example of a big idea concept: **Oxygenation**. Oxygenation is a major concept because it's key to sustaining life, and many health issues are aggravated by inadequate oxygenation. If you have personal in-depth knowledge of oxygenation—why it's needed, the effects of inadequate oxygenation, and what promotes or deters it—learning becomes efficient because you can transfer what you already know about oxygenation to studying *any problem involving oxygenation issues* (e.g., respiratory illnesses, myocardial infarction, and exercise intolerance).

Most people find that even with sentence structure, placing the big ideas before the details promotes understanding. Which of the following sentences—in which *blood* is the big idea—is easier for you to grasp?

- Red blood cells, white blood cells, platelets, and plasma make up blood.
- Blood is made of red blood cells, white blood cells, platelets, and plasma

Conceptual Learning Strategies

Whether you're in class or in the clinical setting, here are some strategies you can use to promote conceptual learning:[2]

- Start by personalizing the information (make it your own); ask questions like:
  - Why do I need to know this?
  - How does this information relate to what I already know?
  - What are the big ideas, or how can I make connections among the facts in a way that the big ideas emerge?
  - What does this information imply, and what questions does it raise for me?
- **Use concept mapping** (Appendix A) or other learning tools to make connections among *professional nursing concepts* (e.g., ethics and teamwork) and *health care concepts* (e.g., oxygenation and mobility).
- **Determine similarities and differences** in the management of patients with different but related health problems (e.g., care of patients with osteoarthritis compared with rheumatoid arthritis).
- **Identify salient points.** Salient points are the most important things that you must learn to accomplish a skill or achieve an outcome. For example, before you can give medications safely, you must know the mathematics involved in calculating drug dosages.
- **When giving patient care, focus on applying principles and concepts** rather than trying to match the exemplars you learned with the current patient situation. For example, ask, "How does the concept of *immobility* apply to *this particular patient?*" instead of, "How does this patient compare with related exemplars we had in class?"
- **Practice conceptual learning strategies by collaborating with your peers to complete unfolding case studies**—studies that discuss how patient situations evolved over time are especially engaging. You can find these studies in books and online or use actual patients you or your peers had. Reflecting on how patient care unfolded in post care conferences is especially helpful.

COMPETENCY-BASED LEARNING

Competency-based learning—an important method to use when teaching anything that requires safety—is now the norm in clinical education. Competence has four interrelated components: knowledge, skills, behavior, and judgment.[3] With competency-based learning, you first work to gain the knowledge and skills you need to work in a given role. Then, before you "pass," you must show that you can *put your knowledge and skills into action*. You must demonstrate that you have (1) the behaviors needed to effectively manage every situation you're likely to encounter in that role and (2) the judgment to address situations when straightforward answers aren't apparent.

For example, let's look at the competency of *using sterile technique*. If you can demonstrate a sterile procedure in a specific situation, but you don't know the underlying principles, you have two issues: (1) you're unprepared to learn other procedures in which sterility is essential, and (2) you're not safe to practice because you won't be able to adapt the procedure when circumstances change (as we all know they do).

> **GUIDING PRINCIPLE**
>
> **Competency—the ability to accomplish specific skills safely and effectively under various circumstances—** isn't just the product of completing required courses, nor is it measured by simply passing a test or completing a checklist. Rather, true competency is confirmed *after* you complete the tests and checklists *and* you consistently display appropriate behaviors and sound judgments at the point of care (e.g., the bedside).

LEARNING, UNLEARNING, AND RELEARNING

To quote Alvin Toffler, author of *Future Shock,* "The illiterate of the twenty-first century will not be those who cannot read and write, but those who cannot learn, unlearn, and relearn."[4] Today's rapid change requires new learning skills—you have to know how to learn efficiently, often having to "unlearn" old ways and replace them with new ones.

Remediation—relearning skills that should have already been mastered—is associated with failure (perhaps because most definitions say that remediation is the process of fixing something bad or defective). Rather than placing blame, we simply must be alert to skills that may not be as sharp as they once were. Relearning is an opportunity to improve, as you can see in the following scenario.

> **SCENARIO SMART IV PUMPS NEED SMART NURSES**
>
> An alert nurse leader of a neonatal intensive care unit noticed that she was hearing a lot of IV smart pump alarms. IV smart pumps have software that sounds an alarm if you enter incorrect information in the dose field. If an alarm goes off, you know to double-check what you entered. To determine why there seemed to be an increase in alarms, the leader ran printouts from all the pumps, detailing what happened when the alarms went off. After analyzing the printouts, she learned that the most common reason for the alarms was that nurses were entering incorrect doses due to decimal point calculation errors. Based on these results, it was clear that the nurses' math skills weren't up to par, and all of them were required to complete a course that included decimal point calculation. The alarm rate decreased dramatically.

> **GUIDING PRINCIPLE**
>
> **Remember: Use it or lose it.** If you don't use skills, you lose them. For example, if you depend on calculators, without ever double-checking the math yourself, you'll forget basic skills such as multiplication and division. Never be afraid to say, "I haven't done this in a while and need to practice before I can be sure I can do it safely today."

What I Learned from *Candy Crush*™

Recently, I experienced the power of remediation when playing the popular game, *Candy Crush*™. I was stuck on the same level for months! I was frustrated with my inability to progress. To regain enjoyment in the game, I decided to play some lower levels. I was amazed how I breezed through the lower levels that had once been a challenge. I realized I had learned a lot after all. Making time to relearn things helps people who feel stuck regain confidence and realize how far they've come. It also ensures that salient points taught early in the process have indeed been learned.

SIMULATION AND DEBRIEFING

Using simulation—computer-based programs, standard patients, and high-fidelity patient simulators (high-tech mannequins that mimic human responses to interventions, such as giving oxygen and IV fluids)—can help you develop communication, clinical reasoning, and decision-making skills in a safe environment. Being able to make a mistake, catch it, and correct it is a powerful way to learn. Using debriefing—discussing what went well, what was challenging, and determining "lessons learned"—is even more powerful.[5]

Testing via simulation can be stressful for even the most competent clinician (listen to the conversations at a cardiopulmonary resuscitation [CPR] session and you may be surprised who is and who isn't nervous). Research on how to best design and implement simulated experiences is ongoing, but we have made significant progress.[6] Educators and simulation specialists continue to streamline the process to promote optimum learning.

Strategies to Make the Most of Simulation

Here are some strategies to make the most of your experience:

1. **Preparing for Simulation (Thinking Ahead).** Preparation can make the difference between *gaining confidence and skills* and *getting stressed, making too many mistakes, and feeling terrible*. With so many things to think about, collaborating with your peers is a good way to prepare. It helps you identify common learner concerns and develop strategies to manage them. Here are some questions you should answer to be prepared:
   - What tools do you have to guide the simulation and debriefing process? (Using a structured, evidence-based tool to guide the experience helps learners and facilitators stay organized and focused on what's most important.)
   - What are the main goals, objectives, or learner outcomes?
   - What procedures will you be doing?
   - What concepts and principles are you likely to apply?
   - Who will you need to communicate with, and how will you do that?
   - What tools and resources will be available to you during this simulation?
   - What knowledge will you need and what skills should you practice before the simulation?
   - What are the safety issues and the most common and bad mistakes you need to avoid?
   - What will you do if things go wrong (What if _____ happens?)? Practicing what to do if things go *wrong* is as important as practicing how to do things *right*. Many pilots credit their survival to the lessons learned in simulators practicing how to respond when things go wrong.

2. **During Simulation (Thinking in Action).** Here are some "do's" and "don'ts":

Do:	Don't:
• Try to stay calm, even when you make mistakes (mistakes are common; that's why you're there).	• Come unprepared.
• Focus on safety; acknowledge and correct your mistakes as soon as possible, then move on.	• Expect yourself to be perfect.
• Think out loud so that the facilitator understands your reasoning.	• Gloss over or hide mistakes.
	• Focus on what you're doing *wrong* (you'll lose confidence because you'll lose sight of what you're doing *right*).

3. **Debriefing (Thinking Back/Reflecting)**
   - Keep in mind that the purpose of debriefing is to reflect on the experience and promote learning by identifying what you did well, what you can do to improve, and the biggest lessons you learned to take with you for the future.
   - Remember that feedback on performance can feel like "stings of criticism"; stay positive and learn how to give and take feedback (Skill 7.4, Chapter 7).
   - If your role is to facilitate the simulation:
     - Use a structured method of debriefing.
     - Encourage learners to analyze what happened and what they thought and felt during the experience (don't judge—just listen).
     - Help learners reflect on the positive aspects of their performance and give positive reinforcement.
     - Have a structured way to discuss how reasoning went during the simulation (e.g., *assess, diagnose, plan, implement and evaluate* or *notice, interpret, respond, and reflect*).
     - Answer questions and expand on what was learned.
     - End by summarizing the experience and giving suggestions for the future.

Simulation Resources

- International Nursing Association for Clinical Simulation and Learning (includes standards and best practices): https://www.inacsl.org
- National League for Nursing Simulation Innovation Resource Center: http://sirc.nln.org
- Society for Simulation in Healthcare (SSH): http://www.ssih.org
- Association for Standardized Patient Educators: http://www.aspeducators.org

PRECEPTORS AND NURSE RESIDENCIES

To keep patients safe, prevent nurse burnout, and develop safe, effective clinicians, using preceptors and nurse residency programs is now best practice. Preceptors—experienced clinicians who are academically and experientially qualified to facilitate critical-thinking skill development—work closely with new nurses to give the type of support that maximizes learning and independence. Nurse residencies—apprenticeship programs that include a series of learning sessions and work experiences aimed at developing essential clinical and professional skills—are also best practice.[7,8] Many new or transitioning nurses (nurses who are moving from one specialty practice to another) choose employment based on whether or not organizations offer preceptors and nurse residency programs.[9] Fig. 3.2 shows how nurse characteristics and preceptor support change as nurses progress through five stages of development (novice to expert). Chapter 4 expands content on novice to expert thinking. You can find links to free resources for preceptors/educators and learners at the Vermont Nurses in Partnership website (http://www.vnip.org).

Clinical Learning Strategies

Clinical learning experiences are challenging because you're often in an unfamiliar environment, there are major concerns about safety, and you have to juggle learning with actual patient care. Here are some strategies to help you deal with the challenges of learning in the clinical setting:
- **Keep in mind that if you're a beginner, you may not know what you don't know.**[7,8] Ask for help if you're not completely sure about something. Proceed with caution if there are risks of patient harm. Before you perform nursing actions, ask yourself, "Do I know why this *particular action, treatment, or medication* is indicated for *this particular patient?*" If you don't, find out.

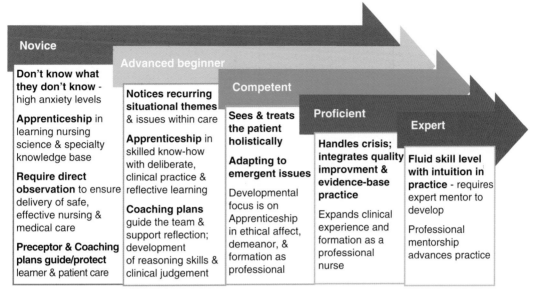

FIG. 3.2 Novice through expert apprenticeship. (© 2016 Boyer, S. All rights reserved.)

- **Develop empowered partnerships (Skill 7.3, Chapter 7).** Learners and preceptors or educators must trust one another and agree about expectations; one person shouldn't be working harder than the other.
- **Ask for a tool that clearly details expectations about content (what's to be learned) and process (how the learning process will progress).** This tool should serve as a "talking point" to promote ongoing dialogue about what's going well and what needs to be improved. (See "Assessing and Evaluating Thinking: Best Practices" later in this chapter).
- **Use a tool to help you pay attention to the most important information and reminders you need during your clinical day.** Fig. 3.3 shows a personal worksheet I created for myself to help me be systematic and complete when I worked in the intensive care unit. If I came to work without it, I was completely disorganized.
- **Keep references—texts, handheld electronic devices, pocket guides, and personal "cheat sheets"—handy.** Until you have a large storehouse of experiential knowledge in your brain, you'll need to refer to these frequently.
- **Learn terminology and concepts.** If you encounter new terms and you don't know what they mean, look them up as you encounter them so that they become part of your long-term memory. Learning terms *in context* helps your brain store information in related groups, rather than as isolated facts.
- **Become familiar with normal findings** (e.g., normal lab values, assessment findings, disease progression, growth, and development) before being concerned with abnormal findings. Once you know what's normal, you'll readily recognize when you encounter information that's *outside the norm* (abnormal).
- **Ask why.** Find out why normal and abnormal findings occur (e.g., "Why is there edema in heart failure, yet none when the heart is functioning normally?").
- **Learn problem-specific facts.** You need to know how health issues usually present themselves (their signs and symptoms), what usually causes them, and how they're managed. Box 3.1 gives questions you need to answer to be prepared for going to the clinical setting.

Name_____	Medical Dx_____
Room_____	PCP_____
Age_____ Religion____	Allergies_____
Culture_____	
Diet_____ Activity_____	
	Medications/IV's:
Neuro:	
Resp:	Potential Complications:
Oxygen:	
Cardiac:	Diagnoses/problems:
Circ:	
Skin:	Test Results
GU:	EKG
GI:	ABG
	Electrolytes
Special today:	Other

FIG. 3.3 Sample clinical worksheet. This is one I used when working in the intensive care unit. Filling in the blanks helps you identify what information you have and what information is missing.

- **As you go through the day, make ADPIE**—*assess, diagnose, plan, implement, and evaluate*—a "guiding mantra" in your head. Assess before you act. Use intuition as a guide, but make judgments based *on evidence.* Evaluate patient responses and change approaches as needed.
- **Use debriefing.** You make the most of your learning when you engage in debriefing and dialogue with your instructor or in groups in post-care conferences. Share your clinical challenges and ask your instructor, preceptor, or peers for insight into what happened and things you should do the next time you're in a similar situation.
- **Seek out role models.** These individuals are often your best teachers.

BOX 3.1   **Preparing for Clinical Learning**

Questions you should answer before going to a clinical setting:
- What common problems are seen in this particular setting?
- What are the signs and symptoms of these problems?
- What risk factors do I know or suspect patients in this setting have?
- What do I assess to determine the status of these signs, symptoms, and risk factors?
- What are the usual causes of these problems?
- What do I assess to determine the status of the causes of the problems?
- How do these problems usually progress, and how are they managed?
- How can these problems be prevented?
- What are the signs and symptoms of potential complications of these problems, and how will I monitor for them?
- How can I be prepared to manage potential complications?
- What medications and treatments are likely to be used, and why?
- What medication-related or treatment-related problems might I encounter, how will I monitor to detect them, and how are they usually managed?
- What population-based factors (e.g., age group, lifestyle, culture, beliefs, and language needs) might have a bearing on health practices related to these health problems?
- What are the key things people need to know to manage these problems independently, and what will I do to ensure that this knowledge is gained?

HELPING OTHERS LEARN: PROMOTING INDEPENDENCE

You may have heard the saying, "Teachers don't empower learners. They encourage them to use the power they were born with." Your role as a facilitator of learning—helping patients, families, and co-workers gain the knowledge and skills they need to be safe and independent—can be one of the most rewarding, time-saving, and cost-effective things you do. Many patients are discharged "quickly and sickly," having to manage complex problems independently at home. They need competent, knowledgeable professionals to help them learn.

The following summarizes key questions you need to answer to stay focused on *learner needs:*
1. What does the learner already know?
2. What does he or she still need to learn?
3. How would he or she like to learn it?
4. What resources can help?

GUIDING PRINCIPLE
You're accountable for ensuring that patients, families, and caregivers you supervise have the knowledge and skills they need to proceed with care safely and effectively. If you don't provide learning that a reasonably prudent nurse in the same situation would have provided and it results in harm, you may be accused of negligence.

Educating Patients and Health Care Consumers

Your role in educating patients and health care consumers is central to avoiding adverse outcomes and costly readmissions. Here are some strategies to help your patients and clients become engaged in their own learning:
- **Consider the learner's health literacy level and ensure clear communication between you and the learner throughout the process**. *Health literacy* is the degree to which individuals are capable of (1) obtaining, processing, and understanding basic health information and (2) accessing and navigating the services needed to make appropriate health decisions.[10] You can find up-to-date information and tools on promoting health literacy at http://www.health.gov.

- **Find out what the person already knows.** Then, together with the learner, determine:
  1. Desired learning outcomes (what exactly the person must be able to do)
  2. How much time you have before the person must be able to do it
  Example: Sam will be able to regulate insulin dosage based on blood glucose readings by discharge.
- **Give a compelling reason to learn.** People are motivated when they know how learning something will make their lives better.
- **Determine readiness to learn** (e.g., "Where would you like to start?" "How do you feel about learning this?" "What are your biggest concerns?"). With patient teaching, be sure you include family and primary caregivers as indicated.
- **Promote curiosity and inquisitiveness.** Say something like, "Feel free to interrupt and ask questions—there are no stupid questions. I want to know what's on your mind."
- **Identify learning barriers** (e.g., consider motivation, personal feelings, and cognitive and developmental issues).
- **Ask about preferred learning styles** (e.g., doing, observing, listening, or reading), and use this information to plan teaching. *Example:* If you're teaching injection technique to doers, start by having them handle a syringe. If they'd rather read, have them read a pamphlet first. Better yet, give them the syringe and pamphlet and tell them they can start either way. Give them some time to learn on their own before you begin to teach.
- **Encourage people to get involved.** *Example:* "Let me know if you have a better way of learning this. Not everyone learns the same way."
- **Reduce anxiety by offering support.** *Example:* "Everyone is nervous when first learning to change dressings, but once you've done it a couple of times, it's much easier."
- **Minimize distractions, and teach at appropriate times.** Pick a quiet room, and choose times when the learners are likely to be comfortable and rested.
- **Use pictures, diagrams, and illustrations** to promote comprehension and retention. Have them draw their own pictures and maps—ask them to explain them to you.
- **Create mental images by using analogies and metaphors.** *Example:* "Insulin is like a key that opens the cell's door to allow sugar to enter. If you don't have the key (insulin), sugar can't get in to feed the cell. The cell starves, and sugar accumulates in the blood, damaging kidneys and vessels."
- **Encourage people to think out loud, using their own words.** For example, a patient may say, "I need to have three things: the soaking-dressing stuff, the scrubbing stuff, and the after-dressing stuff."
- **Keep it simple.** The explain-it-to-me-as-if-I-were-a-10-year-old approach works especially well for complex situations. If you can't make it simple, you're not ready to teach it.
- **Tune in to your learners' responses and change the pace, techniques, or content if needed.** If they don't remember important content, take time to review it; if they don't seem to understand what you're saying, write it down or draw a picture.
- **Summarize main points, and don't leave learners empty-handed.** Give them the important points in print or online so that they can refresh their memory later (many health care organizations now post specific health-teaching videos online).
- **Evaluate what's been learned by asking learners to teach back** what they have learned, as addressed in the following guiding principle.

GUIDING PRINCIPLE

Much of the information patients receive is forgotten immediately, and what is retained is often incorrect.[11] Giving printed guides and using the "teach-back," "show me," or "tell me how you'll handle this at home" approach is central to gaining insight into what the learner understands. This approach isn't a test of the patient's or learner's knowledge. It's a test of how well you explained the concept.[11]

ASSESSING AND EVALUATING THINKING: BEST PRACTICES

While assessing and evaluating thinking is a complex process, this section gives you some best practices. Keep in mind that the terms *assess* and *evaluate* are often used interchangeably.

Evaluating critical thinking is important for two main reasons:

1. You need to know what you're doing well and what you need to work on.
2. Educators, managers, and employers need to determine whether you have the thinking skills necessary to practice safely and effectively in the clinical setting.

Unlike *Star Trek*'s Mr. Spock, we humans can't read minds—understanding what's going on in someone else's head is a challenge. We're all unique, with various personalities and thinking styles. What may seem like reasonable thinking to *you* may seem disorganized and inefficient to someone *else*. Evaluating someone else's thinking is a difficult task that requires knowledge of the many issues related to assessing thinking, as well as a great deal of critical thinking.

Basic Principles of Evaluating Thinking

Valid assessment of someone's thinking depends on three things:

1. **The level of trust in the relationship** (mistrust damages communication and impedes reasoning and evaluation). Open and honest dialogue is key.
2. **Having a shared understanding of exactly what critical thinking behaviors or skills will be assessed.** The person doing the assessment and the person being assessed must be "on the same page." Using the critical thinking indicators (CTIs) in Chapters 1 and 2 (Boxes 1.2, 1.7, and 1.8) is useful for this purpose.
3. **Having several ways of assessing the person's thinking.** Observing behavior; asking the person to explain their reasoning; assessing patient outcomes; and analyzing charting, tests, and other communication.

GUIDING PRINCIPLE

Drawing conclusions about someone's thinking requires focusing on *patterns over time*, not *single incidences*. For example, it's normal to have occasional communication issues, but if these happen frequently, there's a pattern of miscommunication that needs to be investigated.

There are four main things to consider when evaluating reasoning.

1. **Outcomes (results):** Does the person usually achieve desired outcomes?
   - In the clinical setting, this means assessing the nurse's patients directly to determine level of care. When you assess the patients, are they safe, satisfied, and progressing as expected?
   - In class, evaluating outcomes means analyzing test results, projects (e.g., papers and presentations), and classroom participation (e.g., if learners give alternative explanations or ask relevant questions).
2. **Process:** How does the nurse usually go about achieving outcomes? Are you seeing (or not seeing) CTIs? For example, does the nurse:
   - Demonstrate awareness of limits of knowledge and capabilities?
   - Communicate effectively orally and in writing?
   - Include patient and family in decision-making?
3. **Behavior:** What patterns of behavior do you observe in the person? Does the observed behavior send messages of CTIs (e.g., *being accountable and responsible*)? If you're not sure about behavior, ask for an explanation of the *reasoning behind behavior*. For example, "Help me understand what you're trying to accomplish."

4. **Charting and other communications:** Are verbal, written, and electronic communications timely, relevant, clear, and concise? For evaluating electronic charting, see "Thinking with Health Information Technology" in Chapter 4.

> **GUIDING PRINCIPLE**
>
> **Evaluation and feedback should be an ongoing process, not something that happens only during formal evaluations.**

Think how the following principles and strategies apply to you.

- **There are two types of evaluations—formative and summative.** *Formative evaluations are ongoing* and focus on giving feedback about what to do to improve skills. *Summative evaluations* are done at the *end of the learning period* to determine whether learners can have achieved skills, outcomes, and competencies needed to practice independently.
- **Many people find being evaluated to be stressful (it's human nature).** Remind yourself that the purpose of evaluation isn't to judge or point out flaws, but to be sure that you have the feedback needed to develop sound reasoning and practice safely and effectively.
- **Be sure you have a structured tool or coaching plan that specifies goals, expectations, outcomes, and/or behaviors** to serve as a reference point for evaluation. Evaluators and learners must stay focused on common goals and outcomes.[7,8,12]
- **Make the link between critical thinking and the behavior you see (or don't see).** For example, "When you ask lots of questions, you're demonstrating curiosity, a key critical thinking characteristic" or "When I see you constantly having to go back to complete assessments, you're not thinking critically, because if you were, you'd be assessing comprehensively and getting the correct information in the first place."
- **Pay attention to body language and respond accordingly.** *Example*: "I can tell from your body language that you're stressed and unsure of yourself …what's going on?"
- **To understand whether opinions and decisions are based on evidence,** ask questions like, "How do you know?" and "What information do you have to support this?"
- **To determine whether someone is proactive,** ask questions like, "What do you expect to happen when you do this?" "How will you handle this if (fill in the blank) happens?" "What alternatives have you considered?" and "What else is possible here?"
- **Realize that mental blocks occur, even to the best thinker.** When this happens, saying some of the following things can get the thoughts flowing again: "I know I'm putting you on the spot … take your time and try to explain" or "Let's talk later after we reflect on what was going on here."
- **For formative feedback,** find a quiet, private place, or try the "Come walk and talk with me" approach; keep in mind that if people are consistently struggling with clinical reasoning and performance, it may be related to stress in their personal lives (talking about this stress promotes trust and brings insight into real issues).

Skill 7.4, "Giving and Taking Constructive Feedback" in Chapter 7 examines strategies for making the most of feedback.

Self-Assessment, Reflecting on Progress, Initiating Feedback

Assessing your own abilities, reflecting on your progress, and initiating feedback are key to developing sound reasoning. What are you doing well? What areas do you target for improvement? What knowledge, skills, and experiences do you need to gain?

Initiating feedback increases the likelihood of getting timely assessment and advice. It also helps educators, leaders, and preceptors—they have demanding jobs that require them to balance learner and staff needs.[13] It helps them to know that you're someone who reflects on what you're doing, keeps them informed, and asks for their input. Here are examples of things you can say to initiate feedback:

- "When you have time, I need some advice."
- "I'm struggling with _____."
- "I'm feeling overwhelmed."
- "I'm realizing that I need to know more about _____."
- "I learned a lot today."

Critical Thinking and Performance Evaluation

Most organizations do formal performance evaluations every year (for new nurses and those with possible issues, sometimes every 3 to 6 months). Well-designed performance evaluation tools aim to evaluate the most important behaviors and competencies needed for safe, high-quality care in the context of each particular setting (e.g., medical-surgical versus behavioral health areas).

Your clinical performance is linked to your critical thinking and clinical reasoning skills. Critical thinking is what's going on "behind the scenes in your head." It's what drives your decisions. For this reason, if you're meeting expectations on your school's or organization's clinical evaluation tool, then it's likely that you're doing the most important things you need to do to think critically in your particular clinical setting. To help your instructors and managers assess your thinking, learn to "think out loud" and share the rationales behind your actions.

High-Stakes Testing

In recent years, we have paid more attention to high-stakes tests—tests that have significant consequences for learners and teachers (e.g., NCLEX®, certification, and other exams). Using standard tests helps test knowledge and may assess some critical thinking skills. But it's important to consider the following points, summarized from National League for Nurses statements and recommendations on high-stakes testing:[14–16]

- Test accuracy is extremely important when the tests are used to prevent progression or graduation.
- Using only one test to determine learners' progression or graduation can have a profound and harmful effect on that individual.
- Using tests outside of their intended purposes negatively affects all test-takers, especially learners who may be faced with social bias, stereotyping, and poor early preparation.
- Central to these recommendations is a commitment to fair testing practices to ensure that both tests and the decisions based on tests are valid, supported by solid evidence, and fair to all test-takers, regardless of age, gender, disability, race, ethnicity, national origin, religion, sexual orientation, language background, testing style, ability, or other personal characteristics.
- Most available standardized tests provide individual student scores that are linked to a probability of passing the NCLEX-RN®.

While some tests do predict success, they don't necessarily predict ability to think critically in *real* situations. Rather, they indicate ability to apply test-taking strategies and think critically *in the context of that particular test*. If you do poorly on tests, think about how you do in real situations. For example, I sometimes do poorly on timed tests because I like to mull over each question and can be indecisive about the *best* response. However, my indecisiveness on tests doesn't translate into my being indecisive *when it matters*: I was a charge nurse in an intensive care unit and an evening supervisor of a 300-bed hospital. I can make timely clinical decisions as well as anyone.

If you have a track record of success in handling real situations, it's quite likely that you're one of those creative, complex thinkers who struggles with test-taking and needs lots of practice to develop test-taking skills.

- For a practical, complete guide to evaluation and testing, see Oermann's *Evaluation and Testing in Nursing Education.*[12]

IMPROVING GRADES AND PASSING TESTS THE FIRST TIME

Have you heard the saying, "As long as there are tests, there will be prayer in school"? Whether you're a student or an experienced professional, testing is something that can be anxiety producing. We all have been in the position of knowing something well, yet getting confused on a test. Many complex, creative critical thinkers struggle with trying to "match" right answers on a test. As a friend once said to me, "I need to be in real situations to think well." This section helps you use critical thinking to identify the best way to prepare for—and take—tests.

Studying Efficiently

Succeeding on tests begins with knowing how to study efficiently. For many people, this means changing the habit of thinking, *I'll go over this again later* to *I'll make the most of my time by using strategies to make sense of information right now, on the first pass.* Here are some strategies to help you process, manage, and remember information, all central parts of learning:

- **Never read, watch videos, listen to presentations, or engage in class discussions without taking notes—you retain very little**. Making notes helps you process the information so you understand and remember it better. Don't highlight your way through articles—pick out only a few main ideas that stand out from all the others.
- **Remember conceptual learning principles.** Look for big ideas. Think about why the content is important (e.g., Do you need to know it to give safe and effective care? If you'll be tested on the material, what type of questions are you likely to encounter?). In class discussions, it's a good idea to say things like, *I may be missing something, but I'm not clear about this. Can we summarize major points? Can we talk about the most important points we'll apply in the clinical setting (or on the test)?* These types of comments are important for three reasons: (1) they're probably on other people's minds; (2) they spark discussion, clarification, and remembering; and (3) we all learn from one another.
- **To increase understanding after the "first pass" of materials, revise your notes and maps at least once.** Organizing and reorganizing information to find new relationships gives you more in-depth understanding and will help you remember the content better.
- **Learn strategies that boost your memory.** You must be able to *recall* facts to progress to higher levels of thinking, such as *analyzing and applying information.* For example, if you can't recall what *normal* health assessment findings are, you won't be able to analyze your patient's data to decide whether there are any *abnormal* findings.
  - **Review the information in two ways: just before you go to sleep and just after you've had some sleep** (some experts believe your brain moves data into long-term memory better if reviewed late in the day; others point out the benefits of memorizing when your brain is rested and fresh).
  - **Create memory hooks.** For example, suppose you're studying pneumonia in class and you cared for Fred, who had pneumonia when you were doing your clinical experience. Visualize Fred and how he compared with the textbook picture. Fred becomes your memory hook. If you don't have a real situation to connect with, play around with the information until something comes to mind that helps you remember (e.g., a rhyme, a picture, or a story).

- **Use a mnemonic** (a memory jog that makes an association between something that's easy to remember and something that's hard to remember). *Example:* TACIT helps you remember what to assess for medications (**T**herapeutic effect, **A**llergic or **A**dverse reactions, **C**ontraindications, **I**nteractions, **T**oxicity/overdose).
- **Create an acrostic** (a catchy phrase that helps you remember the first letters of the information you're trying to remember). *Example:* **M**aggie **C**hewed **N**uts **E**very **P**lace **S**he **W**ent gives the first letters of things you must assess in neurovascular assessment: **M**ovement, **C**olor, **N**umbness, **E**dema, **P**ulses, **S**ensation, and **W**armth.

GUIDING PRINCIPLE

To test your memory, quiz yourself without your notes. You may think you know the material when you're actually depending on cues from visual materials, not memory

---

Physiological Basis of Test Anxiety

Many people suffer from various levels of test anxiety, from mild to debilitating. Debilitating test anxiety that happens before or during testing situations is accompanied by physiological over-arousal and extreme focus on somatic symptoms (e.g., pain or fatigue). Worry, dread, fear of failure, and catastrophizing are also common.[17]

Yet few realize that there's a physiological basis for the stress they feel. When you're anxious, you feel stressed, and our brain responds by triggering a flood of hormones like cortisol and epinephrine (called the "fight-or-flight" response). These hormones help you in short-term situations like running from danger, but they don't support calm, analytical, or intuitive problem-solving—they inhibit them.[18] With test anxiety, stress becomes a vicious cycle: you feel a bit anxious and the stress hormones kick in, making you feel even more stressed.

A good remedy for test anxiety is to remember that it works against you. Tell yourself to stay calm, take a deep breath, relax your muscles, and just do the best you can. It helps stop the cortisol surge. If you're stressed while studying or on the morning of the test, consider increasing your vitamin C intake. Many stress reduction resources point out that vitamin C mediates the cortisol stress response, thereby helping you stay calm. Manage your stress holistically: eat right, drink lots of fluids, exercise, and avoid situations that interfere with getting enough rest.

Test-Taking Strategies

Keeping up on course work and studying each week—rather than cramming at the end of courses—is the key for doing well on exams. But it isn't the *only* key. Knowing how to reason your way through tests is equally as important. If you struggle with test-taking, don't keep telling yourself that you're terrible at it (this becomes a self-fulfilling prophecy). Instead, accept the fact that you need to learn to "think like the test does" and get the coaching you need to succeed.

This section gives general test-taking strategies to help you reason your way through any test and then specific strategies for taking the NCLEX®.

Preparing for Tests

- **Know yourself.** Identify your usual test-taking behaviors (e.g., Do you get overly anxious? Do you tend to run out of time? Are you better at one type of test than another?). Seek help for areas you'd like to change.

- **Know the test plan.** Find out what types of questions are going to be asked and what information is the most important to study. If the teacher doesn't share this information, review course objectives, text objectives, and summaries—often these will help you decide what's most important.
- **Find out how long you have to take the test,** what resources you're allowed to bring, and whether you get penalized for guessing.
- **Prepare with an attitude of "I can do this—I just have to figure out how."** You are capable. Sometimes you need to remind yourself of this to gain the positive attitude that's so important. Lack of confidence is a self-defeating brain-drain. Take a deep breath and focus on doing the best you can.
- **Get organized and budget your time.** Decide what you need to study, what your resources are (e.g., notes, books, tutors, and peers), and when and how you'll prepare for the test.
- **Join a study group**—be sure the group stays on task and on time.
- **Sign up to receive a practice question each day** at https://www.kaptest.com/nclex/free/nclex-practice
- **Know the parts of a question, how to read questions, and how to make educated guesses** (Boxes 3.2 and 3.3).
- **Practice taking the test under the same conditions you will experience when you actually take it.** For example, if it's a computerized test, practice on the computer.

Taking Tests

- **Arrive early for warm-up.** Give yourself time to calm down, get focused, and scan your review materials. Reviewing practice questions is also a good way to get your brain in test-taking gear.
- **Pay attention to verbal and printed instructions,** and jot down notes to be sure you remember them.

BOX 3.2   **Parts of a Test Question**

1. **The background statement(s):** The statements or phrases that tell you the *context* in which you're expected to answer the question (e.g., the words in italics in the following example).
   Example test question: You're caring for *someone who has severe asthma, is wheezing loudly, is confused,* and *can't sleep.* You check the orders and note that a sedative can be given for sleeplessness. Knowing the possible effects of giving a sedative to an asthmatic, <u>what would you do?</u>
   a. Give the sedative to help the patient relax.
   b. Withhold the sedative, because it aggravates asthma.
   c. Withhold the sedative, and monitor the patient closely.
   d. Give the sedative, but monitor the patient carefully.
2. **The stem:** A phrase that asks or states the intent of the question (e.g., the underlined words above).
3. **Key concepts:** The most important concepts addressed in the background statement(s). In the example above, the key concepts are "severe asthma," "wheezing loudly," and "effects of giving a sedative to an asthmatic."
4. **Key word(s):** The words that specify what's being asked and what's happening. In the example above, the key words are "severe," "loudly," and "confused." These words specify that the asthma problem is severe. "Would you do" specifies that you're being asked for an appropriate action to take.
5. **The options (choices):** These include one correct answer (called the *keyed response*) and three to five distracters (incorrect answers). In the example above, (c) is the keyed response and the rest are distracters.

BOX 3.3   Guidelines for Making Educated Guesses*

Educated guess defined: Using test-taking strategies to choose a right answer when you're unsure from content alone (when none of the options seem to jump out at you).

1. Be sure you understand the test directions.
2. Find out whether you're penalized for guessing.
3. Read the question *twice*, asking yourself the following:
   - **What** does the stem ask? (Box 3.2 defines stem)
   - **Who** is the client? (e.g., age, sex, role)
   - **What** is the problem? (e.g., diagnosis, signs, symptoms, behavior)
   - **What rationale** is offered in the question? (e.g., to prevent respiratory complications … Because the cast is damp …)
   - **What time frame** is being addressed? (e.g., immediately before surgery, on the day of admission)
4. Study all the answers.
   - Eliminate answers you know are outright wrong.
   - Look for answers that are wrong based on the directions.
   - Look for clues in the questions or answers that might help you narrow it down further to the most likely best answer (see strategies 5 and 6 next).
5. Use the following rules together with your knowledge to make educated guesses:
   - **Initial = Assessment.** The word *initial* used in a question usually requires an assessment answer. (What would you assess?)
   - **Essential = Safety.** The word *essential* used in a question usually requires a safety answer. (What's required for safety?) Remember: "Keep them breathing, keep them safe."
   - **Opposites Attract Right Answers.** If you have two answers that are opposite to one another, the *right* answer is usually *one* of the two opposites. *Example:* The correct answer here is likely to be (a) or (b) because they're opposites.
   - **Odd Man Wins.** The option that's most different in length, style, or content is usually the right answer. The *right* answer is often the longest one or the shortest one. *Example:* The correct answer here is likely to be (b) because it's the "odd man."
   - **Same Answer = Neither One.** If two responses say the same thing in different words, they can't both be right, so neither one is right. *Example:* Tachycardia and rapid heartbeat as two answer options.
   - **Repeated Words Means Right One.** If the answer contains the same word (or a synonym) that appears in the question, it's more likely to be a correct response. *Example:* The word *hypotension* in the question, the word *hypotension* or *shock* in the answer.
   - **Absolutely Not.** Answers that use "absolutes" aren't usually the right response. *Example:* always, never, all, none.
   - **Generally So.** Answers that use qualifiers that make the response more "generally so" tend to signify right answers. *Examples:* Usually, frequently, often.
6. When answering questions about setting priorities, remember Maslow's Hierarchy of Needs (See a summary of Maslow in Chapter 6).

*Strategies developed with the help of Judith Miller and Deanne Blach

- **If allowed, skim the whole test and plan your approach.** For example, begin by answering the types of questions you like before tackling types you don't like (you may like matching questions better than essay). Completing what you like and know first reduces anxiety and gets your brain in the test-taking mode before you tackle more difficult questions.
- **Watch your time, and note how the questions are weighted.** If a question is worth 50% of your grade, you might want to save 50% of your time to work on that question.

- **Focus on what you know.**
  - **If allowed, skip difficult questions** and come back to them later. Mark the easy questions and do them first.
  - **For short-answer and essay tests:** Jot down main points you need and ask yourself, "What else can I say?" or "What did I miss?"
- **If you don't understand a question, ask for clarification.** If you're not allowed to ask questions during the test, write something like, "I wasn't sure what you meant, so I'm answering the question assuming you meant …" on your answer sheet, if allowed.
- **When in doubt, don't change answers.** Your first response is more likely to be correct.
- **When being tested using case histories, read the questions first.** Then, look for the answers as you read the case history.
- **If you're stuck on a question**, try sketching a picture, map, or diagram to help you conceptualize the answer.

After Taking Tests

- **If you do poorly, don't think it's the end of the world.** Even the best minds have failed tests (Einstein flunked algebra; Edison was considered unteachable). Instead, do something. Explain your difficulty to your instructor; ask for suggestions on how to prepare better or whether you can do extra-credit work.
- **If there's a test review, be sure to go—you'll learn.** Too many students think that this is an opportunity to skip class because "nothing much will be happening."

NCLEX® FACTS AND STRATEGIES

NCLEX® is based on surveys of skills that new graduates must have to practice safely and effectively (surveys are done every 3 years). It's taken on a computer and takes up to 6 hours. Questions require analysis and application. If you answer easy questions correctly, you move on to higher-level questions. You can't go back and change answers. Don't skip questions—try your best on each one.

As soon as you answer enough questions to predict whether you'll pass or fail, the computer shuts down. You answer a minimum of 75 questions; 15 of these are being tested for reliability and are not a part of your score. The maximum number of questions is 265. Before you take the test, you must go through a short tutorial that explains how to answer alternate-item questions. To get the most out of the tutorial, take a tutorial before going to the testing center (you can find this at www.pearsonvue.com/nclex).

> **GUIDING PRINCIPLE**
>
> **The NCLEX® is a power test, not a speed test.** Work slowly and accurately, rather than rapidly and carelessly. Careless wrong answers can "dig a hole that's hard to climb out of."[19]

While NCLEX is evolving, below is the test plan at the time of this publication (check www.ncsbn.org for most up-to-date plan).

Fast Facts on NCLEX® Test Plan

- **NCLEX® tests five major categories:**
  1. Safe and Effective Care Environment—Management of Care (17% to 23% of the test)
  2. Safe and Effective Care Environment—Safety and Infection Control (9% to 15% of the test)
  3. Health Promotion and Maintenance (6% to 12% of the test)
  4. Psychosocial Integrity (6% to 12% of the test)

    5. Physiological Integrity (around 50% of the test)
       ➢ Basic care and comfort; assistance with activities of daily living (ADLs) (6% to 12% of the test)
       ➢ Pharmacology and IV therapy (12% to 18% of the test)
       ➢ Risk reduction (9% to 15% of the test)
       ➢ Physiological adaptation (11% to 17% of the test)

- **Focuses on four processes throughout:**
  1. Nursing process
  2. Teaching and learning
  3. Caring
  4. Communication and documentation

- **Stresses assessment and monitoring (safe, effective care) throughout:**
  1. Before procedure, during procedure, and after procedure assessment
  2. Before drug administration, during drug administration, and after drug administration assessment
  3. Delegation (what should you delegate, to whom, and when?)
  4. Prioritizing and managing care (what should you do first?)

- **You'll find questions on all major specialties,** as well as advance directives, injury prevention, family systems, cultural diversity, legal rights and responsibilities, error prevention, bioterrorism, disaster response, human sexuality, and mental health. Questions may address clients in acute/critical care, long-term/rehabilitation care, outpatient, and community/home-based settings.

- **Most questions are multiple-choice items that require you to select one best answer.** There are an increasing number of "alternate-item questions." These questions require you to choose one or more responses. They may appear in the following formats: fill in the blank (for calculations); multiple response (select all that apply), ordered response (put in correct order); and click and drag the mouse to select a "hot spot." All items may include charts, tables, or graphs; sound; and video. When questions instruct you to "select all that apply," don't choose all of the answers or just one of the answers. There's no partial credit. All answers are right or wrong.

Tests your ability to:

- Apply infection control (e.g., hand hygiene, aseptic/sterile technique)
- Review pertinent data before medication administration
- Prepare and give medications (calculating doses and applying the five rights of medication administration)
- Provide care within the legal scope of practice
- Maintain patient confidentiality
- Ensure proper patient identification
- Practice in a manner consistent with a code of ethics for a registered nurse
- Protect a patient from injury (falls, malfunctioning equipment, electrical hazards)
- Prioritize individual patient priorities and overall workload to manage time effectively
- Use approved abbreviations and standard terminology when documenting care
- Perform and manage care of patients receiving peritoneal dialysis and hemodialysis
- Provide intrapartum care and education
- Facilitate group sessions
- Identify and report occupational/environmental exposures
- Provide care and support for a patient with non–substance-related dependencies

Source: Summarized from National Council of State Boards of Nursing. 2016 RN-NCLEX test plan. 2016. Retrieved from https://www.ncsbn.org/testplans.htm

Taking the NCLEX®

- Start preparing early; get review books early, and use them as you progress through your program. This helps you be familiar with the types of questions you have to answer. A lot of learning happens when you practice test questions.
- As you do practice questions, increase learning and retention by always reading rationales. If you answered correctly, you want to be sure it was for the right reason; if you answered incorrectly, you need to understand the rationale for the correct answer. There is a wealth of information in the rationales.
- Remember that you must complete a tutorial before the exam: https://www.pearsonvue.com/nclex.
- **Ask your faculty to recommend NCLEX® preparation resources (many schools now have required resources).** Find at least one good source for content review and at least two sources for questions. Using two sources for questions exposes you to more than one style of question (Box 3.4).
- Complete at least 2000 computerized practice questions—this will significantly increase your chances of passing the first time. Practice, practice, practice is the name of the test-taking game. Box 3.4 includes resources for free online practice questions.

BOX 3.4   Studying, Test-Taking, and NCLEX® Resources

General resources
- Test-taking tips for all kinds of tests (essay, multiple choice, short answer, open book): http://www.testtaking-tips.com/
- Study tips, including how to take notes and cram (if you must): http://www.recordnations.com/articles/record-keeping-students/
- Seven dumbest things students do when cramming for tests: http://www.cracked.com/blog/the-7-dumbest-things-students-do-when-cramming-exams/

NCLEX® preparation
- Information about the testing center and practice tutorials: http://www.Pearsonvue.com/nclex
- Help for foreign nurses: http://www.testpreview.com/cgfns_practice.htm
- National Council of State Board of Nursing resources: https://www.ncsbn.org
- Individual state boards of nursing resources: http://www.ncsbn.org (click on "Boards of Nursing")
- Canadian Registered Nurse Examination Preparation: http://www.cno.org/en/become-a-nurse/entry-to-practice-examinations/
- Kaplan Nursing: http://www.kaptest.com/nursing/nclex-prep/
- Tutoring and NCLEX® consulting. http://judymillernclexreview.com; http://www.DeanneBlach.com

Free practice questions
http://www.4tests.com/nclex
http://www.mightynurse.com/nclex-practice-questions/
http://www.kaptest.com/nursing/nclex-prep/free-nclex-prep
http://www.varsitytutors.com/example-nclexrn-problems

Elsevier resources
Silvestri LA. Saunders Comprehensive Review for the NCLEX-RN® Examination.
Silvestri LA. Saunders Q & A Review for the NCLEX-RN® Examination.
Zerwekh J. Illustrated Study Guide for the NCLEX-RN® Exam. For more information and additional resources, go to www.elsevieradvantage.com.

Next-Generation NCLEX® (NGN)

The National Council of State Boards of Nursing (NCSBN) is developing "the next generation of NCLEX®" (NGN), which will include testing of clinical judgment and decision-making skills.[20] Chapters 4 and 6 help you gain virtually all the skills that are likely to be tested in the new exam (e.g., recognizing and analyzing cues, evaluating outcomes, generating hypotheses, judging options, and taking action[20]). For the most up-to-date NGN information, frequently asked questions (both faculty and candidates), and NGN resources, go to https://www.ncsbn.org/.

? CRITICAL THINKING EXERCISES

Find example responses in Appendix I (page 216).

1. **Fill in the following blanks, choosing from the following words:** same, practice, formative, various, details, debriefing, big, calm, ready, know, ideas, preparing
   A. Two main steps to teaching others are finding out what they already (a)_____ and determining whether they are (b)_____ to learn.
   B. You demonstrate competency when you are able to do specific skills safely and effectively under _____ circumstances.
   C. Doing well on a test requires you to not only have the required knowledge but also to (a)_____ taking the test under the (b)_____ conditions you'll experience when you actually take it.
   D. With conceptual learning, you identify the (a)_____ ideas before learning the (b)_____.
   E. You learn more from simulated experiences when you use _____ to reflect on lessons learned.
   F. Initiating feedback helps you get _____feedback and keeps your educators and leaders informed.
   G. Making the most of simulation requires (a)_____for the experience and staying (b)_____during the experience and debriefing.
2. What are your responsibilities related to teaching patients, the caregivers you supervise, and yourself?
3. Why is knowing how to teach others and yourself efficiently essential to meeting nursing outcomes?
4. Drawing from your personal experience, give at least one example of where the "use it or lose it" rule applies; then give strategies you can use to either boost your memory or use the information more frequently.
5. What is the purpose of remediation?
6. Why is it important to have a structured tool for simulation, debriefing, and evaluation?
7. When studying for a test, why is it important to be sure you know the content without looking at your notes?

THINK, PAIR, SHARE

With a partner, in a group, or in a journal entry:

1. Share your best and worst experience with learning, simulation, or evaluation. Identify what made things go well and what made things go poorly. What did you learn from these experiences?
2. Create a health literacy seminar based on the information and tools posted at http://www.health.gov (enter "health literacy tools" into the search field).

3. Apply the ABCD model to evaluating resources in relation to one of your favorite websites.
4. Identify key points of the teach-back method as addressed by the North Carolina Program on Health Literacy at http://www.nchealthliteracy.org/toolkit/tool5.pdf.
5. Discuss the implications of student evaluations in the following article: Turner K, Hatton D, Valiga T. Student evaluations of teachers and courses: time to wake up and shake up. *Nurs Educ Perspect.* 2018;39(3):130–131 doi: 10.1097/01.NEP.0000000000000329.
6. Discuss how positive expectations can influence performance, as addressed in *The Pygmalion Effect: Proving Them Right* available at https://fs.blog/2018/05/pygmalion-effect/.
7. Test your study skills by taking the *Scientific American* quiz at http://www.scientificamerican.com/article/test-your-study-skills-quiz.
8. Share where you stand in relation to understanding the key concepts and achieving the learning outcomes at the beginning of this chapter.
9. Discuss your thoughts on the following Critical Moments and Other Perspectives.

 ## CRITICAL MOMENTS AND OTHER PERSPECTIVES

Learning Proverbs

- *I hear, I forget. I see, I remember. I do, I understand.*
- *A man who asks a question may feel like a fool for 5 minutes. A man who never asks is a fool for life.*
- *Humorous twist on an old proverb: Give a man a fish and he eats for a day—teach a man to fish, and he leaves you alone every weekend.*

What Makes a Good Mentor?

"A mentor is not someone who walks ahead of us to show us how they did it. A mentor walks alongside us to show us what we can do." – Simon Sinek, *Author of Motivating Learners.* When trying to teach or motivate others, use the human instinct to self-focus to your advantage. Ask yourself questions like, "What's in it for them?" and "How can I make this relevant and worth their time?"

Be Sure to Teach "Why"

Knowing *why* something must be done empowers people to solve problems independently. When you stress principles, reasons, and rationales, learners are able to make better decisions about what to do when things don't go as expected.

Teaching Others Helps You Learn

When you want to learn something, offer to teach it to someone else. You learn and recall best what you teach someone *else.*

Most Dangerous Patient Education Mistakes

The most dangerous mistakes in patient education are making assumptions. You assume they can read. You assume they understand. You assume they have no more questions. You assume they can do it. You assume they will do it. —Fran London, MS, RN, author of *No Time to Teach: The Essence of Patient and Family Education for Health Care Providers.*[21]

KEY POINTS/SUMMARY

- Building learning cultures that embrace the motto that "everyone teaches, everyone learns" is central to promoting critical thinking and safety.
- Accessing, analyzing, and applying the best information available is an essential 21st-century skill.
- Concept-based learning helps reduce information overload by guiding you to focus on big ideas before details.
- Competency-based learning—in which nurses focus on achieving certain clinical skills before moving on to learning other clinical skills—is important for any learning in which safety is an important concern.
- Learning, unlearning, and relearning are common challenges; we must all be alert to skills that may not be as sharp as they once were and seek opportunities to improve.
- Critical thinking takes more than memorizing facts—you must know how to *apply* information in the context of various situations.
- Whether you're trying to learn clinical or teamwork skills, simulated experiences—along with debriefing—is a powerful way to learn.
- Practicing what to do when things go wrong is crucial to developing sound reasoning skills.
- Having strong preceptors and educators and participating in nurse residency programs helps you develop sound skills in a supportive environment.
- Competence has four interrelated components—knowledge, skills, behavior, and judgment.[3] The degree to which you're able to display these components under various circumstances determines how clinically competent you are.
- Evaluation can be either formative (ongoing to help you improve) or summative (at the end of a period to test critical thinking and performance).
- Reflecting on your abilities and asking for feedback and help from preceptors and educators is crucial to improving your reasoning skills.
- Helping others learn requires working together with them to identify (1) what must be learned, (2) how they want to learn it, and (3) what resources they can use.
- Learning efficiently requires us to use strategies that help you process, manage, and remember information.
- The NCLEX® is based on surveys of skills that new graduates must have to practice safely and effectively (surveys are done every 3 years).
- Because passing NCLEX®, which is evolving, has very specific rules, requiring you to "think in the way the test questions do," start doing practice questions early; a lot of learning happens when you do practice test questions and read rationales about why you got them right or wrong.
- Scan this chapter to review the illustrations and Guiding Principles throughout.

REFERENCES

1. Forneris S, Fey M. *Critical conversations: the NLN guide for teaching thinking.* Washington, DC: National League for Nursing; 2018.
2. Ignatavicius D. *Teaching and learning in a concept-based curriculum: a how-to best practice approach.* Burlington, MA: Jones & Bartlett; 2019.
3. Wright D. *Competency assessment field guide: a real world guide for implementation and application.* Minneapolis, MN: Creative Health Care Management; 2015.
4. Top 25 Alvin Toffler Quotes. Retrieved from http://www.azquotes.com/author/14696-Alvin_Toffler 1991.
5. International Nursing Association for Clinical Simulation and Learning (INACSL) Standards Committee. INACSL standards of best practices: Simulation debriefing. *Clinical Simulation in Nursing.* 2016;12(5):521–525. https://doi.org/10.1016/j.ecns.2016.09.008.
6. Mariani B, Doolen J. Nursing simulation research: what are the perceived gaps? *Clinical Simulation in Nursing.* 2016;12(1):30–36. https://doi.org/10.1016/j.ecns.2015.11.004.
7. Boyer S, Valdez-Delgado K, Huss J, et al. Impact of a nurse residency program on transition to

specialty practice. *Journal for Nurses in Professional Development*. 2017;33(5):220–227. https://doi.org/10.1097/NND.0000000000000384.

8. Boyer S, Mann-Salinas E, Valdez-Delgado K. Clinical Transition framework: integrating accountability, sampling, and coaching plans in professional practice development. *Journal for Nurses in Professional Development*. 2018;34(2):84–91. https://doi.org/10.1097/NND.0000000000000435.

9. Kennedy M. Nurses wanted—almost everywhere. *AJN*. 2018;118(6):7. https://doi.org/10.1097/01.NAJ.0000534825.57362.96.

10. National Action Plan to Improve Health Literacy. Retrieved from http://www.health.gov.

11. North Carolina Program on Health Literacy. *The Teach-Back Method*. (Website) Retrieved from http://www.nchealthliteracy.org/toolkit/tool5.pdf.

12. Oermann MH, Gaberson K. *Evaluation and testing in nursing education*. 5th ed. New York: Springer; 2017.

13. Oermann M. Reflections on clinical teaching in nursing. *Nurse Educator*. 2016;41(4):165. https://doi.org/10.1097/NNE.0000000000000279.

14. NLN. *The fair testing imperative in nursing education*; 2012. (Website) Retrieved from nln.org; .

15. NLN. *National League for Nursing fair testing guidelines for nursing education*; 2012. (Website) Retrieved from nln.org; .

16. NLN. *NLN CEO update on high stakes testing*; 2017. (Website) Retrieved from nln.org; .

17. Broderson L. Interventions for test anxiety in undergraduate nursing students: an integrative review. *Nursing Education Perspectives*. 2017;38(3):131–137. https://doi.org/10.1097/01.NEP.0000000000000142.

18. Weinberg J. *Uncover the Psycho-emotional Roots of Disease to Tap into the Power of the Mind-Body Connection*. (Website) Retrieved from http://www.jenniferweinbergmd.com; 2017.

19. Miller J, personal communication, 1991

20. NCSBN. *NGN News—Summer 2018*. Retrieved from, www.ncsbn.org; 2018.

21. London F. Personal communication.

Clinical Reasoning, Clinical Judgment, and Decision-Making

LEARNING OUTCOMES

After completing this chapter, you should be able to:

1. Describe key elements of interprofessional, patient, and family-centered practice.
2. Compare and contrast the terms *responsibility* and *accountability*.
3. Describe what it is that nurses think about that's different from other professionals.
4. Explain the relationships among safety, efficiency, patient and family engagement, and clinical reasoning.
5. Apply clinical reasoning principles to develop sound clinical judgment.
6. Compare and contrast nursing and medical models.
7. Discuss the roles of ethics codes, standards, protocols, and laws in clinical decision-making.
8. Describe the process of determining your scope of nursing practice.
9. Compare and contrast novice and expert thinking.
10. Describe the "four steps" and "five rights" of effective delegation.
11. Explain how health information technology (HIT) and electronic health records (EHRs) may promote or inhibit clinical reasoning.
12. Describe the role of intuition and logic in unfolding reasoning.
13. Explain how to use the *predict, prevent, manage, promote* (PPMP) approach.
14. Address how to use critical thinking indicators and the 4-Circle CT Model as tools to develop clinical reasoning skills.

Accountability; compassionate care; care coordination; delegation; emotional comfort; physical comfort; empowerment; hand-offs; health promotion; human response; medical models; medication and treatment management; mobility; nursing models; patient education; practice scope; social determinants of health; surveillance; failure to rescue; system-based practice; population-based care; predictive care models. *See also previous chapters*

NURSES: THE GLUE AND CONSCIENCE OF HEALTH CARE

Consider the words of a parent of an acutely ill child: *Compassion is no substitute for competence. In superficial, short-term encounters, a smiling face and a gentle hand impress. In the long term, it's competence that you value. You find that kindness is a relatively abundant commodity. It's confidence, borne of knowing, that's too often in short supply. Does this mean I found myself disinterested in compassion? Not at all. But I also found it didn't count for much unless it was bundled with competence.*[1]

When you choose to be a nurse, you become part of a profession that's often called "the glue and conscience" of health care. Nurses are "the glue" because they hold care systems together. In many case, nurses are the only regular qualified health care providers consistently available. Through their organizations, nurses are the conscience of health care.[2]

Consumers consistently rank nurses as being the number-one most-trusted professionals.[3] Working on the front line in complex settings—hospitals, specialized centers, home care, long-term care, schools, and communities—nurses spend more time with patients than any other professional does. They promote health, monitor and manage acute and chronic problems, and teach patients and families to do the same.

Your ability to think critically profoundly affects people's lives, often in times of their greatest needs. You must be prepared for a job that's much more than a caring presence. You need to know how to manage resources, prevent complications, and promote physical and mental well-being in diverse patients with complex issues.

Using plain language, this chapter helps you gain the knowledge, insights, and skills needed to develop sound clinical reasoning, decision-making, and judgment. To avoid overwhelming you, leadership, ethics, evidence-based practice, and quality improvement—all important parts of clinical reasoning—are addressed in the next chapter. Chapter 6 gives you opportunities to apply content from this chapter by having you work through case scenarios that are based on real experiences.

GOALS AND OUTCOMES OF NURSING

To better understand nurses' thinking, let's consider the question: "What are the major goals and outcomes of nursing?"

Goals of Nursing

Nurses aim to achieve the following goals in a safe, efficient, and humanistic way:

1. To prevent illness, injury, disability, and complications (and teach people to do the same).
2. To help people—whether they're ill, injured, disabled, or well—to have an optimum quality of life (the best possible function, independence, and sense of well-being).
3. To continually improve patient outcomes, care delivery practices, and nurses' ability to be effective and satisfied in their jobs.

Outcomes of Nursing

Broadly speaking, the following shows the major outcomes that demonstrate the benefits of nursing care.

After receiving individualized, evidence-based care, health care consumers will demonstrate improved physical, mental, and spiritual well-being, as evidenced by the following:

- Absence of (or reduction in) signs, symptoms, and risk factors of illness, disability, or injury
- Use of strategies and behaviors that evidence shows prevent illness and promote health, function, and quality of life
- Documentation of individualized, evidence-based, state-of-the-art care that applies best practices

What Are the Implications?

There are three main implications of the goals and outcomes of nursing:

1. Because the conclusions and decisions we as nurses make affect people's lives, our thinking must be guided by sound reasoning—precise, disciplined thinking that promotes accurate data collection that's as complete and in-depth as the situation warrants.
2. Nursing's ultimate goal is for people to be able to manage their *own* health care to the best of their ability, which means we must stay *focused on patient perceptions, needs, desires, and capabilities.*
3. Because nursing is committed to achieving high-quality outcomes in a cost-effective way, we must constantly seek to improve both our own ability to give nursing care and the overall quality and efficiency of health care delivery. We must work to find answers to questions like: "How can we achieve better outcomes?" "How can we improve satisfaction with our services?" "How can we contain costs, yet maintain high standards?" and "How can we ensure competent nursing practice and retain good nurses?"

INTERPROFESSIONAL, PATIENT, AND FAMILY-CENTERED CARE

We have moved from professionals working alongside one another—like "parallel players," with each one focusing on their own "piece" of the patient—to *interprofessional, patient, and family-centered care* (professionals working *together* with one another and engaging patients and families to ensure individual needs are met).

When nurses, physicians, nutritionists, and other professionals truly work *together,* we are able use the best professional expertise to achieve the best outcomes. For example, pharmacists—who used to be seen only behind the pharmacy counter—now work in emergency departments, preventing errors by reviewing medication orders and making sure that medication records are accurate (medication reconciliation).[4]

21ST-CENTURY SKILLS AND QSEN COMPETENCIES

Chapter 1 details 21st-century nursing skills and Quality and Safety Education for Nurses (QSEN) competencies (patient-centered care, teamwork and collaboration, evidence-based practice, quality improvement, safety, and informatics). Study Fig. 4.1, which shows how these skills and competencies relate to clinical reasoning.

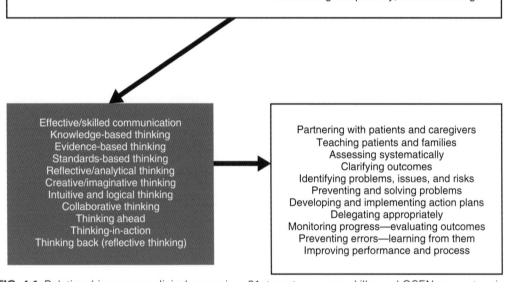

FIG. 4.1 Relationships among clinical reasoning, 21st-century nurse skills, and QSEN competencies.

PRINCIPLES OF CLINICAL REASONING

Understanding clinical reasoning principles gives you the foundation for developing sound thinking habits. This section summarizes major clinical reasoning principles, starting with key points from previous chapters. Keep in mind that Chapter 6 gives details and practice for applying these principles.

- **Engaging patients, families, and caregivers and ensuring their safety and welfare must be top priority** in all reasoning and decision-making.
- **All reasoning depends on the quality of communication.** Has there been *mutual exchange* of information, thoughts, and feelings? Is the information that's been exchanged factual and

complete? Studies show that communication issues cause patient care errors that result in adverse outcomes such as falls and missed care.[5–7]

- **Critical thinking in nursing**—which includes clinical reasoning, judgment, and decision-making—is purposeful, informed, outcome-focused thinking that:
    - **Is guided by standards**, policies, ethics codes, and laws (individual state practice acts and state boards of nursing).
    - **Is driven by patient, family, and community needs**, as well as nurses' needs to give competent and efficient care (e.g., streamlining charting to free nurses for patient care).
    - **Is based on principles of the nursing process, problem-solving, and the scientific method** (requires forming opinions and making decisions based on evidence).
    - **Focuses on safety and quality**, constantly re-evaluating, self-correcting, and striving to improve personal, professional, and system practices.
    - **Carefully identifies the key problems**, issues, and risks involved, including patients, families, and key stakeholders in decision-making early in the process.
    - **Uses logic, intuition, and creativity** and is grounded in specific knowledge, skills, experience, and professional attitudes.
    - **Calls for strategies that make the most of human potential** and compensate for problems created by human nature (e.g., finding ways to prevent errors, use technology, and overcome the powerful influence of personal views).
- **While clinical reasoning centers on *patients and families*, it begins with YOU.** Your personal qualities—your ability to demonstrate *personal* critical thinking indicators (CTIs) as described in Chapter 1 (Box 1.2)—affects your thinking as much as your ability to demonstrate *knowledge and intellectual* skill CTIs in Chapter 2 (Boxes 2.7 and 2.8). Appendix C shows how CTIs relate to the 4-Circle CT Model to target areas you may want to develop.
- **Critical thinking and clinical reasoning are thinking *processes*; clinical judgment is the *result* (outcome) of thinking** (the opinions you form or decisions you make) (Fig. 4.2).

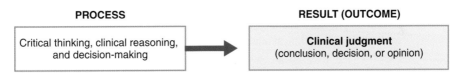

PROCESS	RESULT (OUTCOME)
Critical thinking, clinical reasoning, and decision-making	**Clinical judgment** (conclusion, decision, or opinion)

FIG. 4.2 Clinical judgment—the result of critical thinking, clinical reasoning, and decision-making.

- **While you'll use many resources to gather patient information (e.g., health records, family interviews), always consider your *direct patient assessment* to be the *primary source* of information.** Studies show that *assessment omissions* are a major cause of adverse patient outcomes.[8] For example, several studies examined the concept of *failure to rescue* (when patients die from treatable conditions because nurses failed to detect early signs and symptoms of complications).[9]
- **Clinical reasoning happens in a context of unfolding (evolving) human situations.** It's *fluid and dynamic*, not linear and step by step, requiring systems thinking as described below.

Clinical Reasoning and Systems Thinking[10,11]

- Recognize *relationships among key pieces* of the whole (e.g., How might this patient's heart be affected by suctioning his lungs? How is patient care affected by organizational systems, for example, how is pharmacy operations affecting timely medication administration?).

- Think about the consequences of actions (e.g., What's likely to happen when we stand this patient up after surgery, and what can we do to minimize risks?).
- Gain insight into how things tend to unfold over time (e.g., What's the usual course of recovery for someone who has knee replacement?).

- **The National Council of State Boards of Nursing (NCSBN) describes clinical reasoning as being iterative (repetitive)**, meaning you go through repeated rounds of analysis and actions, fine-tuning information and getting closer to the best results with each repetition.[12] For example, you may identify that a patient has coping issues. It may take several visits to fully understand exactly what's contributing to the coping issues and develop a plan that truly promotes well-being.
- **The most common clinical reasoning framework used** *across health care professionals* **is ADPIE** (*assess, diagnose, plan, implement, evaluate*). The focus of ADPIE changes, depending on the health care professional's role. **Examples:**
  - **Physicians focus on medical problems** (promoting body system functioning, curing diseases, and alleviating symptoms).
  - **Respiratory therapists** focus on promoting lung function.
  - **Nurses focus on nursing concerns** (e.g., monitoring health status and patient responses to health problems; managing treatment regimens; preventing complications; and promoting comfort, mobility, well-being, and independence, as detailed later in this chapter).
- **Using ADPIE guides clinicians to document in a way that clearly communicates care to the interprofessional team, meets legal standards, and provides the data researchers need to develop evidence-based practices.** Some nurses use **A**A**PIE** instead of **A**D**PIE**, naming the second phase, *Analysis.* Calling the second phase *Diagnosis* focuses on the *end result* of analysis: drawing conclusions (diagnosing actual and potential health issues and making care decisions).
- **Studies show that nurses and other health care professionals use a variety of reasoning patterns alone or in combination.**[13] For example, you may use ADPIE together with ABC (airway, breathing, circulation) to set initial priorities. *Maslow's Hierarchy of Human Needs* is also often used to set priorities (see "Setting Priorities," Skill 6.13, Chapter 6). When there are issues with reasoning using other clinical reasoning models, many clinicians revert to asking if the ADPIE phases have been completed (e.g., Did we assess, diagnose, plan, implement, and evaluate well enough?).
- **Broadly speaking, the process of accurately defining health problems requires** *differential diagnosis*. *Differential diagnosis* requires identifying signs and symptoms (cues), creating a list of suspected problems, and weighing the probability of one problem against that of another that's closely related (this is similar to what NCSBN calls *cue recognition and generating and testing hypotheses*).[12] **Examples:** The differential diagnosis of *anxiety* may include considering whether the problem may be better described as a *coping, lack of knowledge,* or *fear* issue. The differential diagnosis of *rhinitis* (runny nose) includes allergic rhinitis (seasonal allergies), nasal decongestants abuse, and the common cold.
- **Tanner describes reasoning patterns as** *noticing, interpreting, responding,* **and** *reflecting.*[13] Fig. 4.3 shows how using ADPIE leads to clinical judgments, including where Tanner's phases fit in.
- **Diagnosis (problem and risk identification) is most of the work of the clinical reasoning process.** Diagnosis is a pivotal point in reasoning: if you miss problems or risks or misunderstand them, the entire plan is likely to be flawed. The National Academy of Medicine's landmark report, *Improving Diagnosis in Health Care,* identifies *diagnostic error* as a major, unaddressed patient safety issue (most people will experience at least one diagnostic error in their lifetime, sometimes with devastating consequences).[14]
- *Diagnosis* **(problem identification) is incomplete until you've determined what's causing or contributing to the problems and risks.** For example, if your patient has pain, and you

PROCESS

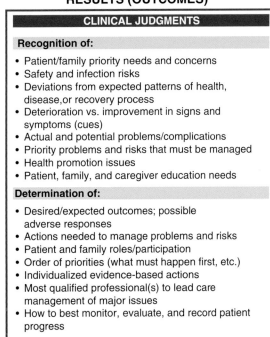

CLINICAL REASONING PHASES

- <u>A</u>ssessing: Detecting/**noticing** cues (signs, symptoms, risks)
- <u>D</u>iagnosing: Analyzing, synthesizing, and **interpreting** data; differential diagnosis (creating a list of suspected problems; weighing the probability of one problem against that of another that's closely related); NCSBN considers this phase to be generating and prioritizing hypotheses.
- <u>P</u>lanning: **Responding**; predicting complications; anticipating consequences; considering actions; setting priorities; decision making
- <u>I</u>mplementing: **Responding**; taking actions; monitoring responses; **reflecting**; making adjustments
- <u>E</u>valuating: **Reflecting;** repeating ADPIE as indicated

RESULTS (OUTCOMES)

CLINICAL JUDGMENTS

Recognition of:

- Patient/family priority needs and concerns
- Safety and infection risks
- Deviations from expected patterns of health, disease, or recovery process
- Deterioration vs. improvement in signs and symptoms (cues)
- Actual and potential problems/complications
- Priority problems and risks that must be managed
- Health promotion issues
- Patient, family, and caregiver education needs

Determination of:

- Desired/expected outcomes; possible adverse responses
- Actions needed to manage problems and risks
- Patient and family roles/participation
- Order of priorities (what must happen first, etc.)
- Individualized evidence-based actions
- Most qualified professional(s) to lead care management of major issues
- How to best monitor, evaluate, and record patient progress

FIG. 4.3 The process and outcomes of clinical reasoning using ADPIE. **Bold terms** indicate Tanner's clinical judgment model (noticing, interpreting, responding, reflecting).[13] (Source: © 2018 http://www.AlfaroTeachSmart.com. No use without permission.)

haven't completely understood what is causing it, how will you know that it's not something serious and what strategies will promote comfort? Box 4.1 summarizes the process of diagnosis (problem identification).

- **Understanding "the why" behind judgments and decisions is crucial to sound reasoning and patient safety.** If you're asked, "Why did you do this?" you should be able to justify your actions. Never do something if you don't understand why you're doing it.

BOX 4.1   Diagnosis (Problem Identification)

- Creating a list of suspected problems/diagnoses (Generating hypotheses)
- Ruling out similar problems/diagnoses
- Naming actual and potential problems/diagnoses and clarifying what's causing or contributing to them
- Determining risk factors that must be managed
- Identifying resources, strengths, and health promotion opportunities

---

- *Assessing and reflecting* play important roles in *all* phases of clinical reasoning. For example, always assess before acting to be sure the environment's safe and the actions are still appropriate; reflect on patient responses after performing actions. **Remember:** *"Assess, act, reassess."*
- **A common clinical reasoning error is *jumping to conclusions*.** Reflect on your thinking to be sure you have factual, complete information. Have some assumptions been made? Think in careful, deliberate ways, and don't accept speculation or guesswork.
- **To prioritize reasoning and think about the most important things first:**
  - **Start by considering whether your patient's signs and symptoms could be related to medical problems, medications, or possible allergies.** Use the memory jog MMA to remember "medical problems, medications, allergies."
  - **Rule out "the bad things" (worst-case scenarios) first.** For example, if your patient has unexplained left ankle pain and swelling, consider whether this may be a blood clot or heart issue that needs to be evaluated by a primary care provider (PCP) before suggesting ice, rest, elevation, and a "wait and watch approach."
  - **After you've ruled out worst-case scenarios, consider the *most common explanations*.** For example, in the above example, unrealized injury or arthritis causing pain and swelling.
- **Developing competence—your ability to reason and make sound judgments while handling complex clinical situations—**requires *on-the-job experiential learning* with guidance from educators, mentors, preceptors, or leaders who know how to coach and support learners.[15,16] Using a common reference as a "talking point" to promote dialogue about what's going well and what needs to be improved is key (many places use coaching plans to facilitate this).

NURSING ACCOUNTABILITY—WHAT DO NURSES DO?

To better understand nurses' thinking, let's examine what nurses are accountable for doing, what happens if they don't do it, and what's the difference between *responsibility* and *accountability*.

Responsibility Versus Accountability

Responsibility and *accountability* are similar concepts, but there is a significant difference:

- **Responsibility** refers to a duty or task that you are legally and morally required to do (e.g., it's your responsibility to maintain optimum patient mobility).
- **Accountability** means not only being responsible but also being *answerable for your actions or inactions* (what you did or didn't do while carrying out your responsibilities). For example, you may accept responsibility for getting a patient out of bed. But if you need help and don't get it and the patient falls, how will you account for not getting help?

Making the shift in thinking from *"I'm responsible"* to *"I'm accountable"* keeps patients safe and helps you be proactive. When you accept accountability, you develop reasoning habits that answer questions like, "How qualified am I to do this?" and "Have I done everything I can do to prevent things from going wrong?"

Keep the concept of accountability in mind as we go on to discuss key nursing roles and responsibilities and how to determine your scope of practice.

Thinking Like a Nurse

Nurses spend more time on the front line in direct patient care than any other profession, making them accountable for many aspects of care. This complex role on the front line makes it difficult to describe what nurses do that's different from what other professions do.

Several organizations—for example, the North American Nursing Diagnosis Association International (NANDA-I)—tried unsuccessfully to develop standard terms that can be widely adopted to reflect the problems that nurses treat independently. While NANDA-I's work was promising, it's no longer widely used for three main reasons: (1) Many nurses find the terms unwieldy and not understood by other nurses or health care providers. (2) Permission to use the terms is costly. (3) Research to support the labels has been missing or weak.

We can expect that standard terms for nursing care to be clarified by analytics (rigorous analysis of data collected from electronic health records [EHRs] over time). Research-based standard terms reflecting nursing responsibilities in relation to diagnoses, interventions, and outcomes will continue to evolve.

Keeping in mind that nursing—like all complex roles and concepts—can't be adequately defined using only *one* definition, this section examines nurses' thinking from two perspectives: (1) major concepts that describe nursing responsibilities and (2) accountability for common nursing and medical problems. Let's start to examine what it means to have a "nursing frame of mind" by considering the following guiding principle.

GUIDING PRINCIPLE

It's not so much *how* nurses think that makes them different from other health care professionals—it's *what* they think *about*. Using a *nursing frame of mind* means staying centered on preventing problems and promoting health by focusing on the *whole person,* identifying individual needs and monitoring responses to interventions (e.g., surgery) and life challenges (e.g., becoming a parent). Nurses' holistic thinking seeks to answer questions like: How are these health issues or challenges affecting *this particular person's* ability to function as a bio-psycho-social human being? For example, a physician may diagnose and treat a fractured hip; as a nurse, it's your responsibility to not only monitor and promote *healing of the hip* but also to monitor the person's *response* to the process *as a whole.* That is, how is the fractured hip repair *affecting the person's health, independence, safety, and ability to function in desired roles* (and what's the best nursing plan to address these issues, prevent complications, and promote health)?

Studying nursing concepts deepens your understanding of what drives nurses' thinking. The following examples of nursing concepts give insight into *what nurses think about* that's different from other health care professionals.

- **Caring, compassionate care.** While technology, documentation requirements, and staffing ratios can overwhelm the best of clinicians, nurses work to keep caring practices in the forefront.[17] In various studies, patients describe caring as vigilance (attentiveness, highly skilled practice, basic care, nurturing, and going the extra mile); mutuality (building relationships among nurses, patients, and families); and healing (lifesaving behaviors and freeing patients from anxiety and concerns).
- **Activities of daily living (ADLs) management.** Promoting independence and assisting with ADLs is a major nursing role.
- **Risk identification, complication prevention, and health promotion.** Monitoring patients to detect risks and implementing plans to manage them (e.g., preventing falls or skin breakdown); promoting health through education; and encouraging healthy behaviors (e.g., exercising, smoking cessation).

- **Surveillance.** Monitoring to detect signs and symptoms (cues) that indicate deviations from expected patterns of health, illness, or recovery; activating the chain of command as indicated.[18] Activating the chain of command means following communication policies for reporting patient issues and *staying with the problems* until the *appropriate qualified professional* has responded. For example: You give medication for incision pain, but the patient has no relief. You try repositioning and other holistic measures, but the person still has no relief. You leave two messages for the doctor to call you about this problem. One hour later, you haven't heard from the doctor, and the patient is still in distress. You're accountable for activating the chain of command and notifying your supervisor about this problem and finding out what to do next.
- **Patient and family education.** Ensuring patients and families have the knowledge and skills they need to successfully manage their health.
- **Mobility promotion.** Ensuring optimum mobility in all patients.
- **Medication and treatment regimen management.** Monitoring for adverse responses to medication and treatment regimens, as well as individualizing the regimens within prescribed parameters to meet individual needs. Nurses aim to ensure that overall medication regimens are as safe, effective, cost-effective, and convenient as possible, considering the persons' age, roles, occupation, and lifestyle. For example, with *pneumonia,* it is asking whether prescribed antibiotics are the best available, considering cost, convenience, and results.
- **Physical and emotional comfort.** Promoting physical comfort through holistic and prescribed strategies (e.g., repositioning patients, managing pain medications); promoting emotional comfort through therapeutic communication.
- **Care coordination.** Coordinating care to ensure treatment regimens meet individual needs (e.g., if you're caring for someone who isn't "a morning person," schedule physical therapy sessions in the afternoon; with complex patients, plan rest periods).
- **Delegation.** Maximizing time and resources by supervising and delegating care to unlicensed assistive personnel (addressed later in detail).
- **Documentation**. Ensuring that patient care is recorded accurately and as completely as needed to communicate the most important aspects of care.
- **Population-based, culturally competent care.** Identifying individual needs of diverse patient populations (e.g., patients of certain cultures, age groups, languages, or sexual orientation). You can download a road map to meeting population-based care standards entitled *Advancing Effective Communication, Cultural Competence and Patient- and Family-Centered Care: A Road Map for Hospitals* from http://www.jointcommission.org/Advancing_Effective_Communication/.

GUIDING PRINCIPLE

Nurses play key roles in monitoring for complications related to medication and treatment regimens. Medication reconciliation—checking to ensure that the patient's medication orders are up-to-date and complete—is the first step to reducing complications. Use **TACIT** to remember the key things you must monitor when caring for patients on various medication and treatment regimens:

Therapeutic effect—Is there a therapeutic effect?

Allergic or adverse reactions—Are there allergic or adverse reaction signs?

Contraindications—Are there contraindications to giving this drug?

Interactions?—Are there possible drug interactions?

Toxicity or overdose—Are there signs of toxicity or overdose?

Nursing Versus Medical Models

Nurses give care that's based on both nursing and medical models. We've moved from "nurses diagnose and treat only nursing diagnoses" to "nurses diagnose and manage various health issues, depending on their qualifications and practice scope" (addressed in the next section).

Box 4.2 gives examples of priority problems nurses are accountable for managing independently. Depending on *problem complexity, nurse qualifications, and practice scope,* nurses are accountable for consulting with primary care providers before determining a plan of care.

Box 4.3 shows common medical problems and their potential complications. Box 4.4 shows complications of treatments and procedures. With the problems listed in these two boxes, nurses are accountable for the following:

1. Surveillance (monitoring to detect reportable signs and symptoms (cues)—those that may indicate the need for additional qualified intervention)
2. Implementing nurse-prescribed interventions to prevent complications (e.g., promoting mobility)
3. Implementing PCP-prescribed nursing interventions

To monitor for medical problems, the body systems approach (Fig. 4.4) is commonly used. To ensure that nursing needs related to ADLs and unique human responses are identified, nursing models are used. For example, *Gordon's 11 Functional Health Patterns* approach, described here, has been widely used.[19]

1. **Health perception–health management pattern:** Perception of health and well-being; knowledge of and adherence to health promotion regimens
2. **Nutritional-metabolic pattern:** Usual food and fluid intake; height, weight, age
3. **Elimination pattern:** Usual bowel and bladder elimination patterns
4. **Activity–exercise pattern:** Usual activity and exercise tolerance
5. **Sleep–rest pattern:** Usual hours' sleep and rest.
6. **Cognitive-perception pattern:** Ability to use all senses to perceive environment; usual way of perceiving environment
7. **Self-perception or self-concept pattern:** Perception of capabilities and self-worth
8. **Role-relationship pattern:** Usual responsibilities and ways of relating to others

(Health patterns 9–11 described on page 89.)

BOX 4.2 Common Priority Nursing Problems (alphabetical list)

NOTE: Depending on problem complexity and nurse qualifications, nurses are accountable for consulting with primary care providers before determining a plan of care.

- Activity intolerance/mobility problems
- Airway and breathing problems
- Behavioral problems management
- Comfort/pain management
- Constipation, diarrhea, and other bowel elimination problems
- Dehydration risks
- Health promotion
- Infection/safety/fall risk management
- Medication and other treatment management
- Nutrition problems
- Oral hygiene†
- Urinary elimination problems
- Patient education
- Pressure ulcer/impaired skin integrity risk management
- Self-care problems (feeding, bathing, dressing, toileting, other ADLs)
- Sleep problems
- Smoking cessation
- Spiritual concerns
- Surveillance (monitoring to detect reportable signs and symptoms)
- Violence or self-harm risks
- Weight management

†Linked with pneumonia incidence

BOX 4.3   Common Medical Problems and Their Potential Complications

Angina/Myocardial Infarction
Dysrhythmias
Congestive heart failure/pulmonary edema
Shock (cardiogenic, hypovolemic)
Infarction, infarction extension
Thrombi/emboli formation (pulmonary emboli, stroke)
Hypoxemia
Electrolyte imbalance
Acid–base imbalance
Pericarditis
Cardiac tamponade
Cardiac arrest
See also Kidney Disease

Lung Diseases (e.g., Asthma, Chronic Obstructive Pulmonary Disease)
Hypoxemia
Acid–base and electrolyte imbalance
Respiratory failure
Infection
See also Pneumonia and Angina/Myocardial Infarction

Pneumonia
Respiratory failure
Dehydration
Sepsis/septic shock
Pulmonary embolus
Pulmonary hypertension
See also Angina/Myocardial Infarction

Diabetes
Hypoglycemia (diabetic shock)
Hyperglycemia (diabetic coma)
Compromised circulation—pressure and leg ulcers
Delayed wound healing
Hypertension
Eye problems (retinal hemorrhage)
Infection
Dehydration
See also Angina/Myocardial Infarction and Kidney Disease

Hypertension
Stroke (cerebrovascular accident)
Transient ischemic attacks
Hypertensive crisis
See also Angina/Myocardial Infarction and Kidney Disease

Kidney Disease
Congestive heart failure
Kidney failure

Edema
Hyperkalemia
Electrolyte/acid–base imbalance
Anemia
See also Hypertension and Urinary Tract Infection

Urinary Tract Infection
Septic shock
Kidney failure

HIV and Immunosuppression
Opportunistic infections (e.g., tuberculosis, herpes, intestinal organisms)
Severe diarrhea
See also Lung Diseases and Pneumonia

Fractures
Bleeding (internal or external)
Bone fragment displacement
Edema/pressure points
Compromised circulation
Nerve compression
Compartment syndrome
Thrombus/embolus formation
Infection

Head Trauma
Respiratory depression
Airway occlusion
Aspiration
Bleeding (internal or external)
Shock
Brain swelling
Increased intracranial pressure
Seizures, coma
Hyperthermia/hypothermia
Infection

Other Trauma
See Anesthesia/Surgical Procedures in Box 4.4

Depression/Psychiatric Disorders
Reality distortion
Dehydration, malnutrition
Suicide
Violence (against self or others)
Self-protection problems
Trauma, death
Medication side effects

Source: Copyright 2019. R. Alfaro-LeFevre. http://www.AlfaroTeachSmart.com.

BOX 4.4 Complications of Treatments and Procedures

Anesthesia: Surgical Procedures
Respiratory depression
Airway management problems
Aspiration
Atelectasis, pneumonia
Bleeding (internal or external)
Hypovolemia/shock
Infection/septic shock
Fluid/electrolyte imbalance
Thrombus/embolus
Paralytic ileus
Urinary retention
Incision complications (infection, poor healing, dehiscence/evisceration)
See also Angina/Myocardial Infarction (Box 4.3)

Cardiac Catheterization: Invasive Monitoring
Bleeding (internal or at insertion site)
Hemopneumothorax
Thrombus/embolus formation
Stroke
Infection/sepsis
See also Angina/Myocardial Infarction (Box 4.3)

Chest Tubes: Thoracentesis
Bleeding (internal or at insertion site)
Hemopneumothorax
Atelectasis
Chest tube malfunction/blockage
Infection/sepsis

Foley Catheter
Infection/sepsis
Catheter malfunction/blockage
Bladder spasms

Intravenous Therapy
Bleeding (internal or at insertion site)
Air embolus
Phlebitis/thrombophlebitis
Infiltration/extravasation/tissue necrosis
Fluid overload
Infection/sepsis

Medications
Adverse reactions (allergic response, exaggerated response, side effects)
Drug interactions
Overdose/toxicity

Nasogastric Suction
Electrolyte imbalance
Tube malfunction/blockage
Aspiration
Bleeding

Paracentesis
Bleeding (internal or at insertion site)
Paralytic ileus
Infection/sepsis

Skeletal Traction/Casts
See Fractures (Box 4.3)

Source: Copyright 2019. R. Alfaro-LeFevre. http://www.AlfaroTeachSmart.com.

(Health patterns continued from page 87.)

9. **Sexuality-reproductive pattern:** Knowledge and perception of sex and reproduction
10. **Coping–stress tolerance pattern:** Ability to manage and tolerate stress
11. **Value–belief pattern:** Values, beliefs, and goals in life; spiritual practices

To gain insight into the difference between nursing and medical models, compare Fig. 4.4 (Body Systems Approach) with Fig. 4.5 (Comprehensive Nursing Assessment Map, page 91).

DECISION-MAKING AND STANDARDS AND PROTOCOLS

Critical thinking and clinical reasoning are guided by professional standards. Think about the following descriptions of *standards*[20]:

- Describe the responsibilities for which its practitioners are accountable.
- Reflect the values and priorities of the profession, and provide direction for professional nursing practice and a framework for the evaluation of this practice.

BODY SYSTEMS ASSESSMENT

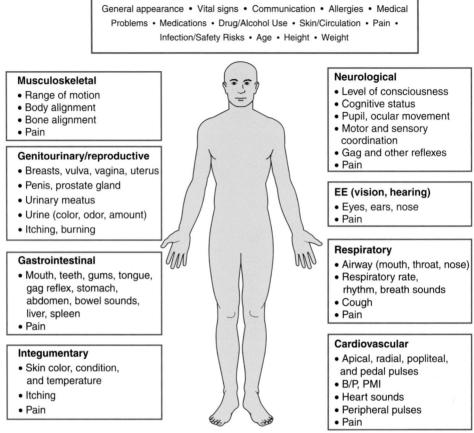

QUICK PRIORITY ASSESSMENT
General appearance • Vital signs • Communication • Allergies • Medical
Problems • Medications • Drug/Alcohol Use • Skin/Circulation • Pain •
Infection/Safety Risks • Age • Height • Weight

Musculoskeletal
• Range of motion
• Body alignment
• Bone alignment
• Pain

Genitourinary/reproductive
• Breasts, vulva, vagina, uterus
• Penis, prostate gland
• Urinary meatus
• Urine (color, odor, amount)
• Itching, burning

Gastrointestinal
• Mouth, teeth, gums, tongue,
  gag reflex, stomach,
  abdomen, bowel sounds,
  liver, spleen
• Pain

Integumentary
• Skin color, condition,
  and temperature
• Itching
• Pain

Neurological
• Level of consciousness
• Cognitive status
• Pupil, ocular movement
• Motor and sensory
  coordination
• Gag and other reflexes
• Pain

EE (vision, hearing)
• Eyes, ears, nose
• Pain

Respiratory
• Airway (mouth, throat, nose)
• Respiratory rate,
  rhythm, breath sounds
• Cough
• Pain

Cardiovascular
• Apical, radial, popliteal,
  and pedal pulses
• B/P, PMI
• Heart sounds
• Peripheral pulses
• Pain

FIG. 4.4 Body systems assessment. To prioritize, go clockwise, starting at 12 o'clock.

• Define the nursing profession's accountability to the public and the outcomes for which registered nurses are responsible.

American Nurses Association (ANA) practice standards—which outline use of the nursing process, summarized in Appendix B—apply to all nursing care. Each specialty organization (e.g., American Association of Critical Care Nurses, Association of Rehabilitation Nurses) develops its own unique standards. The Joint Commission sets many standards for health care organizations. These standards are often tailored to each organization, incorporated into protocols, policies, procedures, and standard plans.

When determining care management, there are three main questions to answer related to standards:

1. Has this facility developed specific standards, guidelines, or policies for the care of this specific situation? For example, if you're caring for someone with a mastectomy, ask, "Has this facility developed guidelines or pathways for someone undergoing a mastectomy?"
2. Are there national or local evidence-based guidelines relating to this particular problem?
3. To what degree do these standards and guidelines apply to my patient's particular situation?

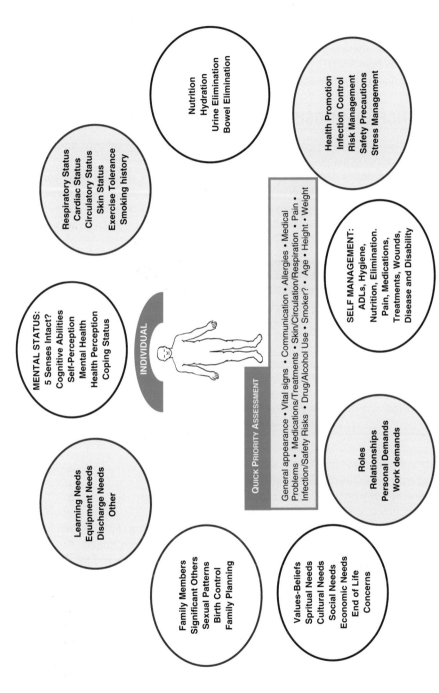

QUICK PRIORITY ASSESSMENT

General appearance • Vital signs • Communication • Allergies • Medical Problems • Medications/Treatments • Skin/Circulation/Respiration • Pain • Infection/Safety Risks • Drug/Alcohol Use • Smoker? • Age • Height • Weight

INDIVIDUAL

MENTAL STATUS:
5 Senses Intact?
Cognitive Abilities
Self-Perception
Mental Health
Health Perception
Coping Status

Respiratory Status
Cardiac Status
Circulatory Status
Skin Status
Exercise Tolerance
Smoking history

Nutrition
Hydration
Urine Elimination
Bowel Elimination

Health Promotion
Infection Control
Risk Management
Safety Precautions
Stress Management

SELF MANAGEMENT:
ADLs, Hygiene,
Nutrition, Elimination.
Pain, Medications,
Treatments, Wounds,
Disease and Disability

Roles
Relationships
Personal Demands
Work demands

Values-Beliefs
Spiritual Needs
Cultural Needs
Social Needs
Economic Needs
End of Life
Concerns

Family Members
Significant Others
Sexual Patterns
Birth Control
Family Planning

Learning Needs
Equipment Needs
Discharge Needs
Other

FIG. 4.5 Comprehensive Nursing Assessment Map. (Source: © 2019 R. Alfaro-LeFevre, http://www.AlfaroTeachSmart.com.)

While practice standards and guidelines are key tools that help you make care decisions, you don't follow them without reflecting and considering whether they apply to your patient's situation. For example, suppose that you're caring for an elderly man after prostate surgery, and protocols call for him to be out of bed twice on the first postoperative day. When you assess the man before getting him out of bed, you find he has chest pain. This finding is significant enough for you to question whether he should indeed get out of bed. Could this man be suffering a complication such as myocardial infarction or pulmonary embolus? In this case, it's your responsibility to keep the man in bed and activate the chain of command.

SCOPE OF PRACTICE, DIAGNOSIS, AND DECISION-MAKING

Keeping patients safe and yourself free from legal suits depends on your understanding of your scope of practice—what you're *accountable* for doing and what you're *prohibited* from doing. Yet making these types of decisions can be difficult when you're new. I'll never forget the horror I felt when I read one of my student's clinical log entries that said, *I didn't know if I was allowed to give the IV drug but I gave it anyway because I did it in my tech job last summer.* This section helps you with making decisions about your scope of practice—when to act independently and when to get help.

GUIDING PRINCIPLE

The terms *diagnose* and *diagnosis* have legal implications. They imply that there's a specific problem that requires management *by a qualified professional.* If you diagnose a problem, it means that you accept accountability for accurately naming and managing it. If you allow signs and symptoms (cues) to persist without ensuring that a *definitive diagnosis—the most correct diagnosis—has been made,* you may cause harm and be accused of negligence. For example, if you deal with *chronic constipation* without determining whether it has been evaluated by a PCP, you may be missing a *major symptom* of *colon or ovarian cancer (constipation).* When you treat signs and symptoms or start people on diet or exercise routines, always ask: "Have these signs and symptoms been evaluated by the primary care provider?" "Does this diet or exercise routine need approval?" Let the caution, "See your primary care provider first" resound in your mind.

Let's consider some important points on how to make decisions about your scope of practice, starting with the following Guiding Principle.

Your scope of practice is determined by five main things:

1. Laws outlined in your state nursing practice act
2. Rules and regulations defined by your state board of nursing (SBN), which is in charge of enforcing the state laws and specifying what nurses may and may not do
3. Professional and organizational standards, policies, procedures, and job descriptions
4. Your qualifications (e.g., your education, certifications, and whether or not you have passed competency tests)
5. Your confidence level (you may have passed competency tests, but if you haven't performed the procedure recently, you may have lost confidence, which is critical to success)

Fig. 4.6 shows a decision tree you can use to make decisions about whether something is within your practice scope or whether you need to get help.

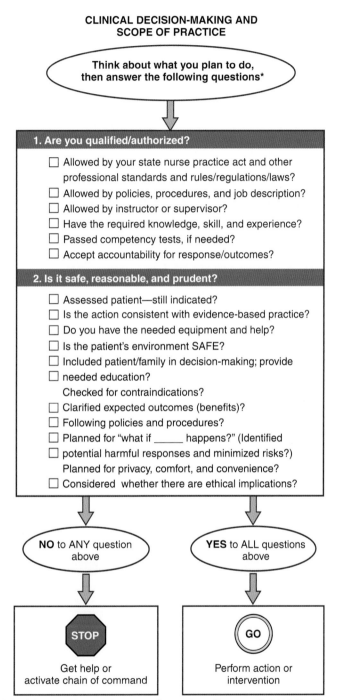

FIG. 4.6 Clinical decision-making and scope of practice. (Source: © 2019 R. Alfaro-LeFevre http://www.AlfaroTeachSmart.com.)

NOVICE VERSUS EXPERT THINKING

Consider the following scenario.

SCENARIO NOVICE VERSUS EXPERT THINKING

A car hits a young man riding his bicycle in the park. Thrown 60 feet, he lies motionless. Within minutes, two park rangers arrive. They put on latex gloves and begin to assess his injuries. An ambulance pulls up, and one ranger yells, "We need airway equipment!" A woman, out for a walk, looks on from a distance. A second woman, riding a bicycle, comes upon the scene. Here's how the conversation goes:

First woman: "This is terrible. I wish the ambulance had gotten here sooner."

Second woman: "Oh?"

First woman: "Yes. He was thrown at least 50 feet. If the ambulance had arrived sooner, they could have done more. I can't believe these two rangers didn't start resuscitation right away. They waited for this ambulance… they should have been breathing for him."

Second woman: "These rangers look like they know what they're doing. They would have started resuscitation if he needed it. This young man has been thrown so far, I'm sure they're concerned about spinal cord injuries. If they tilt his head back to start respirations, they risk severing his spinal cord—they don't want to do that unless it's absolutely necessary."

This scenario is a true story. I was the second woman, on the bicycle. As I talked more with the first woman, I learned she was a student nurse. She thanked me for pointing out something she hadn't thought about. After it was all over, I realized our conversation demonstrated a common difference between expert and novice thinking: the student nurse felt a need to act immediately. As an experienced nurse, I knew the importance of *assessing before acting*.

We're all novices at one time or another. We all know what it's like to be new at something and watch an experienced professional and wonder, "Will I ever know this much?" And almost always, with time and commitment, we soon find ourselves helping someone else who looks at us and thinks, "Will I ever know this much?"

Decide where you stand in relation to novice or expert thinking by studying Box 4.5, which describes the stages novices go through to become experts, and Table 4.1, which compares novice and expert thinking.

BOX 4.5   How Novices Become Experts

According to Patricia Benner, nurses go through the following stages of knowledge and expertise acquisition:

1. **Novices:** Beginners who lack experience in specific situations (e.g., a new graduate with no experience in nursing or an experienced psychiatric nurse who is beginning to work in obstetric nursing)
2. **Advanced beginners:** Those with marginally acceptable performance based on a foundation of experience with real situations (e.g., a nurse who is in the first year of employment or the first year of a new clinical specialty)
3. **Competent:** Those with 2 or 3 years of experience in similar situations (e.g., a nurse who has practiced emergency and intensive care nursing for 2 or 3 years)
4. **Proficient:** Those with broad experience that allows meaning to be understood in terms of the big picture rather than isolated observations (e.g., a nurse who is in charge of making patient assignments)
5. **Expert:** Those with extensive experiences that enable an intuitive grasp of situations and problems (e.g., an experienced nurse who serves as charge nurse, preceptor, or member of a committee)

Source: Data from Benner P. *From novice to expert.* Upper Saddle River, NJ: Prentice Hall; 2001.

TABLE 4.1 Novice Versus Expert Thinking	
NOVICE NURSES	**EXPERT NURSES**
• Often unaware of what they don't know.	• Know the limitations of their own knowledge.
• Knowledge is organized as separate facts. Rely heavily on resources (e.g., texts, notes, preceptors). Lack knowledge gained from experience (e.g., listening to breath sounds).	• Knowledge is organized and structured, making recall of information easier. Have a lot of experiential knowledge (e.g., what abnormal breath sounds are like, what subtle changes look like).
• Focus so much on actions that they tend to forget to assess before acting.	• Assess and think things through before acting.
• Need clear-cut rules.	• Know when to bend the rules.
• Hampered by unawareness of resources.	• Aware of resources and how to use them.
• Hindered by the brain-drains of anxiety and lack of self-confidence.	• Self-confident, less anxious, and more focused.
• Have limited knowledge of suspected problems; therefore they question and collect data more superficially.	• Have a better idea of suspected problems, allowing them to question more deeply and collect more relevant and in-depth data.
• Rely on step-by-step procedures. Tend to focus more on procedures than on the patient response to the procedure.	• Know when it's safe to skip steps or do two steps together. Are able to focus on both the parts (the procedures) and the whole (the patient response).
• Become uncomfortable if patient needs preclude performing procedures exactly as they were learned.	• Comfortable with rethinking procedure if patient needs necessitate modification of the procedure.
• Follow standards and policies by rote.	• Analyze standards and policies, looking for ways to improve them.
• Learn more readily when matched with a supportive, knowledgeable preceptor or mentor.	• Are challenged by novices' questions, clarifying their own thinking when teaching novices.

Source: Copyright © 2018. http://www.AlfaroTeachSmart.com.

PAYING ATTENTION TO CONTEXT

A colleague of mine tells me she knows her students are thinking critically when she asks them questions and they respond, "It depends."

Critical thinking changes depending on context (circumstances). What works in one situation may not work in another. For example, think about the difference between working in pediatrics versus working with adults. Growth and development issues and differences in anatomy and physiology affect many aspects of care. Realize that you may be an expert nurse, but if the circumstances change and you're unfamiliar with giving care under those circumstances, you are more like a novice. Sometimes, you may be familiar with the care but unfamiliar with the patients. Don't be afraid to say, "I'm unfamiliar with dealing with these circumstances and need help."

GUIDING PRINCIPLE

Patients are individuals who may have similar problems but different attitudes, beliefs, and responses. Each person and each situation has a "unique story." Look for differences in patient responses or changes in circumstances—for example, cultural, developmental, physical, or emotional differences—and adjust care as needed.

THINKING WITH HEALTH INFORMATION TECHNOLOGY (HIT)

A new era is here: from using artificial intelligence (computer capabilities) to applying analytics to ensure evidence-based care, HIT affects how clinicians think in many ways, as you'll see in this section.

HIT is a broad concept that includes a wide range of technologies that store, share, and analyze health information. It includes EHRs, prescribing systems, decision support tools, and other electronic tools that aim to improve safety and results, while reducing costs. For example, telehealth is a mainstay for improving access to care, improving outcomes, and reducing costs; patients and care providers use their mobile devices for decision support and communication. Some technology used at the bedside incorporates HIT, sending data directly to the patient record.

A major goal of HIT is achieving *interoperability,* which is the ability of two or more systems to exchange and use the same information. Yet the following scenario shows that we still fall short of that goal.

SCENARIO WHAT WE HAVE HERE IS A FAILURE TO COMMUNICATE

My phone service converts voicemails to text and sends them to my e-mail address. One day, I received the following "readable voicemail": "This is a message from your doctor's office, the mean-sacking snarky primadonna." When I called to listen to the message, I heard an electronic voice say, "This is a message from your doctor's office... para eschuchar este mensaje en Español, oprima uno ...."

HIT—The 21st-Century "Stethoscope"

Leaders stress that nurses must be prepared to make HIT the "stethoscope of the 21st century."[21] Nurses are at the forefront of managing technology—often having to reach around a maze of wires and tubes to get to the human being on the other side.

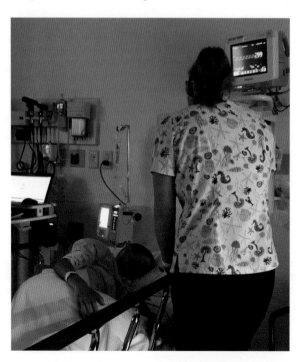

To determine patient status, nurses need to know how to assess both the patient and the technology. For example, if your patient has a pulse oximeter to measure oxygen saturation, you need to know how to assess your patient for signs and symptoms of hypoxia, how to ensure that the device is functioning, and what the readings imply in the context of your particular patient's situation.

Think about the role of HIT and EHR in the following scenario.

SCENARIO HIT EXPEDITES DIAGNOSIS AND TREATMENT

A 65-year-old man arrives at a small rural hospital with persistent high fevers after having the flu for 2 weeks. He is weak, dehydrated, coughing, and has palpitations. His temperature is 103° F. Chest x-rays and initial lab work are inconclusive, but physicians suspect a possible pneumonia. They admit him with the diagnosis of fever of unknown origin (FUO), secondary to possible pneumonia, and start IV antibiotics. Over the next 2 days, the man develops cardiac complications and fluid retention. The fever persists, and the antibiotics don't help.

On the third day—thanks to EHR diagnostic support—the real diagnosis is made: the man has *Anaplasma phagocytophilum* (a tick-borne bacterium) that's treatable with oral doxycycline but may cause death if untreated. While it took 3 days to get the lab work back, it took only one stroke of the keyboard on the day of admission to enter FUO into the health record (which triggered the system to order 16 tests related to febrile illness, including a full panel of tests for various tick-borne diseases). They start the man on doxycycline and give him diuretics and cardiac medications to reverse the cascade of events that happened to his cardiovascular system during the illness. He is discharged 3 days later, taking doxycycline and making a full recovery.

As HIT and EHR become more sophisticated, reliable, and widely adopted, the process described in the previous scenario is likely to be the standard of care, whether the person is admitted to a large city hospital or one in a remote village (remote clinicians will access organizational tools via the Internet).

Evidence-based electronic tools give state-of-the-art standard approaches to help you be systematic and avoid omissions. When you use these tools, several things happen that promote critical thinking, clinical reasoning, decision making, and judgment:

1. As you use the same electronic tools repeatedly in different situations, your brain creates a mental model of what's most important (e.g., how to prioritize assessment, what diagnostic tests are needed, what problems must be ruled out, and what care provider orders are likely).
2. Electronic tools reduce information overload by highlighting and organizing data and allowing users to access critical data quickly.
3. Completed records promote communication among care providers and give a means for recognizing patterns and omissions.

Whatever electronic system you use, remember the following:

GUIDING PRINCIPLE

The accuracy of EHR and decision support systems depends on YOUR ability to assess, interpret, and record your patients' signs and symptoms. Data entry errors—incorrect or missing assessment findings, incorrect medication or treatment documentation, or failure to record patient responses—can *quickly* lead to patient care errors (your incorrect entries may trigger the system and other care providers to give recommendations based on incorrect information).

Guidelines: Using EHR and Other HIT

Keeping in mind that you—not the computer—must be in command, here are some strategies to help you be a safe, effective user of HIT:

- **Focus on the *patient* more than the technology.** While you have to ensure that the technology is working, your primary concern is the *patient*. Your *direct patient assessment* at every opportunity can be the difference between giving care that's based on how your patient is doing *right now* and continuing to give care based on outdated information.

- **Keep an open, active mind, looking for flaws.** For example, determine whether information from technology applies to your patient's *individual circumstances, right now.* HIT recommendations aren't prescriptive for *individual* patient circumstances, and they don't replace the need for you to use clinical judgment. Think about this analogy: how many of us have been advised by a GPS (global positioning system) to make a turn at a point when *circumstances at the moment* make it dangerous or impossible?

- **Follow policies for documentation carefully (e.g., correct errors and omissions as indicated).** Policies and procedures are designed to promote safe and efficient care by ensuring that all caregivers have the data needed to understand the status of the most important patient issues. Standard policies ensure that data within the EHR are understood in the same way across the care team. They also meet legal and third-party payer requirements.

- **Be aware of the following pitfalls:**
  - **Some electronic fields are auto-populated (default data appears automatically).**[22] Pay attention to default data and whether or not it applies to your specific patient situation. For example, a postoperative pain management record may be preset to indicate that the patient receives morphine 5 mg IM for pain. Yet your patient has been ordered a *different* medication or dose. If you forget to change the default values that don't apply, you may cause serious medication errors that cause harm.
  - **Without human interpretation, HIT is prone to errors.** This is a particular risk when patient data are automatically added to the record from another device. For example, be sure that low blood pressure readings noted on the record aren't related to an error in measurement due to an error in the device. If the technology readings are fine but your patient looks distressed, *focus on the patient.* If your patient seems fine but the technology says otherwise, *check the technology.*
  - **Alerts are useful only to the degree that end users read and respond to them.**
  - **Decision support systems are still evolving** and are only as useful as the humans who created them.

- **You can't depend on the system to be aware of the *relationships* among coexisting diseases, issues, and treatments** (for example, in the previous scenario about the man with a tick-borne illness, the man had fever, dehydration, and cardiac issues; these are interrelated). It takes strong clinical reasoning skills to think complex issues through.

- **To improve your knowledge and keep patients safe, always ask, "Why?"** For example, "Why is the system suggesting these tests or treatments for this particular patient?"

- **Because EHR and HIT may cue you to important information, interventions, diagnostic tests, or consultations that should be considered, it's more important than ever to chart as soon as you can.** Timely documentation improves accuracy and helps you notice patterns. When you *think* about what you're about to enter into the record, you can pick up patient problems and recognize things you forgot to do. If you can't get to a patient right away, jot important data down on a personal worksheet (don't rely on memory).

- **Don't just "dump data into the record."** Find ways to reflect on the big picture of patient care (use printouts or summary screens).

- **Be aware that when you're learning HIT, a lot of your brainpower goes toward learning the *technology*.** This decreases your ability to think about *patient care*. We must help staff learn new technology while maintaining patient care standards.
- **HIT may impede thinking in those who are task oriented, rather than thought oriented (a common issue with novice or inexperienced workers).** These individuals complete tasks in a linear way. They don't reflect, evaluate, or change approaches as needed. Sometimes we see staff who are so influenced by knowing the predicted care from the EHR that they rush through assessments and make dangerous assumptions.
- **Think about back up plans.** Electronic devices fail. Plan ahead and think about what you'll do if the device or system fails.
- **Pay attention to cyber security and the possibility of deceptive practices.** Studies show that private patient information is at risk, sometimes to insider threats, such as workers falling for "phishing attacks" (individuals who disguise themselves as being trustworthy so that they can obtain sensitive information such as usernames, passwords, or Social Security numbers). One report indicated that 41% of data breaches were tied to insider errors or wrongdoing.[23]

As a key user of HIT, you have the power to improve it. A lot of what surrounds EHR is medically/legally driven, security driven, or done to maximize reimbursement—don't let nursing get lost in the process (e.g., Where are issues with self-care, communication, immobility, and other human needs addressed?). Report weaknesses within EHR, and communicate suggestions for improvement in efficiency or effectiveness to your leaders and informaticists (health care professionals in charge of implementing HIT).

GUIDING PRINCIPLE

To meet practice standards—regardless of the record-keeping system used—nursing records should reflect use of ADPIE, with special attention to the following:
- **Assessment:** What you assessed in the patient.
- **Diagnosis/Decision/Clinical Judgment:** What you concluded about your patient; be sure the facts that support your conclusions can be found in the record in the appropriate place.
- **Interventions and Evaluation:** What you did, and how the patient responded; remember **AAR** (assess, act, reassess).
- **Safety Measures:** Anything you did to correct or prevent adverse response (e.g., Rates incision pain at 7. Dressing clean and dry. Vital signs normal. Pain med given. Bedrails raised. Call bell given and told to call for help if needed. Reassessed 30 min later and rates pain at 2).

NOTE: To break up chapter reading, complete Exercises 4.1 on starting on page 113.

IS THE CARE PLAN DEAD?

As we continue to use standard plans and HIT, some people wonder, "Is the care plan dead?" The answer is that the care plan is alive and well—it's just changed. Standards mandate that patients have an individualized recorded plan of care that demonstrates that important patient needs and problems are addressed. You may not find the care plan all in one place. Rather, parts of the plan may be addressed in different places of the health record (e.g., assessments may be in one place, routine interventions may be covered in care standards, specific interventions covered in an "add-on" plan, and so on).

Some students wonder why they need to do care plans when so much care is guided by HIT. Here's a few compelling reasons:

- Using an EHR without ever having created care plans on your own is the same as if you used a calculator without understanding the concepts of addition, subtraction, multiplication, and division.
- Creating care plans, maps, and diagrams promotes deep personal learning by making you "think out loud" and identify relationships among health issues, contributing factors, treatment, and outcomes; it helps you learn the concepts and principles you need to apply when thinking in action at the point of care (e.g., bedside).
- Care plans, maps, and diagrams give educators a means to evaluate to what degree students understand major care principles; through this evaluation, they can give feedback on reasoning and give specific suggestions for improvement.

The memory jog **EASE** helps you remember the major care plan components.

Major Care Plan Components

Expected outcomes
Actual/potential problems that must be addressed to reach overall outcomes
Specific interventions designed to achieve the outcomes
Evaluation statements (charting/progress notes)

Intuition, Logic, and Unfolding Reasoning

Let's examine the roles of intuition, logic, and unfolding reasoning. Situations that are unfolding often happen quickly, and we need to use all our abilities to avoid jumping to conclusions. In fact, jumping to conclusions has become such a problem that there's a phrase to describe it: "Ready, fire, aim" (instead of "ready, aim, fire"). This phrase refers to what happens with poor assessment and planning. Critical thinking means not jumping to conclusions or acting on impulse. Time constraints may push you to diagnose issues before they're completely understood. Because of the risks of jumping to conclusions and influencing others to do the same, if you aren't *sure* what the problem or diagnosis is, be prudent and say something like, "There seems to be issues with (whatever), but there's not enough information to completely understand what's going on." *Issues* are problems that are still muddy and not clearly defined.

THINKING-IN-ACTION: UNFOLDING, DYNAMIC REASONING

Thinking-in-action is dynamic reasoning that changes as patient situations unfold. Consider the following scenario.

SCENARIO DYNAMIC, UNFOLDING REASONING

Bob, a medical-surgical nurse, walks into a room. A picture flashes in his mind—his brain assesses the room in an instant. The picture he sees is bed linens in disarray, trash on the floor, and someone who is restless and has a distressed look. Bob's mind jumps to phase 2 of ADPIE (Diagnosis), thinking, *there's a problem here.* Automatically, he goes back to basics—phase 1 (Assessment)—and assesses closely to find out exactly what's going on. He may start thinking, "Something bad is happening here, and I need to get help," or he may simply intervene with a lot of little things, which resolves the *overall problem.* Either way, he is so busy *doing* that he's unaware that his brain is assessing, correlating, and forming opinions as he goes along. In this scenario, Bob is experienced and comfortable in his role. If Bob were a novice, his thinking would be slower—hampered by lack of experience and lack of confidence. He would see a picture of the room, but he'd miss key details. He may also lose brainpower from dealing with his doubts about his own capabilities.

Interplay of Intuition and Logic

Sound clinical reasoning often includes using both intuition (knowing without evidence) and logic (rational thinking based on evidence).

Most agree that intuition—an important part of thinking—is often seen in experts as a result of years of experience and in-depth knowledge of patients. However, there's a concern that encouraging the use of intuition sends the message that it's okay to act on gut feelings without evidence, which is *risky*. To clarify the use of intuition and logic in clinical judgment, it's important to answer two questions:

1. Is the rapid thinking that goes on in experts' heads simply the use of intuition—what many describe as "knowing in your gut"?
2. If you can't explain your thinking, does it mean that you're thinking intuitively?

To the outsider, many experts' actions seem to be based on intuition alone. But rapid thinking is usually the result of "thinking in pictures"—like watching a video—and using intuition and logic *together*. There's a dynamic interplay between intuition and logic. Experts make leaps in thinking with intuitive hunches, then almost at the same time draw on logic and past experience to make well-reasoned conclusions.

Experts who juggle several priorities at once often have trouble explaining their thinking at the very moment it's happening. But if it's really important—for example, if decisions are later challenged in court—they can readily reconstruct the logic of their thinking (and if they can't, they're in trouble).

Clinical reasoning requires using your whole brain—both the intuitive-right and logical-left sides. Use intuitive hunches as guides to search for evidence. Use logic to formulate and double-check your thinking, ensuring that your conclusions are based on the best available facts. In important situations, be careful about acting on intuition alone. Ask questions like, "How do I know I'm right?" and "What could go wrong if I act on intuition alone?"

GUIDING PRINCIPLE

Intuitive thinking is fostered by two things: (1) in-depth knowledge and experience related to the clinical situations at hand and (2) a deep understanding of the patient's normal patterns, circumstances, needs, and desires.

What About Creativity and Innovation?

Creativity and innovation play key roles in critical thinking. Yet creativity and innovation are not the same thing. *Innovation* is a bigger challenge than *creativity* because it requires *transforming* a creative idea into a useful approach that evidence shows improves results. As nurses, we need to promote creativity and innovation in ourselves and our co-workers.

To keep patients safe, use *principle-centered* creativity. When you have a creative idea, determine what principles support or negate it. For example, one nurse tried to warm blood before administering it by putting it in the microwave. This is dangerous creativity. Identifying the principles of what happens to protein in the microwave would have stopped this.

To avoid "reinventing the wheel," ask questions like, "Is this idea (or way) really better or is it just different?" "What does the research say about this idea?" "Is this idea useful to *end users*?"

STANDARD HAND-OFFS: IMPROVING COMMUNICATION

Studies show that hand-offs—when nurses transfer patient care from one nurse to another—are vulnerable to miscommunications that cause errors, missed care, and harm. To improve communication and prevent errors, safety initiatives encourage the use of standard hand-off tools and patient participation in the process. Hand-off tools are great examples of tools that boost human performance: many clinicians struggle to summarize patient information and give specific recommendations. Using standard hand-off tools guides clinicians to quickly determine the most important information that needs to be communicated.

The following summarizes two commonly used hand-off tools:

- **SBAR** (*Situation, Background, Assessment, and R*ecommendation).[24] Some places use **I-SBAR,** putting an *I* at the beginning, which stands for *introduction* (identify yourself, your unit, the patient's name, and date of birth; request the name of the person to whom you are speaking).
- **I-PASS** (*Illness severity, Patient summary, Action list, Situation awareness and contingency planning, and Synthesis*). With *Synthesis*, the person receiving the hand-off gives a summary of what's been communicated, repeating back the most important information. **I-PASS** is included in the Agency for Healthcare Research and Quality's (AHRQ) *Guide to Improving Patient Safety in Primary Care Settings by Engaging Patients and Families.*[25] It's often used in conjunction with "warm hand-offs" (warm hand-offs build trust because they happen transparently, with open honest communication in the presence of patients and families).

To see video examples of using *SBAR, I-PASS*, and *warm hand-offs,* search these terms at www.YouTube.com.

LAWS, STANDARDS, AND TRENDS AFFECTING THINKING

GUIDING PRINCIPLE

In accordance with national safety goals, prevent communication errors by using "Read-Back" and "Repeat-Back" rules.[26] When you receive verbal orders or lab values, write them down and read them back to check for accuracy. When you give lab results or important communications to others, ask, "Can you repeat that back to me to be sure we have it right?"

Health care is changing almost as rapidly as you can say the word *computer.* Some changes are driven by laws, and others are based on standards and evidence. Think about how the following factors may affect clinical reasoning.

Patients' Rights and Privacy Laws

Patients' rights and privacy laws affect virtually all care aspects, from dealing with patients and families on the front line to maintaining EHR. For example, the Health Insurance Portability and Accountability Act (HIPAA) guarantees patients and health care consumer rights to have copies of their medical records (and to keep them private).[27]

Advanced Courses and Certification Improve Care and Job Satisfaction

Studies show that patient outcomes improve when a high percentage of nurses working on a unit have advanced degrees and specialty certification.[28] As a result, many nurses take advanced courses in their specialty practice. Certification isn't only good for patients and health care organizations. It's good for nurses. Certified nurses feel self-empowered and express satisfaction at "owning their practice" and taking their career to the next level. They also stay current on evidence-based best practices and see themselves as being better able to mentor others.[28]

National Safety Goals and High-Reliability Health Care

Health care organizations implement standards aimed at meeting national practice safety goals (NPSGs).[26] They recognize that when systems are poorly designed, patients suffer and staff fail (regardless of how hard they try). The concept of high-reliability organizations (HROs)—organizations that avoid catastrophes in environments where accidents are expected due to risk factors and complexity—is born. Leaders begin the work needed to apply this concept to develop high-reliability health care.[29]

Empowering Patients: Nurses as Stewards for Safe Passage

Two important shifts in thinking empower patients and families to manage their own care:
- Move from "I know what's best for you" to "I want to empower you to make your own decisions."
- Change "I'm here to take care of you" to "I'm here to make sure you know how to take care of yourself when I'm not here."
    Much like a ship's steward—who has the job of protecting passengers on a journey—your job as a nurse is to protect patients and help them navigate safely through the health care system. As a steward, you hold *patients' lives* in your hands, but *they* should be "at the helm," directing where they want to go. The following summarizes *Speak Up initiatives*, which encourage patients to get involved in care decisions[30]:

The Joint Commission Speak Up™ Initiatives[30]

Tell your patients to speak up as follows:

Speak up if you have questions or concerns.
Pay attention to the care you get.
Educate yourself about your illness.
Ask a trusted family member or friend to be your advocate (advisor or supporter).
Know what medicines you take and why you take them.
Use a health care organization that has been carefully checked out.
Participate in all decisions about your treatment

Time-Outs Promote Group Thinking

In today's fast-paced clinical setting, many professionals are involved in giving care to one patient—there are many "cooks stirring the pot." We must ensure that "the right ingredients" go into the "pot" (the patient) at the right time. We need everyone's eyes, ears, and brains to prevent mistakes. Time-outs, in which the entire team stops to become focused and on the same plan of care, are used to prevent errors. There are two kinds of time-outs. One is routine, such as at the beginning of surgeries, when patients' identities and surgical procedures are double- and triple-checked. The other type of time-out is spontaneous. If at any time *any* team member—nurse, nursing aid, respiratory therapist (RT), or physician—recognizes an actual or potential risk for harm to the patient, he or she is responsible for calling a time-out and pointing out the concern (the rest of the team is accountable for listening and deciding how to address it).

Systems-Based Practice and Social Determinants of Health

All health care professionals must be able to function in systems-based practice, recognizing *all* the processes in health care systems that interact to provide quality, cost-effective care.[31] You need to understand how patient care relates to the health care system as a whole to ensure your patients have the best resources for their circumstances. For example, with breast cancer diagnoses, breast health navigators—skilled, experienced nurses who help patients navigate health care systems to make treatment decisions—significantly improve emotional and physical outcomes. Usually, any woman can contact a breast health navigator and no PCP order is needed.

According to the World Health Organization (WHO), achieving quality outcomes requires taking a broad view of patient circumstances, paying attention to social determinants of health (SDH).[32] The WHO defines SDH as "the conditions in which people are born, grow, work, live, and age, as well as the wider set of forces and systems that shape the conditions of daily life." Clinical reasoning requires considering how people's lives are affected by their race/ethnicity, income, education, housing, environment, and whether or not they experience civil unrest. For example, if you have a young boy admitted for asthma, before discharging him you have to consider the circumstances surrounding his life—the air quality at home and in the community, as well as parental education and whether or not they can implement and pay for a home-based treatment regimen.

The WHO continues to study many aspects of SDH, as noted in the following examples[32]:

- How to increase access to health care for socially and economically disadvantaged groups
- Ways to reduce gender-based inequities in health
- How to develop programs that promote early child development (well-established evidence shows that opportunities provided to young children are crucial to shaping lifelong health and development)

Incivility and Violence

As part of maintaining a healthy work environment, organizations develop policies to address incidents of incivility, bullying, and lateral violence (when staff are aggressive to one another because they're unhappy with the circumstances surrounding their work). Nurses in all settings need to be prepared to recognize the potential for violence and be prepared to respond quickly to violence (be sure you know policies and procedures so that you know exactly what you'll do if something happens).

Box 4.6 summarizes other changes and trends affecting nurses' thinking.

BOX 4.6   Changes and Trends Affecting Nurses' Thinking

- **New threats emerge.** Emergence of resistant bacteria such as methicillin-resistant *Staphylococcus aureus* (MRSA) points out the need for meticulous hand hygiene and management of invasive treatments and open wounds. International travel brings threats of pandemics (epidemics over a wide geographic area and affecting a large part of the population). Terrorism, including bioterrorism, is a constant threat, requiring new levels of preparedness and responsiveness.
- **Many people live longer with illnesses and disabilities.** An alarming number of people with obesity and diabetes are major health care concerns because these problems contribute to many other health problems.
- **New diagnostic imaging and treatment modalities** such as vaccine use, stem cell use, and genetic manipulation emerge.
- **Ethical dilemmas grow.** Ethical issues (e.g., end-of-life care, assisted suicide, fertility issues, cloning, stem cell research) require in-depth thinking that's grounded in ethical principles (see Chapter 5).
- **Case management**—the use of collaborative approaches to ensure that the best available resources are used to reach outcomes efficiently—promotes quality. This approach is grounded in prevention and early intervention. Today all nurses are expected to be "case managers," closely monitoring progress toward outcomes to detect delays in progress and intervening as indicated.
- *Healthy People 2020* initiatives guide organizations, businesses, and communities to come together to achieve two major goals: (1) to help people of all ages improve life expectancy and quality of life and (2) to eliminate health disparities among different segments of the population (see http://www.healthypeople.gov/).
- **Holistic and alternative therapies**—for example, diet, exercise, acupuncture, and stress reduction through meditation and aromatherapy—are recognized as key strategies for triggering the body's natural healing powers.

PREDICTIVE CARE MODELS: WHAT IF?

When addressing predictive care models and knowing what to do if something goes wrong, I'm reminded of something that happened to me when I was in Africa: riding in a safari jeep, we stopped to look at a giraffe. Suddenly, to our left, came a raging elephant (photo below). Our guide quickly shifted into reverse and backed away. Pointing to a rifle on the dashboard, someone asked the guide, "Do they teach you how to use that gun?" Our guide responded, "Yes, they do. But even better, they teach us how *not to get into the position of having to use it.*" This is a great example of applying predictive models: You don't wait for problems to happen. You anticipate and prevent them.

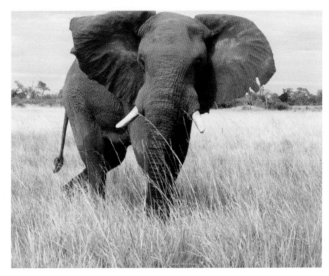

Predict, Prevent, Manage, Promote (PPMP)

Using a predictive care model requires moving from a *diagnose and treat* (DT) approach—which implies that we wait for evidence of problems to start treatment—to a predictive model: *predict, prevent, manage, and promote* (PPMP). PPMP is a proactive approach that aims to predict and manage risk factors *before* problems arise. PPMP is based on evidence. Thanks to research, we can predict when people are at risk for certain problems and, if needed, begin an aggressive prevention plan. Sometimes *prevention* requires *treatment* (called *prophylaxis*). We have evidence-based recommendations for vaccines. For example, with whooping cough (pertussis), to protect the most vulnerable (infants and children), it's recommended that not only children get vaccinated but also their parents, grandparents, and other caregivers.

Here are some more examples of evidence-based recommendations:

- Pulmonary embolism resulting from deep vein thrombosis—collectively referred to as *venous thromboembolism (VTE)*—is the most common preventable cause of hospital deaths. The AHRQ has developed an evidence-based tool kit to help clinicians prevent VTE through pharmacological intervention and use of other strategies, such as applying pulsating antiemboli stockings during and after many surgeries.[33]
- For those with significant exposure to the human immunodeficiency virus (HIV), treatment begins immediately, before there's evidence of the virus in the blood. We also have pre-exposure prophylaxis (PrEP), meaning that there are recommendations to give people who are at substantial risk of getting HIV preventive medications.[34]

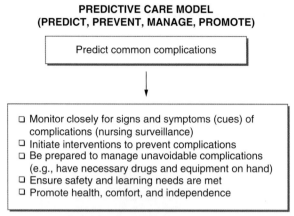

FIG. 4.7 Predictive care model.

Fig. 4.7 maps nursing responsibilities in relation to the PPMP model. For a case example on risk management, study the following scenario. For online resources on risk management, health screening, and health promotion, go to *Healthy People 2020* initiatives (http://www.healthypeople.gov), the Harvard Center For Risk Analysis (http://www.hcra.harvard.edu/), the Centers for Disease Control and Prevention (http://www.cdc.gov/), and the U.S. Preventive Services Task Force (http://www.uspreventiveservicestaskforce.org).

SCENARIO PREDICTING, PREVENTING, AND MANAGING DEHYDRATION

Living in Florida, where we have heat, humidity, and a lot of elderly people, I learned the need to prevent and manage dehydration firsthand. Many health care providers tell people to walk to gain strength. Sometimes these instructions backfire, and people faint in the heat. If you or someone else is going to exercise, improve performance by pacing yourself and ensuring adequate hydration. Teach people about risk factors (obesity, alcohol or caffeine use, use of some medications like diuretics, and being very young or old will put you at risk). Teach the signs of heatstroke (i.e., weakness, nausea, vomiting, chills, confusion, disorientation, hallucinations). Stress the importance of improving ability to exercise by drinking water *before* exercising (so they start out well hydrated), wearing loose-fitting clothes, avoiding the hotter parts of the day, avoiding tea or caffeine (they act as diuretics), and replacing fluids during exercise (water is best; with extreme sweating, consider that there's electrolyte loss, and Gatorade may help). If you suspect heatstroke, manage it by cooling down the person immediately (place the person near an air conditioner, or place damp towels all over the body, especially to the temples and wrists, where blood vessels are near the skin). If the person can tolerate liquids, offer cool drinks. If the person becomes dazed, confused, or has stopped sweating, head to the emergency department because dehydration is severe, requiring immediate medical management.

Quick Priority Assessments (QPAs)

With predictive models and rapidly unfolding situations, it's important to know how to do a quick priority assessment (QPA). These are short, focused assessments that you do to gain the *most important information* you need to have *first* (Table 4.2).

QPAs are important for two reasons:
1. These assessments often "flag" key problems and risks.
2. The information you gain often affects *every aspect of care*, including how you proceed with your assessment. For example, if your patient shows signs of a communicable disease, you need to immediately consider what precautions to take before going on with the rest of the assessment.

TABLE 4.2 **Quick Priority Assessment (QPA)**	
Assessment Priorities	**Rationale**
• General appearance; cognitive awareness; risks for infection, injury, or violence.	General appearance (e.g., distress level) and cognitive awareness flags the urgency of presenting problems. Infection control and keeping patients, yourself, and others safe is top priority.
• Problems (or risks) with breathing, circulation, pain, or communication	Problems and risks in these areas should be dealt with *early* and may point to problems in *other areas* (e.g., pain usually flags a problem that needs to be dealt with).
• Chief complaint • Vital signs, age, weight • Allergies • Medications/treatments • Current and past health problems • Smoking history • Alcohol or drug abuse	All the bullets on the left here, beginning with "chief complaint" flag known problems and risks and significantly affect decisions about initiating certain treatments.

Source: © 2018 R. Alfaro-LeFevre. www.AlfaroTeachSmart.com.

Disease and Disability Management

Disease and disability management—care that focuses on keeping people with chronic diseases and disabilities as healthy and independent as possible—is an important part of the PPMP approach. With PPMP, you *manage* chronic conditions over time rather than waiting for episodes of relapse or crisis. For example, with asthma, you don't just keep *treating* asthma attacks. You *manage* it by promoting healthy behaviors and fine-tuning medications and inhalers to keep the patient symptom-free.

With chronic diseases, the goal of treatment may be to manage symptoms rather than cure the disease (cure may be impossible). We can expect nursing roles related to disease and disability management to grow as nurse-led care significantly improves the condition and quality of life of patients with multiple chronic illnesses.[35]

Rapid Response Teams and Code H (Help)

Rapid response teams (RRTs) and Code H (help) are great examples of using the whole team's brainpower to ensure early intervention. The complexity of care today makes it difficult for nurses to balance their patient load. If a nurse is worried that someone's condition is deteriorating, he or she calls the RRT to do an assessment. RRTs are usually staffed by nurse managers, house physicians, respiratory therapists, critical care nurses, and pharmacists. Code H was developed after 18-month-old Josie King died when her family was unable to get her the attention they felt she needed.[36] With Code H, patients, families, and visitors can trigger levels of rapid response. For example, patients and visitors can call a code number, which goes directly to hospital operators. The operators are trained to ask questions according to an algorithm. Callers who report something important, such as bleeding or chest pain, are routed immediately to the RRT. If the call is about problems like delays in getting pain medications, lack of communication, or some issue that doesn't require the RRT, the operator triggers a Code H. In this case, only the nurse manager responds (within minutes of the call). Even if the Code H turns out to be something very mild, families feel reassured to know that they will be heard. Using RRT and Code H saves lives and improves job satisfaction because nurses get help when they need it.

Monitoring for Dangerous Situations

While Skill 7.8 (Chapter 7) details "Preventing and Dealing With Mistakes Constructively," this section addresses the role of front-line nurses in monitoring for dangerous situations. Think about the following strategies that research shows nurses use to prevent and correct mistakes.

Strategies to Identify, Interrupt, and Correct Errors

The following strategies will help you identify and manage errors[37]:

- **Error identification strategies:** Knowing the patient, knowing the "players," knowing the plan of care, surveillance, knowing policy/procedure, double-checking, using systematic processes, and questioning.
- **Error interruption strategies:** Offering help, clarifying, and verbally interrupting.
- **Error correction strategies:** Persevering, being physically present, reviewing or confirming the plan of care, offering options, referencing standards or experts, and involving another nurse or physician.

Fig. 4.8 shows how monitoring closely for dangerous situations and creating safety nets promote early intervention and keep patients safe.

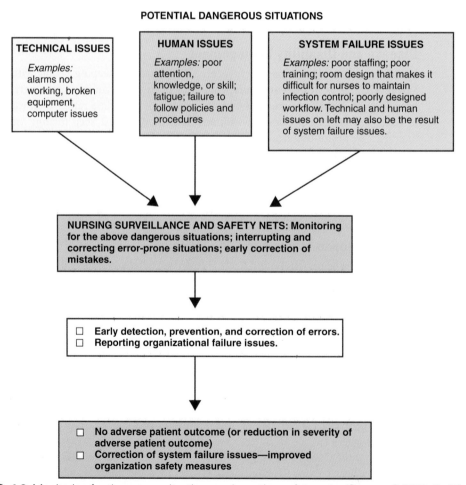

FIG. 4.8 Monitoring for dangerous situations and creating safety nets. (Source: © 2019, R. Alfaro-LeFevre. http://www.AlfaroTeachSmart.com.)

DELEGATING SAFELY AND EFFECTIVELY

Knowing how to delegate—defined as *authorizing someone to perform a selected task in a selected situation, while retaining accountability for results*—is an important part of managing time and resources.[38] Delegation is a skill that's developed over time with experience. It takes significant critical thinking and judgment because it requires you to understand *both* patients' needs and workers' capabilities. Keep this in mind as you read this section.

GUIDING PRINCIPLE

When you delegate tasks, you're accountable for decisions made, actions taken, and patient responses during the course of delegation. When you delegate tasks, teach and supervise as needed. Follow up after tasks are done by assessing patient responses yourself. This does two things: (1) you have firsthand knowledge of how the patient responded to care; and (2) when workers know that you check results directly with the patient, they're more likely to do a good job.

The following summarizes when it's safe to delegate, as well as the four and five "rights" of delegation.[39]

When Is It Safe to Delegate?

Delegate when:
- The patient is stable.
- The task is within the worker's job description and capabilities.
- You're able to do the teaching and supervision the worker needs.
- You've planned how to monitor patient results yourself.

Don't delegate when:
- Complex assessment, thinking, and judgment are required.
- The outcome of the task is unpredictable.
- There's increased risk for harm (e.g., arterial puncture can cause more severe complications than venous puncture).
- Problem-solving and creativity are required.

Four Steps of Delegation

1. **Assess and Plan:** Consider the patient, the task, and worker competencies to make a plan for what tasks you will assign to whom.
2. **Communicate:** Give clear, concise, complete directions about what must done, how it must be done, what needs reporting, and when to touch base with you (verify that worker understands directions).
3. **Ensure Surveillance and Supervision:** Monitor the patient and worker performance as frequently as needed based on the earlier items.
4. **Evaluate and Give Feedback:** Evaluate the effectiveness of the delegation by assessing patient response yourself. Decide whether you need to make changes in the patient's plan of care or how the worker is completing the task. Evaluate the worker's performance, and give teaching and feedback as needed (this helps the worker improve skills and ultimately frees you for other important work).

Five "Rights" of Delegation

Delegate (1) the right task; (2) in the right situation; (3) to the right worker; (4) with the right direction and communication; and (5) the right teaching, supervision, and evaluation.

OUTCOME-FOCUSED, EVIDENCE-BASED CARE

From professional and economic perspectives, the care we give must focus on outcomes and be driven by the best available evidence. We must be able to answer questions like:

- Exactly what does the patient, family, client, or group need to achieve?
- Have the best-qualified professionals decided what, realistically, based on circumstances, can be achieved?
- Have the key stakeholders been included in decision-making?
- What evidence indicates that the outcomes are likely to be achieved in this particular situation?
  "Determining Patient-Centered (Client-Centered) Outcomes" (Skill 6.14, Chapter 6) gives detailed information on how to determine outcomes.

Clinical, Functional, and Other Outcomes

Determining overall care quality requires you to examine outcomes from *several* perspectives. Study the following types of outcomes listed in the context of how they apply to a surgical repair of a fractured hip. Think about the importance of considering all the outcomes to determine overall care quality.

- **Clinical outcomes:** To what degree are the patient's health problems resolved? For example, is the hip healed?
- **Functional outcomes:** To what degree is the patient able to function independently, physically, cognitively, and socially? For example, is the person able to do required daily activities without help? Are there problems with cognitive function?
- **Symptom severity and quality-of-life outcomes:** To what degree is the patient free of symptoms and able to do desired, as well as required, activities? For example, is there any hip pain, and is the person able to meet physical work requirements and do favorite activities?
- **Risk reduction outcomes:** To what degree is the patient able to demonstrate ways to reduce health risks? For example, is he or she able to explain ways of improving safety, such as using a cane when fatigued? Does he or she keep the home free from hazards that may cause falls?
- **Protective factor outcomes:** To what degree does the patient's environment protect against deteriorating health? For example, when bedridden, are bedrails up as needed and skin care protocols followed?
- **Therapeutic alliance outcomes:** To what degree does the patient express a positive relationship between himself or herself and health care professionals? For example, when asked, does he or she state that he or she feels free to ask questions?
- **Satisfaction outcomes:** To what degree do the patient and family express satisfaction with care given? For example, when asked, do they state that they had competent, efficient treatment? Were services convenient?
- **Use of services outcomes:** To what degree were appropriate nursing services used? For example, was a case manager used if needed?

GUIDING PRINCIPLE

Outcome-focused thinking means more than "fixing the problems." It means fixing the problems in ways that you get the *best results* in terms of cost, time, and patient satisfaction perspectives.

Dynamic Relationship of Problems and Outcomes

There's a close, dynamic relationship between problems and outcomes. Sometimes you'll find yourself focusing on *problems* and sometimes on *outcomes,* depending on the situation. For instance, imagine that you're working with a patient on a respirator, and the desired outcome is that the patient has *adequate ventilation*. You see that the patient seems to be struggling for air. You check the tubing and see a lot of water from condensation. You empty the water. If the patient is still struggling, you continue to look for other problems that might be interfering with *adequate ventilation*. For example, you assess breath sounds and help the patient get in a position to cough and clear mucus.

Clinical reasoning requires focusing on *both* problems and outcomes. Together, they serve as a compass that promotes sound decision making in each unique patient situation.

STRATEGIES FOR DEVELOPING CLINICAL JUDGMENT

By now, you should have a good understanding of what clinical reasoning, judgment, and decision-making entail. Let's finish this chapter by considering strategies you can use to navigate the journey to developing sound clinical judgment.

- **Work on becoming a confident learner** (getting stressed reduces your brainpower). Remember that beginners often don't know what they don't know. When in doubt, get help from a qualified professional. Asking questions or getting help is "the default solution" for uncertainty.[16]
- **Be a self-starter,** identifying experiences you would like to have (e.g., "I haven't looked after someone in traction and would like to have the opportunity to do this").
- **Learn the "big ideas"—the major principles and concepts—first.** Review "Principles of Clinical Reasoning" earlier in this chapter. To gain understanding of the details of clinical reasoning skills, complete Chapter 6, "Practicing Clinical Reasoning Skills."
- **Keep references—texts, handheld devices, pocket guides, and personal "cheat sheets"—handy, and be sure that you:**
  - **Learn terminology and concepts.** If you encounter words like *embolus, thrombus,* or *phlebitis* and you don't know what they mean, look them up as you encounter them so that they become part of your long-term memory. Learning terms *in context* helps your brain store information in related groups rather than as isolated facts.
  - **Become familiar with normal findings** (e.g., normal lab values, assessment findings, disease progression, growth and development) before being concerned with abnormal findings. Once you know what's normal, you'll readily recognize when you encounter information that's *outside the norm* (abnormal).
  - **Ask, "Why?"** Find out why normal and abnormal findings occur (e.g., "Why is there edema in heart failure, yet none when the heart is functioning normally?").
- **Turn errors into learning opportunities.** If you aren't making mistakes, maybe you're not trying new things.
- **To develop sound reasoning habits, consistently use approaches that help you think in organized ways.** For example, let ADPIE resound in your head and reflect on it to decide whether you've considered each phase.
- **Don't just enter data into the computer.** *Reflect* on what you entered, looking for patterns and things you may have forgotten to do. Keep your own personal notes or use a worksheet to keep track of information, stay organized, and jog your mind (brain overload in the clinical setting is a common issue that needs solutions).
- **Practice your assessment skills and learn from your peers' experiences.** Collaborating with peers is a win-win situation. Asking questions like "What did you look for in that patient?" "How did you know?" and "What was the biggest thing you learned?" helps your peer clarify their knowledge and helps you learn from being involved in real situations. (Don't use names or talk about patients in public places such as cafeterias or elevators, or you may violate privacy laws.)

- **When planning time for nursing care, consider the time required** for (a) direct care interventions (things you do directly for or with the patient, such as helping someone walk) and (b) indirect care interventions (things you do away from the patient, such as consulting with the pharmacist or analyzing lab study results).
- **Consider the importance of asking the questions in Fig. 4.9.**

Finish this chapter by completing the following critical thinking exercises and reviewing the "Key Points/Summary" section.

---

10 KEY QUESTIONS

1. What **major outcomes** (*observable* beneficial results) do you and key stakeholders—those with a vested interest in how care is given and what results are achieved (e.g., patient, family, care providers)—expect to observe in the patient after care is complete?
2. What **problems**, **issues**, or **risks** must be addressed to achieve the major outcomes?
3. What are the **circumstances** (**context**) in this particular patient situation?
4. What **knowledge and skills** are required to care for this patient?
5. How much room is there for **error**?
6. How much **time** do you have?
7. What human and information **resources** can help?
8. What or whose **perspectives** must be considered (e.g., patient and caregiver viewpoints, both medical and nursing concerns)?
9. What's **influencing thinking** (your own and others')?
10. What **must be done** to monitor, prevent, manage, or eliminate the problems, issues, and risks identified above in #2 (and **who's accountable** for doing it)?

REFLECT ON THE ABOVE — DETERMINE THE BELOW

- Patient's environment **SAFE** ?
- Patient participation was at an optimum level?
- Patient/family educational needs identified and met?
- Health assessment data is current, accurate, and complete?
- Assumptions were identified and conclusions were based on facts (evidence)?
- Considered relevant policies, procedures, and standard plans?
- Alternate diagnoses, conclusions, ideas, and solutions were considered?
- Identified contraindications and adjusted plan accordingly?
- Consulted the best-qualified professionals as needed?
- Best evidence and qualified professional's information reliable and applicable to *current situation and patient*?
- Key stakeholders agree about the expected outcomes of care?

FIG. 4.9 Reflecting on thinking: 10 key questions.

❓ CRITICAL THINKING EXERCISES 4.1. Clinical Reasoning Principles, Thinking Like a Nurse, Decision-Making, and Thinking With Hit

Find example responses in Appendix I (page 216).

1. **Fill in the following blanks, choosing from the following words:** broad; your; pivotal; whole person; flawed; about; interpret; responses; scope; analyze
    A. It's not so much how nurses think that makes them different from other professionals, it's what they think_____.
    B. Having a nursing frame of mind means staying centered on preventing problems and promoting health by focusing on the (a) _____, identifying individual needs and monitoring (b) _____ to interventions and life challenges.
    C. Diagnosis is a (a) _____ point in reasoning: if you miss problems or risks or misunderstand them, the entire plan is likely to be (b) _____.
    D. Nurses diagnose and manage various health issues, depending on their practice _____.
    E. HIT, which includes EHR, is a (a) _____concept that includes a wide range of technologies that store, share, and (b) _____ health information.
    F. The accuracy of EHR and decision support systems depends on (a) _____ ability to assess, (b) _____, and record your patients' signs and symptoms.
2. In relation to HIT, why is *interoperability* important?
3. How does surveillance relate to nursing responsibilities?
4. Describe five major nursing concepts that illustrate what nurses think about.
5. How do standards, policies, ethics codes, and laws (individual state practice acts and state boards of nursing) relate to clinical reasoning, decision making, and judgment?
6. Why do you start a differential diagnosis with ruling out "the bad things" (worst-case scenarios) first?

👥 THINK, PAIR, SHARE

With a partner, in a group, or in a journal entry:

1. Discuss where you stand in relation to novice versus expert thinking (see Table 4.1 and Box 4.5).
2. Address the impact of effective communication and cultural competence as described in *Advancing Effective Communication, Cultural Competence and Patient- and Family-Centered Care: A Road Map for Hospitals* (http://www.jointcommission.org/Advancing_Effective_Communication/).
3. Gain insight into what information is missing when you assess someone using only a body systems approach, without using a guide for *nursing* concerns. Compare Fig. 4.4 (body systems approach) and Fig. 4.5 (nursing assessment map). Determine what information would be missing if you only used the body systems approach.
4. Describe key concepts that drive nurses' thinking—what makes nurses think differently from other health care professionals?
5. Discuss nursing responsibilities in relation to the problems listed in Box 4.2, Box 4.3, and Box 4.4.
6. After reading *Reducing Medical Mistakes, Talking with Your Clinician, Getting Medical Tests, Planning for Surgery, Getting a Prescription, and Build Your Question List* posted at http://www.ahrq.gov/questionsaretheanswer/, discuss ways to encourage patients to be proactive and involved in their care.
7. Share your thoughts on the following *Critical Moments and Other Perspectives.*

CRITICAL MOMENTS AND OTHER PERSPECTIVES

What Good Nursing Looks Like

When my father almost died, he had a seamless hospital experience, marked by a world-class nursing staff that was ranked as Magnet by the American Nurses Credentialing Center. Throughout a long weekend the nurses kept my family involved with Dad's progress through flexible visiting hours, countless phone calls, and e-mails—even in the middle of the night. —Robert Hess, RN, PhD, FAAN[40]

Clinical Judgment: A Sixth Sense?

Critical judgment is like a "sixth sense" that's developed over time from an accumulation of years of knowledge and experience—both personal and what you've learned from others. When you do a job for years, you learn what to look for and what to do. In almost a split second, you evaluate what you see, correlate it with what you've learned, and take appropriate action. —Doris Alfaro, SRN, class of 1944, Chesterfield Royal Hospital

Deconstructing Thinking Improves Reasoning

When you deconstruct your thinking—reflect on it and break it down into what was going on in your head at certain points in time—you can identify "pieces of thinking" that you're doing well and "pieces" you need to correct (lessons learned). For example, one nurse I know deconstructed her thinking like this: I came to work very tired because I had been up with a sick child. We were very busy and I was handling several priorities. The computer froze again and I had to deal with that. I got so behind that I couldn't get one of my patients to x-ray within the 1-hour time frame required by protocols. I probably should have gotten help. The thing that bothers me the most, though, is that I made some assumptions that I shouldn't have. We all make assumptions, but I'll assess more carefully next time, even when it seems to be a straightforward problem.

Elderly and Chronically Ill: Don't Assume

When dealing with elderly and chronically ill clients, be especially careful of the human tendency to make assumptions. The complexity of their health status often hides problems that might otherwise be obvious. For example, we had a 70-year-old man with chronic back pain. He complained of increasing pain for weeks before someone said, "Maybe it's not his back. Has anyone checked his kidneys?" Only then were kidney stones diagnosed. Clinical reasoning requires *differential diagnosis,* which includes considering alternative problems and explanations for presenting signs and symptoms. The more alternative problems (or hypotheses), explanations, and solutions you consider, the more likely it is that you're thinking critically.

❓ CRITICAL THINKING EXERCISES 4.2. Care Planning, Hand-Offs, Predictive Care Models, Delegating Effectively, and Outcome-Focused Care

Find example responses in Appendix I (page 217).
1. **Fill in the following blanks, choosing from the following words:** assessment and planning; care omissions; decisions; created; concepts; outcomes, PPMP; principles, EASE; logic; intuition; falls
   A. Using EHR without ever having _____ care plans on your own is the same as if you used a calculator without understanding the concept of addition, subtraction, multiplication, or division.

B. Creating care plans and maps promotes deep personal learning and helps you learn the (a) _____and (b) _____ you need to apply when thinking-in-action.

C. _____ helps you remember the major care plan components.

D. "Ready, fire, aim" refers to what happens with poor_____.

E. Clinical reasoning requires using both (a) _____and (b) _____.

F. Predictive care models such as _____ aim to predict and manage risk factors before problems arise.

G. Communication issues during hand-offs are major causes of mistakes and adverse outcomes such as (a) _____ and (b) _____.

H. When you delegate tasks, you're accountable for (a) _____ made, actions taken, and patient (b) _____.

2. In three to five sentences and giving examples, describe system-based practice.

3. Imagine that you're caring for a 4-year-old diabetic child who is being raised by his 60-year-old single grandmother. The grandmother, who never finished high school, is on food stamps and has no car. How does understanding the concept of social determinants of health apply to identifying this child's health needs?

4. Using your own words and giving examples or drawing a map, explain how you use the PPMP approach to health care delivery.

5. An important part of developing clinical judgment is recognizing when you don't have enough information to draw valid conclusions. How does this relate to the statements made by the following off-going nurse?
On-coming nurse: "How is the family doing?"
Off-going nurse: "They seem to be fine. They don't say much, but they're sticking to visiting hours and have been here 15 minutes this morning and 15 minutes this afternoon."

6. How do you use the memory jogs MMA and EASE?

7. Using the *clinical decision-making scope of practice* guide (Fig. 4.6, page 93), decide whether you're allowed to insert a nasogastric tube in your current clinical setting.

THINK, PAIR, SHARE

With a partner, in a group, or in a journal entry:

1. Imagine that you're considering delegating the task of getting a patient out of bed to an unlicensed assistive personnel. Applying the "four steps" and "five rights" of delegation, how would you decide if it's safe to delegate this task?

2. Discuss the challenges of delegating effectively as addressed in this chapter.

3. Address how your specific state practice act influences your reasoning (find links to individual state practice acts at https://www.ncsbn.org/npa.htm).

4. Determine whether you are more intuitive than logical or vice versa. Then discuss how intuitive and logical reasoning complement one another.

5. Discuss why it's important to consider clinical, functional, and satisfaction outcomes when developing a plan of care.

6. Address how to use time-outs to promote safe clinical practices.

7. Discuss where you stand in relation to understanding the key concepts and achieving the learning outcomes at the beginning of this chapter.

8. Share your thoughts on the following *Critical Moments and Other Perspectives*.

CRITICAL MOMENTS AND OTHER PERSPECTIVES

"No Pain, No Gain" Can Damage

While the "No pain, no gain" rule may be true during physical therapy, it can backfire on you. For example, I started lifting weights to strengthen my arm muscles. I began to have shoulder pain and told myself to "work through the pain." The result was a damaged shoulder joint. Never work through pain (or allow a patient to do it) without checking with a doctor or physical therapist.

Reporting Issues Keeps Patients Safe

There's something to be said for reporting system issues and organizational failure. This includes alarms not working, broken equipment, [and] incompetent colleagues (knowledge or skill deficit). I think individual accountability by the nurse is also key... what are YOU, the staff nurse, doing to keep the patient safe? Keeping patients safe involves following standard procedures (keeping the alarms on, washing those hands, and other infection control activities), identifying patient needs, and doing something about them (implementing falls precautions or measures to prevent pressure ulcers). —Nancy Konzelmann, MS, RN-BC, CPHQ[41]

Dealing With Families and Privacy Laws

Maintaining patient privacy is important. But sometimes patients' families need information before it's officially released. In this case, I use my judgment and say something like, "Because of privacy laws, I can't tell you what's going on with your family member. I can tell you what typically happens in situations like this, but I can't be sure that this is what will happen now." —Matthew Riley, Psy.D.[42]

Overheard in the Emergency Department

"Why do you think you passed out?" "Because when I woke up I was on the floor."
"How do you know this is a tick bite?" "Because when I pulled it out, I looked at it."
"Do you have a dog?" "No. Should we?"

KEY POINTS/SUMMARY

- Nurses spend more time in direct patient care than any other profession, making them accountable for many aspects of care; like all complex concepts, nursing can't be adequately defined using only *one* definition.
- Your ability to reason and make sound judgments profoundly affects people's lives.
- With interprofessional, patient- and family-centered care, professionals work together to engage patients to ensure individual needs are met.
- Clinical reasoning is guided by standards, policies, ethics codes, and laws (individual state practice acts and state boards of nursing).
- Understanding clinical reasoning principles as addressed in this chapter gives you the foundation for developing sound thinking habits.
- Clinical reasoning requires developing personal CTIs and knowledge and intellectual CTIs.

- Clinical reasoning happens in the context of unfolding human situations; it's fluid and dynamic, not linear and step by step.
- While nurses and other health care professionals use a variety of reasoning patterns alone or in combination, the most common reasoning model is ADPIE.
- Accurately defining health problems requires differential diagnosis (identifying signs and symptoms, creating a list of suspected problems, and weighing the probability of one problem against that of another that's closely related).
- Assessing and reflecting play important roles in *all* phases of clinical reasoning.
- Nurses give care that's based on both nursing and medical models; nurses diagnose and manage various health issues, depending on their practice scope and qualifications.

- Depending on problem complexity and nurse qualifications, nurses are accountable for consulting with primary care providers before determining a plan of care.
- Keeping patients safe depends on your understanding of your scope of practice—what you're accountable for doing and what you're prohibited from doing.
- A major HIT goal is interoperability (the ability of two or more systems to exchange and use the same information); when using HIT, *focus on the patient* more than the technology.
- Your direct patient assessment can be the difference between giving care that's based on how your patient is doing *right now* and continuing to give care based on outdated information.
- Follow policies for documentation carefully (e.g., correct errors and omissions as indicated).
- Using EHR without ever having creating care plans on your own is the same as if you used a calculator without ever having learned what it means to add, subtract, multiply, and divide (impossible).
- Clinical reasoning requires using your whole brain—both the intuitive-right and logical-left sides.
- Hand-offs are vulnerable to miscommunications that cause errors, missed care, and harm.
- Nurses must be able to function in systems-based practice, recognizing all the processes in health care systems that interact to give quality, cost-effective care.
- Clinical reasoning requires considering social determinants of health.
- Predictive care models such as PPMP aim to predict and manage risk factors before problems arise.
- Delegation, a crucial nursing skill, takes significant critical thinking because it requires you to understand both patients' needs and workers' capabilities.
- Scan this chapter to review the illustrations and Guiding Principles throughout.

REFERENCES

1. Beckman, D. Andrew's not-so-excellent adventure. Retrieved from http://www.beckhamco.com (Website).
2. Florence Nightingale International Foundation (Website). Retrieved from http://www.fnif.org/support.htm.
3. Riffkin R. *Americans rate nurses highest on honesty, ethical standards*. Retrieved from, news.gallup.com/poll/224639/nurses-keep-healthy-lead-honest-ethical-profession.aspx; 2017.
4. Laggase J. *Medication errors reduced when pharmacy staff take drug histories in ER*. http://www.healthcarefinancenews.com/news/medication-errors-reduced-when-pharmacy-staff-take-drug-histories-er; 2017.
5. Agency for Healthcare Research and Quality. *Guide to Improving Patient Safety in Primary Care Settings by Engaging Patients and Families*. Retrieved from: http://www.ahrq.gov/professionals/quality; 2017.
6. *The healthcare leader's guide: Preventing patient harm through better communications*. Retrieved from (Website), www.spok.com.
7. Maxfield. D. Grenny, J. McMillan, K, et. al. (2005). Silence kills: the seven crucial conversations in healthcare. Retrieved from https://psnet.ahrq.gov/resources/resource/1149.
8. Kalisch B. *Errors of Omission*. Silver Springs, MD, Nursesbooks.org; 2015.
9. Agency for Healthcare Research and Quality (AHRQ). *Failure to rescue*. Retrieved from, psnet.ahrq.gov/primers/primer/38/failure-to-rescue; 2017.
10. Dolansky MA, Moore SM. Quality and Safety Education for Nurses (QSEN): The Key is Systems Thinking. *OJIN: The Online Journal of Issues in Nursing Vol. 18, No. 3, Manuscript 1*. September 30, 2013. https://doi.org/10.3912/OJIN.Vol18No03Man01.
11. Senge P, Fritz R, Wheattly M. *Learning organizations: The promise and the possibilities*. Retrieved from, https://thesystemsthinker.com/learning-organizations-the-promise-and-the-possibilities/; 2018.
12. National Council of State Boards of Nursing. Measuring the right things. In: *Focus (Winter)*; 2018. P. 12.
13. Tanner CA. Thinking like a nurse: a research-based model of clinical judgment in nursing. *Journal of Nursing Education*. 2006;45(6):204–211.
14. National Academies of Sciences, Engineering, and Medicine; Institute of Medicine; Board on Health Care Services; Committee on Diagnostic Error in Health Care. *Improving diagnosis in healthcare*; 2016. Retrieved from, https://www.nap.edu/download/21794. DOI: https://doi.org/10.17226/21794.

15. Boyer S, Valdez-Delgado K, Huss J, et al. Impact of a nurse residency program on transition to specialty practice. *Journal for Nurses in Professional Development*. 2017;33(5):220–227. https://doi.org/10.1097/NND.0000000000000384.

16. Boyer S, Mann-Salinas E, Valdez-Delgado K. Clinical transition framework: integrating accountability, sampling, and coaching plans in professional practice development. *Journal for Nurses in Professional Development*. 2018;34(2):84–91. https://doi.org/10.1097/NND.0000000000000435.

17. Hassmiller S. Bringing compassion back to the forefront of care. *Journal of Nursing Administration*. 2018;48(4):175–176. https://doi.org/10.1097/NNA.0000000000000594.

18. Lasater Kathie. Clinical judgment development: using simulation to create an assessment rubric. *The Journal of nursing education*. 2007;46:496–503.

19. Gordon M. *Manual of nursing diagnosis*. 13th ed. Sudbury, MA: Jones Bartlett; 2015.

20. American Nurses Association. (Website). Retrieved from http://www.nursingworld.org.

21. *The TIGER Initiatives*. Retrieved from, http://www.himss.org/professionaldevelopment/tiger-initiative; 2018.

22. Intelligence EHR. *EHR defaults cause medication, patient safety errors*. Retrieved from (Website), https://ehrintelligence.com; 2018.

23. Sweeney E. *Healthcare data breaches haven't slowed down in 2017, and insiders are mostly to blame*. Retrieved from, https://www.fiercehealthcare.com/privacy-security/healthcare-data-breaches-haven-t-slowed-down-2017-and-insiders-are-mostly-to-blame; 2017.

24. SBAR (Situation; Background; Assessment; Recommendation). Retrieved from European Union Network for Patient Safety and Quality of Care (Website). http://www.pasq.eu/Wiki/SCP/WorkPackage5ToolBoxes/SurgicalSafetyChecklist/SpecificTools/SBAR.aspx.

25. Agency for Healthcare Research and Quality. *Guide to Improving Patient Safety in Primary Care Settings by Engaging Patients and Families*. Retrieved from: http://www.ahrq.gov/professionals/quality; 2017.

26. The Joint Commission. *National patient safety goals*. Retrieved from (Website), https://www.jointcommission.org; 2017.

27. Summary of HIPAA Privacy Rule. Retrieved from (Website) https://www.hhs.gov/hipaa/for-professionals/privacy/laws-regulations/index.html.

28. Sherman R. *Why certification matters*. Retrieved from (Website) http://www.emergingrnleader.com/why-certification-in-nursing-matters/; 2018.

29. Hines S, Luna K, Lofthus J, Marquardt M, Stelmokas D. *Becoming a high reliability organization: Operational advice for hospital leaders (AHRQ Publication No. 08–0022)*. Rockville, MD: Agency for Healthcare Research and Quality; 2008. Retrieved from (Website), https://archive.ahrq.gov/professionals/qualitypatient-safety/quality-resources/tools/hroadvice/hroadvice.pdf.

30. Commision The Joint. *Facts about Speak Up*. Retrieved from (Website), https://www.jointcommission.org; 2017.

31. Beauvais A, Kazer M, Aronson B, et al. After the gap analysis: education and practice changes to prepare nurses of the future. *Nursing Education Perspectives*. 2017;8(5):250–254. https://doi.org/10.1097/01.NEP.0000000000000196.

32. World Health Organization. *Social Determinants of Health*. Retrieved from (Website) http://www.who.int/social_determinants/sdh_definition/en/; 2018.

33. AHRQ. *Preventing Hospital-Associated Venous Thromboembolism AHRQ. A Guide for Effective Quality Improvement*. Retrieved from, https://www.ahrq.gov/professionals/quality-patient-safety/patient-safety-resources/resources/vtguide/index.html; 2018.

34. Center for Disease Control and Prevention. *Pre-Esposure Prophylaxis:HIV Risk and Prevention*. Retrieved from (Website), www.cdc.gov/hiv/risk/prep; 2018.

35. Salmond S, Echevarria M. Healthcare transformation and changing roles for nursing. *Orthop Nurs*. 2017;36(1):12–25. https://doi.org/10.1097/NOR.0000000000000308.

36. Josey King Foundation. (Website) Retrieved from http://www.josieking.org/.

37. Gaffney T, Hatcher B, Milligan R, Trickey A. Enhancing patient safety: factors influencing medical error recovery among medical-surgical nurses. *OJIN: The Online Journal of Issues in Nursing*. 2016;21(3):https://doi.org/10.3912/OJIN.Vol21No03Man06. Manuscript 6.

38. American Nurses Association. (Website) Retrieved from http://www.nursingworld.org.

39. American Nurses Association & National Council of State Boards of Nursing. *Joint statement on delegation*. Retrieved from (Website), https://www.ncsbn.org; 2006.

40. Hess, R. Personal communication.

41. Konzelmann, N. Personal communication.

42. Riley, M. Personal communication.

Ethical Reasoning, Professionalism, Evidence-Based Practice, and Quality Improvement

LEARNING OUTCOMES

After completing this chapter, you should be able to:

1. Compare and contrast moral reasoning and ethical reasoning.
2. Describe five ethical principles.
3. Determine how well your personal values align with your school or employment values.
4. Compare and contrast the utilitarian and deontological ethics approach.
5. Address how patients' and nurses' bills of rights affect health care delivery.
6. Apply ADPIE principles to make ethically sound decisions.
7. Describe your role in relation to advocacy, professionalism, and leadership.

8. Explain the relationships among research, evidence-based practice (EBP), and quality improvement (QI).
9. Compare and contrast qualitative research and quantitative research.
10. Address the relationships among clinical outcomes, patient satisfaction outcomes, and QI.
11. Explain why QI studies should examine outcomes, process, and structure.
12. Describe your responsibilities for research, EBP, and QI.

KEY CONCEPTS

Ethical reasoning; moral reasoning; values clarification; research; evidence-based practice; quality improvement; patient satisfaction; professionalism; nursing-sensitive indicators; value-based care. *See also previous chapters*

SWEEPING CHANGES

Sweeping changes in health care—treatment advances, longer life spans, expanding nursing roles, and an increased focus on patient outcomes, cost containment, and organizational accountability—are creating unprecedented challenges. Knowing how to navigate these challenges to give ethical care, ensure evidence-based practice (EBP), and maintain professionalism is central to your ability to think critically. This chapter gives strategies for moral and ethical reasoning, maintaining professionalism, and ensuring EBP that focuses on quality improvement (QI).

MORAL AND ETHICAL REASONING

Faced with conflicting values and beliefs of patients and health care providers, today's nurses face complex ethical dilemmas related to the beginning of life, end of life, and quality of life. How do you support patient and family values when they conflict with your own? What are your responsibilities when patients refuse treatment? This section explores how to reason your way through moral and ethical issues. Having an *ethics compass* that's based on professional standards of right and wrong gives you direction and peace of mind that you're making decisions that are in your patients' best interest.

Moral Versus Ethical Reasoning

The terms *moral reasoning* and *ethical reasoning* are sometimes used interchangeably. However, consider the difference between the two following descriptions:

- **Moral reasoning:** Thinking that's guided by *personal* standards of right and wrong (e.g., "I personally believe it's okay to tell 'white lies' now and then.").
- **Ethical reasoning:** Thinking that's guided by *professional* standards derived from the formal study of what criteria should be used to determine whether actions are justified (e.g., "In my nursing role, I don't tell *any* lies because the *American Nurses Association [ANA] Code of Ethics* stresses that I must be honest and tell the truth.").[1]

To understand the difference between moral and ethical reasoning, imagine that you're caring for a woman who is freely and knowledgeably asking for her tubes to be tied to prevent pregnancy. Morally (according to your personal standards), you believe sterilization is wrong. However, you know that professional standards and ethics codes stress that people have the right to make their own choices, based on their own beliefs. It's unethical for you, as a nurse, to tell her that sterilization is wrong.

Clarifying Values

Clarifying values is an important starting point for moral and ethical reasoning. Your values and beliefs affect your thinking at a subconscious level. Unless you spend considerable time getting in touch with your deep personal beliefs—and the implications of these beliefs—you're making "gut," not ethical, decisions.

There are two main ways of looking at values:

1. **Personal values:** These are the beliefs, qualities, and standards that you're passionate about—things you hold "near and dear," for example, your sense of right and wrong. We all have significant emotional investment in our personal values. Yet it often takes "serious thinking" to get in touch with them. Once you clarify what you believe, why you believe it, and how it affects your ability to be objective in various situations, you improve your ability to deal with moral and ethical issues.
2. **Organizational values:** These are deeply held beliefs within an organization (e.g., a school or hospital). These values are expected to be demonstrated through the day-to-day behaviors of all organizational members. Examples of common organizational values are leadership, collaboration, honesty, integrity, dedication to customer service, and respect for diversity.

Think about what's important to you as a person and nurse. What are your beliefs about managing terminal illness? What rights and responsibilities should patients have? Reflect on the values of your school or hospital. Are they compatible with your own values? How committed are you to giving nursing care that's based on the following from nursing codes of ethics?[1,2]

- Ethical care requires respecting individual uniqueness, personal relationships, and the dynamic nature of life.
- Compassion, collaboration, accountability, and trust are central to giving ethical care.

Many people are unaware of their own ethical frameworks. As a colleague of mine says, "We all need to clarify our ethical frameworks before we're faced with dilemmas. Just as we're too late if we're flipping through our advanced life support book during a code, we can make some regrettable decisions if we haven't given thought to how we'll respond to difficult situations."[3]

How Do You Decide?

So how do you make decisions about moral and ethical issues? The answer is that it's not easy. These types of issues are rarely simple. Let's look at how to handle situations that have no clear "right" answers—when each answer has its own merits and drawbacks, and it's hard to say that one is better than another.

Moral and ethical problems are divided into three categories:

- **Moral uncertainty:** You're not sure which moral or ethical principles apply. *Example:* A patient asks you whether you think his or her doctor is a good doctor. You don't think the doctor is very competent. Do you tell the patient this?
- **Moral dilemma:** You're faced with a situation in which you have two (or more) choices available, but neither (or none) of them seems satisfactory. *Example:* A doctor takes you aside and tells you that your friend's blood work indicates probable *leukemia*. But the doctor tells your friend, "I won't know anything until the lab work is complete next week." When your friend begs you to tell him or her what the doctor knows, what do you do?
- **Moral distress:** You know the right thing to do, but institutional constraints make it nearly impossible to do what is right. *Example:* You think a patient isn't ready for discharge because his wife is unprepared to care for him. When you report this problem to the physician, you're told the hospital has "no choice" but to discharge him. What do you do?

Think about the ethical issues in the following scenario.

SCENARIO UNHEARD SCREAMS

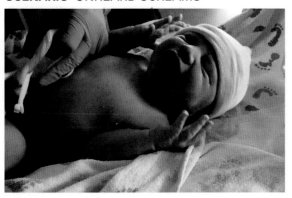

I was working in a clinic and trying to persuade a pregnant teenager who tested positive for HIV to agree to take antiviral medications. After taking a deep breath to calm my emotions, I said, "I can't tell you what to do. I can only support your decision. But I can tell you that infants have a much worse time dealing with HIV than adults. Whatever difficulties you have with the virus or the medication, multiply them and think about your baby having them. You must be prepared to deal with the consequences of whatever choice you make." The doctor and I waited for a response. There was none. The young woman snatched the prescriptions and left the room. In that quiet room, I felt that there were silent screams. The patient was screaming her fear. I was screaming my anger. The physician was screaming his frustration. I imagined the unborn baby's screams. As loud as our screams were, in that little room you couldn't hear a sound.[4]

Do you know what you would do in the preceding examples and scenario? If so, on what would you base your decisions? Gut feelings? Personal values? Professional standards? Are there laws you need to consider?

GUIDING PRINCIPLE

Recognize the difference between legal and ethical aspects of care. Legal aspects of care are guided by local, state, and national laws (if you go against laws, you face legal consequences). Ethics is guided by ethics codes (what you *should* do, not what you *must* do, as required by law). When you're determining ethical courses of action, always ask: "What are the laws related to these actions?"

Five Ethics Principles

There are five ethical principles you should apply when making ethical decisions[5]:

1. **Autonomy.** People have the right to make legally acceptable decisions based on personal values and beliefs, adequate information that's given free from coercion, and sound reasoning that considers all the alternatives.
2. **Nonmaleficence** (pronounced non-mal-FEE-sents): Avoid harm.
3. **Beneficence.** Aim to benefit others; balance benefits against risks and harm.
4. **Justice.** Treat all people fairly, and give what is due or owed.
5. **Fidelity.** Keep promises, and don't make promises you can't keep. Maintain confidentiality. Be honest and tell the truth (called *veracity*). Accept responsibility for the consequences of your actions. Never leave patients without first ensuring their needs will be met.

Ethics Approaches

There are two main ethics approaches that guide your actions[5]:

1. **Utilitarian approach:** Whether actions are right or wrong depends on *the consequences* of the actions. *Example:* You decide that it's right to stop a biological mother from seeing her son because his condition is unstable and you've been told that he's afraid of her.
2. **Deontological approach:** Whether actions are right or wrong depends on a rule that's *independent* of the consequences. *Example:* You decide that the biological mother should be allowed to see her child because you believe in the rule that "mothers shouldn't be separated from their children."

GUIDING PRINCIPLE

Ensuring ethical care—identifying issues and taking responsibility and advocating for what's right—is a key feature of competent nursing practice. With the **utilitarian** ethics approach, actions are right when they promote the greater good and wrong when they don't. The **deontological** approach views actions as right or wrong, regardless of consequences.[5]

Standards, Ethics Codes, and Patients' Rights

Standards, ethics codes, and statements of patients' rights also influence how you conduct yourself as a nurse. For example, the American Nursing Association's (ANA) Code of Ethics stress that nurses must[1]:

- **Practice with compassion and respect for each person's dignity, worth, and unique individuality.** This applies to co-workers, families, and patients, regardless of the nature of health problems present, socioeconomic status, or culture.

- **Keep your primary commitment to consumers (patients, families, and communities).** It's your responsibility to promote, advocate, and protect the health, safety, privacy, and rights of consumers.
- **Promote, advocate for, and protect the health, safety, and rights of patients.**
- **Acknowledge that nurses have the authority, accountability, and responsibility for individual nursing practice.** This includes delegating tasks appropriately to provide optimum care.
- **Respect your own worth and dignity.** Keep yourself healthy and safe. Strive to grow personally and professionally. Maintain competence by broadening your knowledge and seeking out learning experiences.
- **Participate in establishing, maintaining, and improving the health care environment for both patients and workers.** The environment should support the development of moral virtues (qualities needed to make moral decisions—for example, having the courage to do the right thing). Nurses must work to ensure that the physical environment and employment conditions are conducive to providing high-quality health care.
- **Advance the profession** through research and scholarly inquiry, professional standards development, and the generation of both nursing and health policy.
- **Collaborate with other professionals** to protect human rights, promote health diplomacy, and reduce disparities. Work with the public to promote community, national, and international efforts to meet health needs.
- **Work with nursing professional organizations** to articulate nursing values, maintain the integrity of the profession, and integrate principles of social justice into nursing and health policy. Principles of social justice stress the need to treat all people fairly, regardless of economic status, ethnicity, age, citizenship, disability, or sexual orientation.

Advance directives (Box 5.1) help you make decisions about cardiac resuscitation and other end-of-life treatments. When there are no advance directives or patients are unable to communicate, help their families make end-of-life decisions by saying something like, "You need to speak *for* your family member. It's not what *you* want, but what you predict *he (or she)* would want."

Appendix D gives an example patients' bill of rights and the ANA's Nurses' Bill of Rights. There are other bills of rights (e.g., a pregnant patient's bill of rights and a nursing home resident's bill of rights) that may guide how you respond to ethical issues.

ADPIE Applied to Ethical Reasoning

Just as with clinical reasoning, ethical reasoning requires you to be systematic, planful, and complete. Here's a summary of how to use ADPIE to guide ethical reasoning.

BOX 5.1   What Are Advance Directives?

Advance directives include two documents, which may be combined into one document, called a *combination directive:*

1. **Living will:** Designates the types of medical treatments you would or wouldn't want in specific instances (e.g., whether you want to continue ventilator support if you become permanently unconscious).
2. **Durable power of attorney for health care:** Identifies who you want to make treatment decisions if there comes a time when you aren't able to do so for yourself.

   Don't wait too late: Too many people wait until it's too late to address advance directives. Encourage people to talk with loved ones about what they would want if they were unable to speak for themselves. This eases the burden of making tough decisions about whether to refuse aggressive treatment that merely prolongs dying.

Assess

Gather the information you need to identify the ethical issues. What are the patient's cognitive abilities and sense of physical and emotional well-being (Competent? Incompetent? In pain? Afraid?)? If the patient is unable to make decisions, who are the designated decision-makers? What decision is the patient and family trying to make? What are their values and beliefs? What conflicts exist? What resources do you have to help?

Diagnose

Analyze the information, make a list of possible problems (hypotheses), and determine:

1. **The main ethical issues** based on the perspectives of the patient and family. For example, Mrs. Morris, an elderly woman who lives alone, tells you she doesn't want her leg amputated and that she'd rather die than live as an amputee. Mrs. Morris's daughter tells you her mother is incompetent to make this decision. Who has the legal right to make this decision? Is Mrs. Morris competent? Does she have the right to refuse surgery? Does the daughter have the right to overrule her mother?
2. **The key stakeholders**—the people who will be most affected by care (patients and families) or from whom requirements will be drawn (caregivers, insurance companies, third-party payers, health care organizations).

Plan

Clarify your personal values and how they influence your ability to participate in decision-making. For example, in Mrs. Morris's case, do you believe that no one has the right to refuse lifesaving surgery? If so, how would this affect your ability to help Mrs. Morris with this decision? If you can't be objective, let your supervisor know so that another caregiver can assist with decision-making.

1. **Decide what your role will be.** Does this family rely heavily on your judgment? Do you just need to listen and help them sort out their thoughts? Who else will be involved in helping make decisions (e.g., chaplain or case manager)?
2. **Determine possible courses of action** (go "out of the box"—think about as many alternatives as you can). Would it be possible to have the daughter come in to discuss caring for her mother? Could social services help? Should you request an ethics consult?
3. **Determine the outcomes (consequences) of each of the courses of actions you thought about.** For example, what would happen if the daughter is incapable of caring for her mother—what role could the daughter have in this case?
4. **List the courses of action, and rate them according to which choice is most likely to produce an outcome that gives the greatest balance of benefits over possible harm.** To do so, don't consider "good" versus "bad." Instead, ask where each choice fits on the following scale.

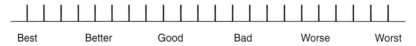

5. **Together with the key stakeholders,** develop a plan of action aimed at achieving the best outcomes based on the circumstances.

Implement and Evaluate

Put the plan into action, monitoring patient and family responses closely; modify approaches as needed.

Ethics Resources
- American Nurses Association, Center for Ethics and Human Rights: http://www.nursing-world.org/ethics/
- National Reference Center for Bioethics Literature: http://bioethics.georgetown.edu/
- American Society of Law and Ethics: http://www.aslme.org
- American Society of Bioethics and Humanities: http://www.asbh.org
- Nursing Ethics of Canada: http://www.nursingethics.ca
- Markkula Center for Applied Ethics: https://www.scu.edu/ethics/

ADVOCACY, PROFESSIONALISM, AND BOUNDARIES

Your understanding of *advocacy, professionalism, and professional boundaries* significantly affects ethical reasoning. Think about your responsibilities in relation to the following descriptions:
- **Advocacy:** Taking actions to support your patients', co-workers', and your own needs.
- **Professionalism:** Conducting yourself in ways that uphold professional standards (e.g., keeping yourself informed, following ethics and conduct codes). A study to determine professional behaviors that students must learn in the classroom ranks *communication* as being the most important, followed by *self-awareness*.[6] *Prioritizing, expecting change, learning from failure,* and *conflict resolution*—all addressed in Chapters 6 and 7—are also listed as important.[6]
- **Professional boundaries:** Limiting the relationship between you and the people in your care— and between you and your co-workers—to ways that promote safe, therapeutic connections. You're accountable for upholding professional standards and advocating for your patients' rights. If you witnesses unsafe care, you have a duty to address or report it. This includes informing leaders if you have concerns about any of the following[5]:
- Short staffing, incivility, or harassment
- Unprofessional, incompetent, unethical, or illegal practices (on the part of physicians, nurses, or anyone else).

Ensuring safe ethical care may involve *whistle-blowing* (telling the authorities or the public that the organization you work for is doing something immoral or illegal).

Maintaining professionalism and professional boundaries serves you, your patients, and your co-workers well. It not only guards you from being accused of inappropriate conduct; it promotes trust and protects your patients' dignity, autonomy, and privacy.[7] You can find excellent information and helpful videos on maintaining professional boundaries at https://www.ncsbn.org/ (put *professional boundaries* in the search field).

Leadership

Leadership—knowing how to motivate and empower patients, families, peers, and co-workers to achieve common goals—is a vital 21st-century skill for students and practicing nurses alike.

Seeing yourself as a leader and developing leadership skills—for example, knowing how to propose new ideas, advocate, and stay "calm under fire"—significantly affect your nursing career. It can make the difference between feeling frustrated and stressed and reaping the rewards of achieving your goals and knowing you contributed to the success of those around you.

Regardless of your role or practice setting, you'll be called upon to lead. As we continue to "grow" nursing leaders, keep in mind that there's a difference between managers and leaders[8]:

Managers typically are in authority positions and have power and control ("I'm in charge and you should be doing what I told you to do."). Managers are expected to keep an eye on "the bottom line" and focus on "here and now," ensuring efficiency and task completion. For example, you may manage patient care by controlling assignments (e.g., you do some of the care yourself and assign some tasks to unlicensed assistants), and you can only do what your budget allows. Managers without knowledge of leadership principles look *to their boss* for direction and approval *more than their co-workers*.

Leaders aren't necessarily tied to positions of authority. You can find them anywhere—from managerial positions, to front-line nurses, to students. True leaders have a "leadership frame of mind." They seize opportunities and have a vision of the future and what needs to be done to create and shape it. They build relationships with their staff and empower and engage those around them (called circle of influence). Rather than focusing only on the "bottom line" and the "here and now," leaders think ahead and use things like improved patient outcomes, nurse job satisfaction, and reduction in *long-term costs* as indicators of success. For example, there may be an investment needed to provide nurses with education; leaders know that the cost is likely to be recovered in terms of staff retention and improved patient outcomes.

Few people are born leaders. Rather, they become leaders by making the commitment to develop leadership qualities and skills. The qualities listed in the personal CTIs (Box 1.2, Chapter 1) are often listed as leadership qualities. Chapter 7 also covers key skills needed for leadership. The following are additional leadership resources.

- Grossman S, Valiga T. The new leadership challenge: creating the future of nursing[8]
- Dr. Rose O. Sherman's blog (www.emergingRNleader.com)—Published twice a week; helps nurses interested in nursing leadership as a career path; includes free leadership resources.
- Nurse Leader (https://www.nurseleader.com/): Journal published bimonthly; provides the vision, skills, and tools needed by nurses currently in, or aspiring to, leadership positions.
- ANA (https://www.nursingworld.org/): Enter "leadership resources" into the search field.

RESEARCH, EVIDENCE-BASED PRACTICE, AND QUALITY IMPROVEMENT

Thanks to informatics and the hard work of committed researchers, care has shifted from practices based in tradition ("We do it this way because that's the way it's always been done") to EBP ("We do it this way because the most current research shows we get the best outcomes when we do it this way").

Nursing Research

Nursing research—the foundation for EBP and QI—requires highly developed critical thinking skills, from knowing how to clearly define the issue(s) to be studied, to determining the best way to collect meaningful data, to analyzing and interpreting statistical data.[9] Broadly speaking, there are two main research methods:

- **Qualitative research**—studies that are exploratory and aim to uncover underlying reasons, opinions, and motivations. These studies often have a small sample size and are less structured than quantitative methods (see the next bullet). Common methods of data collection include focus groups and individual interviews. Qualitative studies may be the first step to quantitative studies. **Example:** Interviewing the staff on a specific unit by using a tool that guides the researcher to ask specific questions about their opinion on what things can be done to improve efficiency.
- **Quantitative research**—studies that emphasize objective measurement and statistical or numerical analysis. Common methods of data collection include polls, questionnaires, and surveys and manipulating preexisting statistical data using computational techniques. **Example:** Keeping a log of how long patients wait in the waiting room before seeing the care provider, then analyzing the log to determine average patient wait times on various days.

How Research, EBP, and QI Are Related

Understanding how research, EBP, and QI are related clarifies the process of improving care. Study Fig. 5.1, which describes these terms and shows the relationships among them. Then study Fig. 5.2, which shows questions that are central to critical thinking and QI.

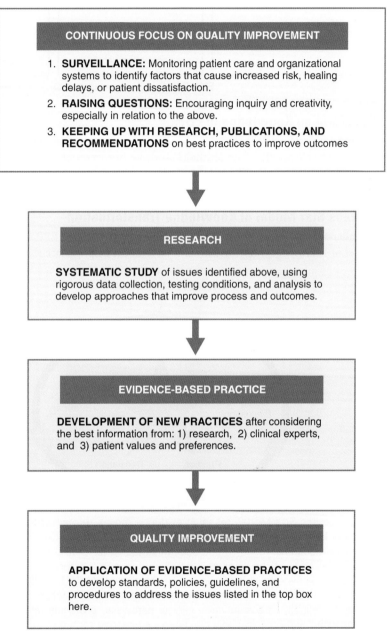

CONTINUOUS FOCUS ON QUALITY IMPROVEMENT

1. **SURVEILLANCE:** Monitoring patient care and organizational systems to identify factors that cause increased risk, healing delays, or patient dissatisfaction.
2. **RAISING QUESTIONS:** Encouraging inquiry and creativity, especially in relation to the above.
3. **KEEPING UP WITH RESEARCH, PUBLICATIONS, AND RECOMMENDATIONS** on best practices to improve outcomes

RESEARCH

SYSTEMATIC STUDY of issues identified above, using rigorous data collection, testing conditions, and analysis to develop approaches that improve process and outcomes.

EVIDENCE-BASED PRACTICE

DEVELOPMENT OF NEW PRACTICES after considering the best information from: 1) research, 2) clinical experts, and 3) patient values and preferences.

QUALITY IMPROVEMENT

APPLICATION OF EVIDENCE-BASED PRACTICES to develop standards, policies, guidelines, and procedures to address the issues listed in the top box here.

FIG. 5.1 Continually raising questions related to QI leads to research, which is then transformed into EBP. EBP is then incorporated into care practices, leading to actual QI. (Source: © 2019 http://www.AlfaroTeachSmart.com.)

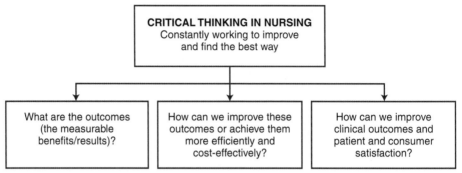

FIG. 5.2 Critical thinking and QI.

Transforming Knowledge to EBP

EBP requires that knowledge be transformed by the systematic study of how evidence from research can best be applied to practice. Transforming knowledge from research to practice is something you don't do alone. The volume of scientific information is such that no one can do it all. You need the collaborative knowledge of a team of experts to interpret the data and decide how it can best be applied to practice.

Stevens Star Model of Knowledge Transformation

To understand how knowledge is transformed from research to EBP, study Fig. 5.3, the Stevens Star Model of Knowledge Transformation.[10] This model helps ensure that care is driven by evidence,

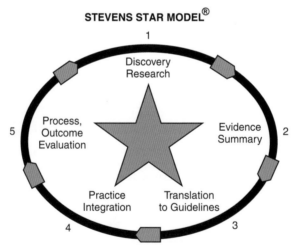

FIG. 5.3 With the Stevens Star Model, research evidence moves through the following cycles and then is combined with other knowledge and integrated into practice. (1) DISCOVERY RESEARCH: New knowledge is discovered through traditional research and scientific inquiry. (2) EVIDENCE SUMMARY: A single, meaningful statement of the state of the science is developed (this is a complex task that takes a lot of critical thinking on the part of knowledgeable experts). (3) TRANSLATION INTO GUIDELINES: Evidence summaries are translated into practice recommendations and integrated into practice. Recommendations are made in clinical practice guidelines, care standards, clinical pathways, protocols, and algorithms. (4) PRACTICE INTEGRATION: Individual and organizational practices are changed through formal and informal channels. (5) PROCESS OUTCOME EVALUATION: The impact on patient health outcomes, provider and patient satisfaction, efficacy, efficiency, and economic costs is continually examined. (Source: © 2015 Used with expressed permission. Retrieved from http://nursing.uthscsa.edu/onrs/starmodel/star-model.asp.)

BOX 5.2   Clinical Practice Guidelines and Practice Standards

1. **What are clinical practice guidelines (CPGs)?** CPGs are recommendations for how to manage care in specific diseases, problems, or situations (e.g., how to best manage smoking cessation or neonate umbilical cord care). CPGs are developed for specific use and designed by a collaborative panel of clinical and scientific experts. When scientific evidence is sufficient, practice guidelines are obvious and clear. When scientific evidence is insufficient, other sources of knowledge—for example, wisdom gained from clinical experts or specific cases—must be brought to bear on the recommendations to fill in the gaps in the research evidence. Evidence summaries and CPGs are the essence of evidence-based practice (EBP). EBP provides mechanisms for fulfilling our social responsibility to provide the best care in the most effective and affordable way. You will find many helpful links and resources at http://www.acestar.uthscsa.edu/.
2. **What are the best EBP websites for updating practice standards?**
   - **For evidence summaries:** The Agency for Healthcare Research and Quality (http://www.ahrq.gov) and the Cochrane Library (http://www.cochrane.org).
   - **For CPGs:** National Guideline Clearinghouse (http://www.guideline.gov/index.aspx). The Cochrane Library produces systematic reviews, which give a single statement that summarizes the state of the science and draws on all research on a given topic. A systematic review is the strongest level of evidence for clinical decisions.

---

rather than tradition. It combines the best of what we know from research with the best of what we know from clinical practice to give current information that's clinically relevant.

Box 5.2 gives resources for finding the most up-to-date information on clinical practice guidelines and EBP. Remember that Chapter 3 gives guidelines for evaluating the accuracy of information gained from online and other resources.

Clinical Summaries and Practice Alerts

Because reading and critiquing research studies is time consuming and requires significant expertise, clinical summaries are now a common way to make research more useable. Many organizations send out EBP alerts via e-mail. Practice alerts summarize cutting-edge research that may change current practices. For example, I received at least four e-mails letting me know that guidelines for care of patients with strokes were changed based on clinician feedback.[11] Signing up for alerts specific to your interests and clinical practice simplifies staying up to date on evidence-based recommendations.

RESEARCH, EBP, AND QI: ALL NURSES PLAY A PART

All nurses play key roles in research, EBP, and QI. To give care that's based on the best available evidence, we must question current practices and develop new knowledge through research. From studying how to improve patient and nurse environments to examining how to get the best outcomes for patients with specific health issues—for example, asthma, wound healing, or depression—nurses, educators, and leaders together can provide the evidence needed to promote safety and efficiency for all.

Students and Staff Nurses' Roles

Whether you're a student who brings a fresh, questioning mind or a staff nurse who's deeply entrenched in the realities of daily practices, you should see yourself as a key player in nursing research. While you're unlikely to actually *do* the research yourself, paying attention to care practices, raising questions, and participating in research projects by diligently recording patient information significantly improves EBP.

Front-line nurses are in the unique position of being able to identify overall system problems that affect patient care. They bring important insights into deciding whether care practices are practical, consistent, and timely. For example, in one case, nurses noted that medications were always arriving late from the pharmacy. They did a study that showed that delays in medication administration increased the length of hospital stays. As a result, policies and procedures were changed to ensure that medications came to the units in a timely way, ultimately shortening patients' length of stay.

To gain insight into staff nurses' roles related to research and QI, study the following frequently asked questions.

Frequently Asked Questions on Staff Nurses' Roles

Q. If I'm a student or staff nurse, what are my responsibilities related to research and EBP?

A.   You have five main responsibilities:

1.   **Reflect on your daily practices,** thinking analytically about the patients and situations you encounter—seek out evidence of findings that might improve nursing care. For example, if you're caring for someone with leg edema after heart surgery, you should be asking, "I wonder if there are any new studies explaining why this happens and what can be done about it?"
2.   **Know the rationale behind your actions and the level of evidence that supports it.** For example, are the rationales behind your actions supported by clinical practice guidelines? A textbook? Your instructor or another clinical expert?

GUIDING PRINCIPLE

As shown in Fig. 5.4**, different levels of evidence may support clinical practices**—from expert opinion to meta-analysis (analysis of data from all studies on a certain topic) and clinical practice guidelines (a collaborative panel of clinical and scientific experts gives recommendations for how to manage care in specific diseases, problems, or circumstances to achieve the best outcomes, from safety, efficiency, cost, and satisfaction perspectives).

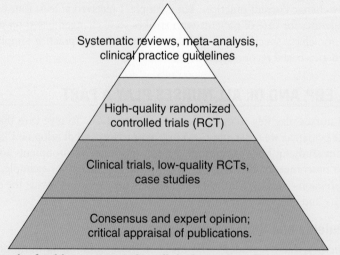

Systematic reviews, meta-analysis, clinical practice guidelines

High-quality randomized controlled trials (RCT)

Clinical trials, low-quality RCTs, case studies

Consensus and expert opinion; critical appraisal of publications.

FIG. 5.4 Strength of evidence supporting clinical practices. The lowest tier of the pyramid is weakest strength, moving up to the top tier, which is the strongest. The most definitive source for clinical practice guidelines (CPGs) is the National Guideline Clearinghouse. CPGs may also come from the AHRQ Evidence-Based Practice Center or from clinical specialty organizations. (Source: Data from various EBP publications.)

> **GUIDING PRINCIPLE**
>
> **Evidence-level supporting practices aren't equally persuasive** in making the case that a specific practice should become part of recommended care for specific problems or populations. If the clinical practices affect patient outcomes in major or unchanging ways, you need rigorous, scientific evidence to support their use. If the outcomes aren't significant or can readily be changed, you can apply studies with less scientific rigor. For example, care practices for postoperative cardiac patients need supporting evidence that is much stronger than care practices related to delivering meals to patients efficiently.

3. **Raise questions that might prompt researchers to formulate questions to guide a study.** For example, you could ask your manager, "Because we seem to be having an increase in infections again, should we revisit our hand-sanitizing procedures?"

4. **Help researchers collect data.** If you're asked to complete a questionnaire or to chart specific data for research purposes, it's your professional responsibility to do so, diligently and accurately, as long as it doesn't interfere with nursing care.

5. **Acquire and share knowledge related to research and EBP.** We must constantly ask ourselves questions like, "Am I making time to become familiar with EBP related to the clinical situations in which I'm involved?" and "Do I interact with others (peers, educators) to learn more about research and EBP?" If you find reading research articles tedious, get started by talking with peers and educators or perhaps joining a journal club. This helps you learn in a dynamic, stimulating environment. Once you learn the basics, reading research articles becomes easier, more interesting, and even an enjoyable challenge!

Q.   If I have limited knowledge of research, how do I know whether there are results from research studies that I should be using in my practice?

A.   As a student or staff nurse, it's important that you ask your leaders and educators for help with finding and using research articles. However, be sure that you understand the following basic facts about choosing useful research articles and information:

1. Choose refereed or peer-reviewed publications (articles are reviewed for accuracy).

2. Remember that only a small percentage of the published literature contains strong evidence that's ready for clinical application. Very few ideas make it through all of the trials and the research stages.

3. Always ask, "How valid and reliable are these results?" "How sure am I that this study was conducted in a way that I can trust that the results are accurate?" and "How does this information compare with what other publications say about this topic?" Consider whether there's vested interest on the part of the researchers or publishers. For example, how often have you heard a commercial that proclaims, "In a recent research study, our product was proved to be more effective than the other leading products"? Do you believe every one of these commercials? Probably not. Think independently, and ask questions.

Reading Research Articles Efficiently

Applying research to practice requires reading a lot of research articles. Knowing how to scan research articles saves you time. You can quickly eliminate irrelevant articles, giving you more time to focus on ones that are relevant. Here are some steps to systematically scan articles so you can choose the ones most relevant to your needs.

1. **Read the abstract first:** This summarizes the issues, the methods, and the results. If the abstract isn't applicable to your clinical problem, you might choose to read no further.

2. **If the abstract seems applicable, skip to the end of the article,** and then scan the article by reading the content under the following headings, in the order listed here:
   - Summary (may also be listed as Conclusions)
   - Discussion

- Nursing Implications
- Suggestions for Further Research
  You may be able to eliminate articles just by reading the content under any of these headings.

3. **If what you scanned is relevant, go on to read the entire study.** Give yourself plenty of time, and don't be discouraged if you find sections you don't understand. Instead, take notes on what you do understand. Come back to the more difficult sections at another time, after getting help from an expert or textbook (or both).

4. **After you read the article, ask yourself whether you understand the following:**
   - What's already known about the topic?
   - What did the researchers study, and why and how did they study it?
   - What did they find out, and are the results valid?
   - What do the results imply, and how do they apply to my particular clinical situation?
   - Might the study be biased (e.g., when drug companies fund a study, there may be a vested interest)?
   - How do the results of the study compare with the results of other, similar studies? If other studies produced similar findings, the probability that the results are reliable increases.

Questioning Practices: Promoting Inquiry and Creativity

Too few nurses think "out of the box" and question care practices. Don't settle for the status quo. Question what you do, why you do it, what your patients' experiences are, and how patient care and nurses' jobs can be improved. Use the following strategies to promote inquiry and creativity:
- On a bulletin board, post a blank paper with "What Do You Want to Know?" at the top. For example, someone might write, "Does anyone know the best programs on managing wound infections?"
- Make reading research articles convenient. If you find a good article, post it on the bulletin board, and ask people to initial that they've read it. Reward nurses who find useful literature.
- Encourage nurses to critique practice protocols and make suggestions for improvement.
- Keep a suggestion box (virtual or real). On performance evaluations, recognize nurses who raise questions or come up with creative, practical solutions.
- Join an Internet listserv on which nurses with common interests. Share questions and information.

QUALITY IMPROVEMENT

Changes in how Medicare and other insurance companies reimburse care providers makes QI more important today than ever before: if your organization doesn't demonstrate QI, not only will the patients and nurses suffer but the organization will suffer financial consequences as well. Read on to find out why.

Value-Based Programs

QI is now tied to reimbursement for patient care in the form of value-based programs. With value-based programs, Medicare and other insurance programs reward care providers with payments based on care *quality* instead of *quantity* (the numbers of patients they treat).[12]

Aiming to achieve better care for individuals and specific populations while reducing cost and encouraging use of best practices, value-based programs are designed to promote[12]:
- Better teamwork and coordination across health care settings
- More attention to population health
- Using the power of health care information

Value-based programs are coordinated with priorities from the Agency for Healthcare Research and Quality's (AHRQ) National Quality Strategy, measuring quality in four domains: safety, clinical care, efficiency, and patient experience.[11] These domains are measured using specific indicators (e.g., whether or not patients are readmitted after discharge or if a patient is treated for a hospital-acquired infection, such as a catheter-associated urinary tract infection [CAUTI]).

Patient experience and satisfaction are measured by HCAHPS (pronounced H-Caps) scores. HCAHPS stands for *Hospital Consumer Assessment of Healthcare Providers and Systems*. These surveys gain information about overall patient experiences by measuring patient satisfaction with specific aspects of care (e.g., pain control, promptness of care delivery, communication, discharge instructions, room and facility cleanliness, and whether the patients felt they were treated with courtesy and respect). These surveys help hospitals target areas of improvement.

There are specific value-based programs among different settings (e.g., skilled nursing facilities and home health) and for chronic diseases (e.g., end-stage renal disease).[12] You can find the most up-to-date information on value-based programs at https://www.cms.gov/Medicare/Quality-Initiatives-Patient-Assessment-Instruments/Value-Based-Programs/Value-Based-Programs.html.

Three Approaches to QI Studies

To ensure comprehensive ways of examining how we can improve care practices, QI studies examine three different aspects of care: outcomes, process, and structure:

1. **Outcomes evaluation (studies results).** *Example:* Studying the number of respiratory complications in postoperative patients.
2. **Process evaluation (studies how care was given).** *Example:* Studying how frequently the respiratory status of patients was assessed and whether care was managed by a registered nurse (RN).
3. **Structure evaluation (studies the setting in which care was given).** *Example:* Studying the locations of the rooms of patients who had respiratory complications in relation to closeness to the nurses' station.

Studying all three of these aspects gives you a comprehensive analysis that helps you improve practice. If you only examine outcomes, you won't be able to improve efficiency. You could be getting great outcomes, but there may be more efficient, cost-effective ways to achieve them.

Nursing-Sensitive Indicators: Improving Patient Outcomes

Studying nursing-sensitive indicators (NSI) is also a key part of QI. NSI are patient outcomes that are known to improve if there's a greater quantity or quality of nursing care (e.g., pressure ulcers, falls, and intravenous infiltrations).[13] With NSI, the structure of nursing care is indicated by the supply, skill level, and education/certification of nursing staff. Process indicators measure nursing care such as assessment, intervention, and RN job satisfaction. You can find out more about NSI in The National Database of Nursing Quality Indicators (NDNQI), where significant, cutting-edge research related to the impact of nursing care is being done.[13]

You Can Make a Difference

Research, EBP, and QI are essential pieces of critical thinking in nursing. You can make significant contributions to these processes, not only improving patient care but also improving the care you and your family experience. Your contributions can help show nursing's value to health care, providing the basis to gain the resources patients and communities need to improve their own health. Make the commitment to question what needs to be done to enhance clinical outcomes and patient satisfaction while containing costs and retaining good nurses. You can find tools and resources for QI at http://www.ahrq.gov/ncepcr/research-qi-practice/index.html.

? CRITICAL THINKING EXERCISES

Find example responses in Appendix I (page 218).

Critical Thinking Exercises 5.1. Moral and Ethical Reasoning, Professionalism, and Leadership

1. **Fill in the following blanks, choosing from the following words:** consequences, deontological, good, utilitarian, virtues, accountability, confidentiality, veracity, fidelity, justice, beneficence, autonomy, personal, professional.

   a. Ethical reasoning differs from moral reasoning in that it requires you to apply _____ standards rather than _____ standards.

   b. The principle of _____ focuses on individuals' right to self-determination and to make legally acceptable decisions based on their own values and adequate information that's given free from coercion.

   c. The principle of _____ aims to benefit others and avoid harm.

   d. Treating all people fairly and giving what is due applies the principle of _____.

   e. _____ has to do with keeping promises and not making promises you can't keep.

   f. Being honest and telling the truth applies the principle of _____.

   g. Keeping information private applies the principle of _____.

   h. Accepting responsibility for the consequences of your actions applies the principle of _____.

   i. Qualities needed to do the right thing—for example, having the courage to advocate for your patients under difficult circumstances—are called moral _____.

   j. Applying the _____ ethics approach means deciding that actions are right when they promote the greater _____ and wrong when they don't.

   k. Applying the _____ approach means deciding that actions are right or wrong based on a rule and views, regardless of _____.

2. The following scenario is a true story of what happened to me when my father was admitted to the intensive care unit (ICU). What would you do if you had been me in the following scenario?

SCENARIO CODE OR NO CODE: WHAT WOULD YOU DO?

Soon after my father was admitted to the ICU after a cardiac arrest, I was approached by a physician, who asked, "Do you want us to resuscitate him if he arrests again?" My father never talked about this, and I didn't know what he wanted. I knew that my mother, not me, should make this decision, so I called her. Here's how the conversation went:

Me: "Mom, they want to know if they should resuscitate Dad if he arrests again."

Mom: "You don't know what you're asking me."

Me: "Yes, I do. I know it's hard, but you're supposed to speak in his voice. Not what you want—what you think *he* wants."

Mom: "That's the problem. All my life when I've tried to guess his decisions, he's always done just the opposite. Even when I made decisions by choosing the opposite of what I think he'd want, I've still been wrong."

---

3. How does maintaining professional conduct protect you and your patients?
4. Name two things that make leaders different from managers.

THINK, PAIR, SHARE

With a partner, in a group, or in a journal entry:

1. Discuss the information and videos on maintaining professional boundaries at https://www .ncsbn.org/ (put *professional boundaries* in the search field).
2. Shared governance—an innovative leadership approach that gives nurses control over their practice and influence over areas previously controlled only by managers—improves patient outcomes and nurses' job satisfaction. Discuss some of the resources posted at the Forum for Shared Governance website (http://sharedgovernance.org/).
3. Decide where you stand in relation to achieving the learning outcomes 1 to 7 at the beginning of this chapter.
4. Share your thoughts on the following *Critical moments and other perspectives.*

CRITICAL MOMENTS AND OTHER PERSPECTIVES

Two Wolves in Each of Us

An old Indian tells his grandson, "There's a battle between two 'wolves' inside all of us. One is Evil. It is anger, envy, jealousy, sorrow, regret, greed, arrogance, self-pity, guilt, resentment, inferiority, lies, false pride, superiority, and ego. The other is Good. It is joy, peace, love, hope, serenity, humility, kindness, empathy, generosity, truth, compassion, and faith." The boy thinks about it and asks, "Which wolf wins?" The old Indian replies, "The one you feed."

In Crises, Silence Is Golden!

Giving ethical care means working to do the best thing for your patients, giving them control, and allowing them to work through their own issues. I see too many basic errors in handling crisis situations. Simple principles such as providing enough space and time for patients to de-escalate are often ignored. Two common mistakes I've noticed when staff respond to patients or clients in crisis are the use of too much verbal interaction and premature use of intrusive intervention strategies. Our first instinct is to talk to a client; however, silence can be an extremely effective strategy to de-escalate a crisis situation. When I train staff, I stress that they should never try to force a situation to resolution if time and space may solve the problem. Many people intervene before it is necessary instead of allowing time to solve the problem. — Matt Riley, Psy.D., BCBA[14]

Critical Thinking Exercises 5.2. Research, EBP, and QI

1. **Fill in the following blanks, choosing from the following words:** domains, improve, evidence, transformed, rigorous, surveys, satisfaction, unchanging.
   a. Research is an objective, orderly process that uses _____ data collection and testing conditions.
   b. Aiming to improve safety, efficiency, satisfaction while reducing costs, EBP integrates knowledge from clinical experts, research, and patient _____.
   c. EBP requires that knowledge be _____ by the systematic study of how evidence from research can best be applied in clinical practice.
   d. If the clinical practices affect patient outcomes in major or_____ ways, you need strong scientific evidence to support their use.
   e. QI focuses on continuous improvement by applying _____to practice.

    f. Nursing-sensitive indicators are outcomes that _____ if there's a greater quantity or quality of nursing care.

    g. Value-based programs measure quality in four _____: safety, clinical care, efficiency, and patient experience.

    h. HCAHPS surveys measure patient_____ with experience.

2. What is the purpose of clinical summaries and practice alerts?

3. Is the following statement true or false, and why? Staff nurses must make finding and critiquing applicable research results a part of their daily work.

4. Which of the following needs the strongest evidence to support changing clinical practices, and why?

    a. Identifying strategies to improve patient satisfaction with surgical experience

    b. Developing protocols to manage postoperative complications

THINK, PAIR, SHARE

With a partner, in a group, or in a journal entry:

1. Draw the Stevens Star Model (see Fig. 5.3) and then discuss the process of each point on the star.

2. To achieve EBP, two main hurdles must be addressed: (1) knowledge complexity and volume and (2) the form of available knowledge.[15] Go to http://www.acestar.uthscsa.edu/ace-star-model.asp and discuss the solutions to these hurdles described there.

3. Find a research article on a topic you find interesting. Then discuss the following:
   - What did the researchers study?
   - What were the key points listed in the discussion, nursing interventions, and summary sections?
   - What questions does this article raise?
   - How do you feel about applying the results to your practice?
   - Where can you find out more about this topic?

4. Choose one of the following websites, and discuss how you might be able to use the information found there:
   - Organizing your social science research paper: http://libguides.usc.edu/writingguide/purpose
   - Evaluating the Evidence – Evidence-Based Practice for Nursing: http://libguides.ecu.edu/c.php?g=17486&p=97640
   - Nursing Resources: A Self-Paced Tutorial and Refresher (Beginner's Research Guide): https://guides.nyu.edu/c.php?g=276860&p=1846275
   - AHRQ Quality Indicators: http://www.qualityindicators.ahrq.gov/
   - National Institute of Nursing Research: http://www.nih.gov/about/almanac/organization/NINR.htm
   - National Database of Nursing Quality Indicators: http://www.pressganey.com/solutions/clinical-quality/nursing-quality
   - The Joint Commission (enter "evidence-based practice" into the search field): http://www.jointcommision.org
   - Joanna Briggs Institute: http://www.joannabriggs.org

5. Discuss where you stand in relation to understanding the key concepts and achieving the learning outcomes at the beginning of this chapter.

6. Share your thoughts on the following *Critical moments and other perspectives.*

CRITICAL MOMENTS AND OTHER PERSPECTIVES

Supporting Research and Inquiry

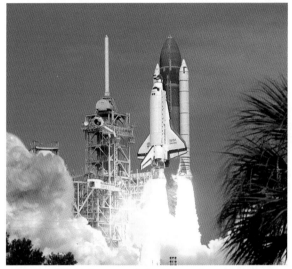

Source: NASA Images Gallery, http://www.nasa.gov

Being curious and inquisitive is a hallmark of critical thinking. Inquisitive researchers have a challenging mission that's worth supporting. You never know what knowledge their work will bring—studying one thing for a specific purpose often brings knowledge for another. For example, the following are just a few of the spin-off technologies we gained from National Aeronautics and Space Administration (NASA) research: heart monitors, laparoscopes, voice-controlled wheelchairs, portable x-rays, magnetic resonance imaging (MRI), ultrasound, automatic insulin pumps, and light-emitting diode (LED) lights (give light for laparoscopes and are being studied for use in promoting bone growth and removing tumors that are hard to reach).[16]

Trial and Error: A Continuous Process

Trial and error is an important learning experience. It takes a lot of critical thinking. Call it what you want, but individuals and health care organizations must continue to interact with the world, learn from experience, and then use that experience to improve care quality. —Workshop participant, a quality improvement expert

KEY POINTS/SUMMARY

- Moral reasoning is guided by *personal* standards; ethical reasoning is guided by *professional* standards.
- Clarifying personal and organizational values is a key starting point for moral and ethical reasoning.

- Moral problems are divided into three categories: moral uncertainty, moral dilemma, and moral distress.
- Five principles form a foundation for ethical reasoning: autonomy, beneficence, justice, fidelity, and veracity.

- Practice standards, ethics codes, and bills of rights guide ethical conduct. The following are common values addressed in ethical codes and standards: maintaining client confidentiality; acting as client advocate; delivering care in a nonjudgmental and nondiscriminatory way; being sensitive to diversity and culture; promoting autonomy, dignity, and rights; and seeking resources for solving ethical dilemmas.
- Developing the leadership skills you need to advocate for your patients and yourself and maintaining professionalism is central to nursing practice.
- Leaders aren't necessarily tied to authority positions, as managers are. Managers tend to control their staff ("you should do as I say"); leaders build relationships with their staff and empower and engage those around them (called circle of influence).
- Understanding the big picture of how research, EBP, and QI are related clarifies the process of improving care.
- Research, the cornerstone of QI, is a rigorous, disciplined use of critical thinking. It requires highly developed critical thinking skills—from knowing how to clearly identify the issue to be studied, to determining the best way to collect meaningful data, to analyzing and interpreting statistical data.
- EBP requires that knowledge be transformed by the systematic study of how evidence from research can be best applied in practice; it combines the best of what we know from research with the best of what we know from clinical practice to give current information that's clinically relevant.
- If the clinical practices affect patient outcomes in major or unchanging ways, you need rigorous, scientific evidence to support their use. If not, you can apply studies with less scientific rigor
- To ensure comprehensive studies of how to improve care practices, QI studies three different aspects of care: outcomes, process, and structure.
- QI is now tied to reimbursement for patient care through value-based programs (programs that focus on *quality* of care, rather *quantity* of patients treated).
- HCAHPS surveys measure patient satisfaction with specific aspects of care (e.g., pain control, promptness of care delivery, communication, discharge instructions, room and facility cleanliness, and whether the patients felt they were treated with courtesy and respect).
- NCNQ maintains the database for nursing-sensitive indicators (outcomes that are known to improve if there's a greater quantity or quality of nursing care).
- Scan this chapter to review the illustrations and Guiding Principles throughout.

REFERENCES

1. American Nurses Association. *Code of ethics for nurses with interpretive statements.* Retrieved from, http://nursingworld.org/DocumentVault/Ethics-1/Code-of-Ethics-for-Nurses.html; 2015.
2. American Association of Critical Care Nurses. *AACN Standards for establishing and sustaining healthy work environments.* 2nd ed 2015. Retrieved from, https://www.aacn.org/wd/hwe/docs/hwestandards.pdf.
3. Riley, M. Personal communication.
4. Scipio-Bannerman, J. Personal communication.
5. Taylor C, Lillis C, Lemone P, Lynn PL. *Fundamentals of nursing: the art and science of nursing care.* 9th ed. Philadelphia: Lippincott Williams & Wilkins; 2019.
6. Sortedahl C, Persinger S, Sobtzak K, et al. Essential professional behaviors of nursing. Students and new nurses: hospital nurse leader perspectives survey. *Nursing Education Perspectives.*
   2017;38(6):297–303. https://doi.org/10.1097/01.NEP.0000000000000240.
7. NCSBN. A nurse's guide to professional boundaries. (Website). www.ncsbn.org.
8. Grossman S, Valiga T. *The new leadership challenge: creating the future of nursing.* 5th ed. Philadelphia: F.A. Davis; 2016.
9. Burns N, Grove S. *Understanding nursing research: building an evidence-based practice.* 8th ed. Philadelphia: Saunders; 2018.
10. Academic Center for Evidence-Based Practice. (Website). http://www.acestar.uthscsa.edu.
11. *Correction to 2018 guidelines for the early management of patients with ischemic stroke.* Retrieved from, https://www.dailyrounds.org/library/correction-to-2018-guidelines-for-the-early-management-of-patients-with-acute-ischemic-stroke.

12. Center for Medicare and Medicaid Services. *What are the value-based care programs? (Website).* https://www.cms.gov; 2018.

13. National Database of Nursing Quality Indicators (NDNQI®). (Website) http://www.pressganey.com/solutions/clinical-quality/nursing-quality

14. Riley, Matt. Personal communication.

15. Star Model Background. Retrieved from http://www.acestar.uthscsa.edu/acestar-model.asp

16. Health and Medicine. NASA spin offs. (Website). http://www.thespaceplace.com/nasa/spinoffs.html#health.

Practicing Clinical Reasoning, Clinical Judgment, and Decision-Making Skills

THIS CHAPTER AT A GLANCE

LEARNING OUTCOMES

After completing this chapter, you should be able to:

1. Explain why each skill in this chapter is needed for clinical reasoning.
2. Describe how to do each of the skills listed in this chapter.
3. Analyze and improve your clinical reasoning and decision-making skills.
4. Develop a comprehensive, patient-centered plan of care.

KEY CONCEPTS

Systematic; validation; health patterns inference; cues; signs and symptoms; relevance; prioritization; client-centered outcomes; self-regulation; *See also previous chapters.*

CLINICAL REASONING SKILLS: DYNAMIC AND INTERRELATED (ITERATIVE)

Using scenarios based on actual experiences, this chapter helps you practice interrelated clinical reasoning and decision-making skills. Keep in mind that these skills depend on—and facilitate—each other (in other words, they are *iterative*). For example, you may recognize inconsistencies (Skill 6.8) in how someone responds to your care. This should trigger you to wonder, "Did I identify assumptions (Skill 6.1)?" These are the skills you need to develop to reason well in clinical practice, simulations, and testing situations. Since use of electronic health record (EHR) and decision support tools is now standard practice, the following Guiding Principle is worth repeating.

> **GUIDING PRINCIPLE**
>
> **Using EHR and decision support tools without developing the clinical reasoning and decision-making skills detailed in this chapter is like using a calculator without ever having learned what it means to add, subtract, multiply, and divide.** To give safe and effective care, you must know (1) how to assess, interpret, and record signs and symptoms (cues) and (2) what to do to manage symptoms and risk factors, prevent complications, and promote well-being.

Organized in logical progression according to how the skills might be used in the clinical reasoning and decision-making process, each skill is presented in the following format: (1) name of the skill, (2) definition of the skill, (3) why the skill is needed for clinical reasoning, (4) how to accomplish the skill, and (5) Clinical Reasoning Exercises.

HOW TO GET THE MOST OUT OF THIS CHAPTER

To get the most out of these exercises, review "Principles of Clinical Reasoning" in Chapter 4, starting on page 80, before going on to read about the individual skills. Realize that some of these exercises, as in real life, are time consuming. Take your time and get in touch with your thinking. If possible, get at least one other person to complete the exercises with you. You learn more by discussing the skills with others.

If you have trouble with an exercise, read on and come back to it later. Explanations and exercises in later sections may help you. If you encounter diseases or drugs you don't know, look them up right away. This helps you build your own mental storehouse of problem-specific facts, because you apply the information to the exercise.

Before starting this chapter, be sure you have a good understanding of the following terms, which are listed in order of how to best learn them (you need to know the first term to understand the second term, and so on).

REQUIRED VOCABULARY

Diagnosis: (1) The *process* of working to identify the specific health problem(s) indicated by the patient's signs and symptoms (cues). (2) The *opinion or conclusion* reached by this process (usually refers to naming the disease or health problem). The terms *diagnosis* and *problem identification* are sometimes used interchangeably.

   Definitive diagnosis: The most specific, most correct diagnosis. For example, someone is admitted with an initial diagnosis of respiratory distress. Then, after studies are completed, the definitive diagnosis is congestive heart failure. To identify the best treatment, you must determine the most specific diagnosis.

Risk factor: Something known to cause, or be associated with, a specific problem. For example, smoking is a risk factor for cancer; *having a history of frequent falls* is a risk factor for falls.

Related factor: Something known to be associated with a specific problem (often used interchangeably with *risk factor*).

Potential problem or diagnosis: A problem or diagnosis that may occur because certain risk factors are present. For example, someone who's on prolonged bed rest has a potential (or risk for) pressure ulcer.

Data: Pieces of information about health status. *Example:* Vital signs.

Objective data: Information that you can clearly *observe* or *measure*. *Example:* A pulse of 140 beats/min. To remember this term, remember:

$$\textbf{O} - \textbf{O} : \textbf{O}\text{bjective data} = \textbf{O}\text{bservable data.}$$

Subjective data: Information the patient *states* or *communicates*. These are the patient's perceptions. *Example:* My heart feels like it's racing. To remember this term, remember this:

$$\textbf{S} - \textbf{S} : \textbf{S}\text{ubjective data} = \textbf{S}\text{tated (or communicated) data.}$$

Signs and symptoms (cues): Abnormal data that prompt you to suspect a health problem. Signs are objective data. Symptoms are subjective data. For example, fever is a sign of infection; chest pain is a symptom of heart disease.

Baseline data: Information collected before treatment begins.

Database assessment: Comprehensive data collection performed to gain complete information about all aspects of health status (e.g., respiratory status, neurological status, circulatory status).

Focus assessment: Data collection that aims to gain specific (focused) information about only one aspect of health status (e.g., neurological status).

Infer: To draw a conclusion or to attach meaning to a cue. *Example:* If an infant doesn't stop crying, no matter what's done for him or her, you might infer <u>that he or she is in pain.</u>

Inference: Something we suspect to be true, based on a logical conclusion. *Example:* The underlined words in the preceding definition.

SKILL 6.1:   Identifying Assumptions

Definition

Recognizing when something is taken for granted or presented as fact without supporting evidence (e.g., you might assume a woman on a maternity unit has just had a baby *when,* in fact, she has just lost one).

Why This Skill Is Needed for Clinical Reasoning

As humans, we all have preconceived notions and tend to make assumptions, especially in unfamiliar circumstances. Sound clinical reasoning requires that you make judgments based on the best available evidence. This means double-checking your thinking to overcome your brain's natural tendency to grasp things at an intuitive (gut) level. By identifying assumptions, you apply logic and avoid jumping to conclusions and making judgment errors. *Identifying assumptions* is placed at the top of the list in this section because it's one of the most commonly addressed skills in the critical thinking literature (both nursing and non-nursing).

Guidelines: How to Identify Assumptions

The best way to identify assumptions is to *look for them* by asking questions like, "What's being taken for granted here?" and "How do I know that I've got the facts right?" To identify assumptions, make sure that you have a complete picture of what's going on with the patient (addressed in the next skill, "Assessing Systematically and Comprehensively"). Other skills that help you identify assumptions are "Checking Accuracy and Reliability (Validating Data)" (Skill 6.3), "Recognizing Inconsistencies" (Skill 6.8), "Identifying Patterns" (Skill 6.9), and "Identifying Missing Information" (Skill 6.10).

☀ CLINICAL REASONING EXERCISES

Find example responses in Appendix I (page 218).
1. Explain why the following statement is an assumption: "We need to teach this patient how to stick to a low-salt diet because he eats whatever he wants."
2. What could happen if you planned nursing care based on the preceding assumption?
3. Read the following scenarios and then answer the questions that follow them.

SCENARIO ONE
Anita plans to teach Jeff about diabetes today. She's well prepared and decides she'll create a positive attitude for Jeff by telling him about all the advances in diabetes care. She doesn't have much time, so she introduces herself and starts telling him how much easier it is to manage diabetes than it used to be. She goes on to explain how easy it is to learn the required diet, monitor blood sugar, and take insulin. Jeff listens to all Anita has to say, asks a few questions, and then leaves with his wife. As they drive off, he says to his wife in a discouraged tone, "She sure is a know-it-all, isn't she?"

a. In the preceding scenario, what assumption does it seem Anita made about creating a positive attitude?
b. What key thing did Anita forget to do that might have helped her avoid making this assumption?
c. Why do you think Jeff said Anita is a know-it-all?

SCENARIO TWO
Four-year-old Bobby is in the emergency department with his mother. He fell off his bike and had an initial period of unconsciousness lasting about a minute. He's been examined, has no skull fracture, and is now awake and alert and ready to go home with his mother. The nurse gives his mother a computer printout of instructions for checking Bobby's neurological status and says, "Let me know if you have questions."

a. In the preceding scenario, what assumption does it seem the nurse has made?
b. What might happen if the nurse's assumption is incorrect?

SCENARIO THREE
I was working evenings in the emergency department of a seaside hospital. We admitted a 54-year-old man, whom I'll call Mr. Schmidt. He told me, "I just got here for vacation, and I'm not feeling so great. I had pneumonia at home, got treated, and thought I was better. Now my

breathing feels lousy again." A check of his vital signs while he was sitting quietly revealed the following: T 99° C, P 138 beats/min, R 36 breaths per minute, BP 168/80 mm Hg. As I helped him to the stretcher, he became significantly more short of breath. I checked his lung sounds and heard a lot of congestion. I notified the doctor and voiced my concern that Mr. Schmidt seemed quite ill. The doctor examined him and ordered an electrocardiograph and chest x-ray study. During this time we got very busy. I was helping another patient when the doctor came to me and said, "I want you to give Mr. Schmidt 80 mg of furosemide (a diuretic) IV now and discharge him." I looked at him skeptically and said, "Discharge him?" He said, "Yes. I'm sure the diuretic will help him get rid of this fluid." Tactfully, I asked, "Can we give him some time to see how he responds?" The doctor said, "No. This place is wild. I'm sending him home. He's going to a private physician in the morning. He'll be fine once he gets rid of some fluid. Discharge him with instructions to call if he doesn't feel better." I gave Mr. Schmidt the furosemide, but still had trouble with the idea of sending this man home before knowing his response to the IV diuretic. Then I decided to use my own clout as a nurse: I had established a rapport with the Schmidts, and they trusted me. I said to them, "I realize the doctor has discharged you, but I'd be interested to see if there's any change in blood pressure after you get rid of some fluid. How would you feel about sitting in the waiting room, and I'll check your blood pressure in an hour?" The Schmidts thought this was a good idea and went off to the waiting room. Only 45 minutes had passed when there was a shout for help. I ran to the waiting room and found Mr. Schmidt on the floor having a grand mal seizure. He then stopped breathing. We were able to resuscitate him and he was admitted to the hospital, diagnosed with electrolyte imbalance and heart failure, and discharged a week later.

a. In the preceding scenario, what assumption does it seem the physician made about Mr. Schmidt's response to the furosemide?
b. Why do you think the nurse was so concerned about the assumption the physician made?
c. What assumption does it seem the nurse made about how the physician would respond to her if she cautioned him about discharging Mr. Schmidt?

SKILL 6.2:   Assessing Systematically and Comprehensively

Definition

Using an organized, systematic approach that enhances your ability to discover all the information needed to fully understand a person's health status (e.g., "What are the risk factors and actual and potential problems? What needs aren't being met? What are the priority problems? What are the person's strengths and resources?").

Why This Skill Is Needed for Clinical Reasoning

Making judgments or decisions *based on incomplete information* is a leading cause of mistakes. Having an organized approach to assessment prevents you from forgetting something. For example, you might be interrupted while doing a physical assessment. If you use a tool to record your assessment, you know exactly where you left off and where to continue. If you consistently use the same organized approach, you form habits that help you be systematic and complete.

Guidelines: How to Assess Systematically and Comprehensively

Being purposeful and focused is the key to knowing how to assess systemically and comprehensively. You must decide the purpose of your assessment and use an approach that gets the information needed to achieve your purpose. For example, in Chapter 4, Figs. 4.4 and 4.5 show the difference between medically focused assessments and nursing-focused assessments (keep in mind that nurses use *both* medical and nursing approaches).

GUIDING PRINCIPLE

Always consider your direct assessment of the patient to be the primary source of information. Also collect information from secondary resources (patient records, caregivers, significant others, and print and electronic references, e.g., using drug references to determine side effects of patients' medications).

In most cases, you'll be using electronic tools to guide assessment. Some tools are designed for *database assessment*. Others are designed for *focus assessment* (see the Neurological Focus Assessment Guide in Fig. 6.1). The following are some points that can help you develop clinical reasoning skills related to assessment:

- Make connections between *what information you're required to record* and *why it's relevant*. For example, if you use a neurological focus assessment tool that requires you to record how the pupils react to light, ask, "Why do I need to check the pupils, and what is the significance of how pupils react to light in the context of determining neurological status?"
- Consider both subjective data (patient's perceptions) and objective data (your observations).
- After you interview and examine your patient, ask, "What other resources might provide additional information about this person's health status (e.g., medical and nursing records, significant others, other health care professionals)?"
- Change your approach to assessment, depending on the person's health status:
  1. If the person is acutely ill, assess urgent problems first (see Skill 6.13, "Setting Priorities").
  2. If the person has a specific complaint, assess that problem first and then go on to complete the assessment in the same way you would if the person were healthy (see next point).
  3. If the person is generally healthy, follow the electronic guide or choose the method that meets your purpose and is most convenient. For example, use the head-to-toe approach or the body systems approach.
  4. Keep in mind that a body systems approach to assessment helps you collect data about *medical problems*. Be sure that the tool(s) you use to guide assessment include data related to *nursing problems* (e.g., human function, activities of daily living, and human responses).
- **Consider the "seven major vital signs":** temperature, pulse, respirations, blood pressure, pain, cough, and pulse oximetry. Ask about the presence of pain or discomfort, and assess closely as indicated. Ask the person to cough. Although asking the person to cough doesn't replace a thorough lung assessment, you can learn a lot from brief encounters. Say something like, "Can you cough for me so I can hear how it sounds?" The person's ability (or inability) to comply with this request gives you a lot of information (e.g., whether the person has pain with coughing, whether there's congestion, or whether the person coughs well enough to clear the airway). These brief encounters can flag patients that need more in-depth monitoring and assessment.

⍰ CLINICAL REASONING EXERCISES

Find example responses in Appendix I (page 219).
1. Imagine you're a school nurse and have been asked to do physical exams to screen students for possible medical problems. Identify an organized, comprehensive approach to assessing for signs and symptoms of medical problems. (Exercises continue after Fig. 4.2)

NEUROLOGIC FOCUS ASSESSMENT GUIDE

VITAL SIGNS Temp.＿＿ Pulse＿＿ Resp.＿＿ BP＿＿
(Check the boxes that apply below)

EYE OPENING
☐ Spontaneous ☐ To command ☐ To pain ☐ No response

MOTOR RESPONSE
☐ Obeys commands ☐ Localizes pain ☐ Flexion withdrawal
☐ Abnormal flexion ☐ Abnormal extension ☐ No response

BEST VERBAL RESPONSE
☐ Oriented ☐ Confused ☐ Inappropriate words
☐ Incomprehensible words ☐ No response

PUPIL REACTION
☐ Right eye:＿＿ Size of pupil＿＿ Reaction to light (brisk, sluggish)
☐ Left eye:＿＿ Size of pupil＿＿ Reaction to light (brisk, sluggish)

GAG REFLEX
☐ Present ☐ Absent ☐ Weak

PURPOSEFUL LIMB MOVEMENT

Right arm
☐ Spontaneous ☐ To command ☐ Paralysis
☐ Visible muscle contraction but no movement
☐ Weak contraction; not enough to overcome gravity
☐ Moves against gravity, not to external resistance
☐ Normal range of motion; can be overcome by increased gravity
☐ Normal muscle strength

Right leg
☐ Spontaneous ☐ To command ☐ Paralysis
☐ Visible muscle contraction but no movement
☐ Weak contraction; not enough to overcome gravity
☐ Moves against gravity, not to external resistance
☐ Normal range of motion; can be overcome by increased gravity
☐ Normal muscle strength

Left arm
☐ Spontaneous ☐ To command ☐ Paralysis
☐ Visible muscle contraction but no movement
☐ Weak contraction; not enough to overcome gravity
☐ Moves against gravity, not to external resistance
☐ Normal range of motion; can be overcome by increased gravity
☐ Normal muscle strength

Left leg
☐ Spontaneous ☐ To command ☐ Paralysis
☐ Visible muscle contraction but no movement
☐ Weak contraction; not enough to overcome gravity
☐ Moves against gravity, not to external resistance
☐ Normal range of motion; can be overcome by increased gravity
☐ Normal muscle strength

Limb Sensation (prick limb with sterile needle)
Right arm: ☐ Normal ☐ Decreased ☐ Absent
Right leg: ☐ Normal ☐ Decreased ☐ Absent
Left arm: ☐ Normal ☐ Decreased ☐ Absent
Left leg: ☐ Normal ☐ Decreased ☐ Absent
Seizure Activity: Describe in nurse's notes.

FIG. 6.1 Neurological Focus Assessment Tool.

2. Suppose you make a home visit to a woman who has a newborn child and seven other children younger than 12 years old. Both the baby and the mother are healthy. Identify an organized and comprehensive approach to assessing for nursing and medical problems.

3. Consider the following scenarios and answer the questions that follow them.

SCENARIO ONE

Pearl, an 89-year-old grandmother, is admitted with a fractured ankle. She has surgery, and a cast is applied. The cast goes from her toes to the knee. Her toes are visible, and she can wiggle them freely. A small window was cut in the cast over the dorsalis pedis pulse. Routine hospital protocols state that anyone with a cast must have neurovascular checks every 2 hours. You have a standard tool to follow for neurovascular checks, but you also want to remember assessment parameters for a classroom test you're going to take.

a. Use the following memory jog to remember the things you need to check when performing a neurovascular assessment:

Maggie **C**hewed **N**uts **E**very **P**lace **S**he **W**ent, which stands for this :

Movement, **C**olor, **N**umbness, **E**dema, **P**ulses, **S**ensation, **W**armth

b. Based on the preceding memory jog, how would you assess the neurovascular status of Pearl's injured leg?
c. Why is it necessary to monitor each of the assessment parameters listed in the memory jog to determine neurovascular status?
d. What would you do if Pearl told you her toes felt numb and cold?

SCENARIO TWO

You have to give Mr. Wu digoxin by mouth. You know that using the following memory jog (TACIT) helps you remember what you need to monitor in patients taking medications:

- **T**herapeutic effect (Is there a therapeutic effect?)
- **A**llergic or adverse reactions (Are there signs of allergic or adverse reactions?)
- **C**ontraindications (Are there contraindications to giving this drug?)
- **I**nteractions? (Are there possible drug interactions?)
- **T**oxicity or overdose (Are there signs of toxicity or overdose?)

Assuming that you followed medication reconciliation standards (i.e., you made sure that Mr. Wu's drug regimen is correct and up to date), use TACIT to systematically gather information about how Mr. Wu is responding to the digoxin, and answer the following questions:
   a. What, specifically, would you assess to decide whether to give the digoxin?
   b. Why is it important to determine all of the things listed in the mnemonic TACIT?

SCENARIO THREE

You just admitted Gerome, who fell off his bike, hit his head, and had a short period of unconsciousness. He is now awake and alert but is admitted for 24 hours of neurological monitoring. The physician orders neurological assessments every hour.

Using the Neurological Focus Assessment Guide (see Fig. 6.1), respond to the following questions:
   a. How would you assess Gerome to determine the status of each of the neurological assessment parameters addressed in the guide?
   b. Why is each piece of data on the focus assessment guide relevant to determining neurological status?
   c. What would you do if, on admission, Gerome demonstrates normal neurological assessment findings but 2 hours later demonstrates extreme drowsiness (i.e., he awakens only if you shake him and call his name)?

d. What would you do if one pupil started to become more sluggish in its response to light than the other?

e. What would you do if you noted a general pattern of the pulse getting slower than the baseline pulse?

SKILL 6.3: Checking Accuracy and Reliability (validating data)

Definition

Collecting additional data to verify (validate) whether information you gathered is correct and complete.

Why This Skill Is Needed for Clinical Reasoning

Clinical reasoning and judgments must be based on evidence. Verifying that your information is accurate, factual, and complete helps you avoid making assumptions and identifying problems and making decisions based on incorrect or incomplete data.

Guidelines: How to Check Accuracy and Reliability

1. Review the data you gathered and ask questions like these:
   - Do the *objective data* (what you observed) support the *subjective data* (what the patient stated)? For example, if the patient complains of rib pain, how are the breath sounds and are recent x-ray films posted on the record?
   - How do I know this information is reliable?
   - How does this information compare with similar data collected in a different way or at another time (e.g., how does an oral temperature compare with a rectal temperature)?
2. Focus your assessment to gain more information about whether your information is correct. For example, an elderly person may have told you that she took her medicine. To verify this, interview significant others or caregivers, check pill containers to see if pills are gone, and ask whether there is any record kept when pills are taken.

GUIDING PRINCIPLE

More than one source, more likely of course. The more information you have coming from different sources, indicating the same thing, the more likely it is that your information is valid and reliable. For example, verify what your patient says by checking with family members and patient records.

❓ CLINICAL REASONING EXERCISES

Find example responses in Appendix I (page 220).

For each of the following, determine how to validate whether the information is accurate and reliable:

1. The off-going nurse tells you that Mrs. Molina is depressed and angry about being in the hospital.
2. Mr. Nola tells you his blood sugar was 240 when he tested it an hour ago.
3. You take a blood pressure from the left arm and find it to be abnormally high.
4. A team member tells you that Mr. McGwire needs teaching about diabetic foot care because this is his third admission for foot ulcers.

SKILL 6.4: Distinguishing Normal from Abnormal—Detecting Signs and Symptoms (Cues)

Definition

Recognizing/noticing deterioration in patient status. Analyzing patient information to determine (1) what data are *within* normal range, (2) what data are *outside* of normal range, and (3) whether abnormal data may be signs or symptoms of a specific problem. *Example:* If a 62-year-old man who takes no medications has a pulse of 42 beats/min, this is abnormal because a normal pulse rate rarely drops below 55 to 60 beats/min (this may be a sign of a cardiac issue).

Why This Skill Is Needed for Clinical Reasoning

Recognizing abnormal data (signs and symptoms) is the first step to problem identification. Signs and symptoms are like red flags that prompt you to suspect a problem. If you miss these red flags, you allow problems to go untreated. If you miss *subtle* signs and symptoms, which may indicate impending complications, your patient may die from complications that he or she would have otherwise survived (this is called *failure to rescue* as described in Chapter 4).

> **GUIDING PRINCIPLE**
>
> **If you identify signs and symptoms but are unsure about what they indicate,** activate the chain of command (report them to your instructor, supervisor, or appropriate care provider).

Guidelines: How to Distinguish Normal From Abnormal and Detect Signs and Symptoms (Cues)

Detecting signs and symptoms requires you to apply knowledge of what are considered to be normal findings. If your patient's findings are outside the normal range, then you have identified an abnormality—a possible sign or symptom. Use all your senses (sight, hearing, touch, and smell) to gain all the relevant information you need (e.g., if you see cloudy urine, smell it to check its odor).

  Ask the following questions:
1. **How does my patient's information compare with accepted standards for normal** for someone of this age, culture, disease process, and lifestyle? If the patient's information isn't within normal accepted standards, this is a possible sign or symptom of a problem.
2. **Does my patient take any medications or have any chronic conditions that change normal function?** For example, if someone is taking a medication that lowers heart rate, this abnormally low heart rate may be normal for him or her. Check the action and side effects of all medications.
3. **How does my patient's current information compare with the previously collected data?** This question is especially helpful in situations in which the patient has chronic signs and symptoms and you need to decide whether the signs and symptoms are getting worse. For example, an asthmatic always may be slightly wheezy. However, if this same person is now wheezier than before, this increased wheezing is a sign of increasing problems.

🔎 CLINICAL REASONING EXERCISES

Find example responses in Appendix I (page 221).
1. Place an **S** next to the data in the following list that are signs or symptoms (cues) of a possible problem. Place an **O** if it's neither a sign nor a symptom. Place a question mark if you need more information to decide.
  _____a. Temperature of 99.68° F.
  _____b. Bilateral pulmonary rales.

_____c. Someone tells you she rarely sleeps more than 3 hours at a time.

_____d. Someone's nasogastric drainage has turned from brown to red.

_____e. Someone's abdominal incision is slightly red around the sutures.

_____f. A 2-year-old child is inconsolable when his mother leaves the room.

_____g. Someone with no health problems has developed ankle edema.

_____h. Someone tells you he bathes every other week.

_____i. Someone on kidney dialysis never urinates.

_____j. Pulse rate of 54 beats/min.

2. For each question mark you placed in the previous question, what else do you want to know before you decide whether the information is abnormal (and therefore a sign or a symptom)?

SKILL 6.5   Making Inferences (Drawing Valid Conclusions)

Definition

Forming opinions and judgments that follow logically, based on patient signs and symptoms (cues).

Examples of Cues and Inferences

Cue	Corresponding Inference
Frowning	Seems worried
White blood cell count = 14,000	Probable infection
Deaf	Probable communication problems

Why This Skill Is Needed for Clinical Reasoning

Your ability to interpret data and draw valid conclusions is key to determining health status. If you draw incorrect conclusions, your clinical judgments will be flawed, which may cause the entire treatment plan to be flawed.

Making correct inferences helps you focus your assessment to look for additional relevant information. For example, if you infer that an elevated white blood cell count may indicate an infection, you know to look for signs and symptoms of infection (or vice versa).

Guidelines: How to Make Inferences (Draw Valid Conclusions)

1. Making correct inferences requires knowledge of:
   - Signs and symptoms of common complications and health problems
   - The common needs of certain age groups (e.g., elderly versus young)
   - Cultural and spiritual influences
   - Knowledge of the patient as a person
   - Anatomy, pathophysiology, pharmacology, medical-surgical nursing, and specialty nursing practice (e.g., pediatrics or gerontology)

   For example, to make the inference of probable infection, you must know the signs and symptoms of infection. To draw conclusions about someone's lack of eye contact, you must know how eye contact is used in his or her particular culture (in some cultures, direct eye contact may be disrespectful). To draw conclusions about how to help a diabetic manage his or her care, you need to know what's important to him or her as a person.

2. **To avoid jumping to conclusions**, begin your statements about inferences by saying, "I suspect this information indicates...." Using this phrase reinforces that you need to collect more

data to decide if your suspicions are correct. Once you have enough evidence to support your inference, you can know that you are probably correct.

3. **Think about alternative conclusions (hypotheses). What other issues could the data suggest?** If you make an inference, try to think of other things you could also reasonably infer. Consider worse case scenarios (could someone's headache be related to impending stroke rather than tension?).

4. **When drawing conclusions**, always consider whether signs and symptoms could be related to medications, medical problems, or allergic responses; remember **"MMA"** (**M**edications, **M**edical problems, **A**llergies).

GUIDING PRINCIPLE

Remember: **"More than one cue, more likely it's true—more than one source, more likely of course."** Avoid making inferences based on only one cue or only one source (the more facts and sources you have to support your inference, the more likely it is that your inference is correct).

❓ CLINICAL REASONING EXERCISES

Find example responses in Appendix I (page 221).

Make an inference about each of the following data (begin your inference by saying, "I suspect this information indicates...").

1. A patient has a temperature of 102.8° F for 3 days.
2. A mother tells you she can't afford prenatal care.
3. A patient with diabetes is 100 pounds overweight and says his blood sugar is always out of control, even though he watches his food intake and takes his insulin regularly.
4. A 6-year-old child whose mother told you he broke his leg falling down the stairs keeps looking at his mother before answering your questions.
5. A usually active, alert grandmother has an unkempt appearance and seems a bit confused.

SKILL 6.6:   Clustering Related Cues (Signs and Symptoms)

Definition

Grouping data together in a way that you can see patterns and relationships among the data. *Example:* Suppose you grouped the following cues together: 2 years old; temperature 100.8° F; pulse 150 beats/min; rash all over trunk; recent measles exposure; never had measles; screaming that he wants his mother. If you consider the relationship among these data, you should suspect that the child's rapid pulse is related to his screaming and elevated temperature rather than a sign of cardiac problems. If you consider all of the data, you'll probably suspect that these symptoms indicate the child may have measles.

Why This Skill Is Needed for Clinical Reasoning

Grouping information applies the scientific principle of classifying information to enhance the ability to see relationships between and among data. It helps you get a beginning picture of patterns of health or illness. A good way to remember the importance of clustering related data is to think about what you do when you begin to put together a picture puzzle: you put all the edges of the picture in one pile, all the pieces of a certain color in another pile, and so on. Putting the pieces in piles helps you begin to see patterns. The same principle applies to health assessment data, but in health care you put together (cluster) signs and symptoms (cues).

Guidelines: How to Cluster Related Cues

1. How you cluster data depends on your purpose:
   - If you're trying to determine the status of medical problems or physiological responses, cluster the data according to body systems (see Fig. 4.4, page 90).
   - If you're trying to determine the status of nursing problems, cluster the data according to a nursing framework (e.g., Functional Health Patterns on page 87, or the Comprehensive Nursing Assessment Map on page 91).
2. Using concept mapping is especially helpful to identify relationships.

CLINICAL REASONING EXERCISES

Find example responses in Appendix I (page 221).

Read the following scenarios and then complete the instructions that follow them.
Cluster the information in the preceding scenario that helps you determine the following:

SCENARIO ONE

The babysitter next door calls and tells you that Jack, the 8-year-old she's watching, was stung by a bee on the ear an hour ago. She tells you the ear is swollen and asks you to come and check him. You go over and examine the child. He asks you if he might die "like the kid on TV did." The babysitter tells you she's afraid because she doesn't know where the mother is. You check the ear and find it red, swollen, and free of the stinger. When asked, Jack tells you he was stung before but that it wasn't as scary. Jack has no rash and no wheezing. He asks if he could have a Popsicle and watch TV. His pulse and respirations are normal.

a. Jack's physical health status
b. Jack's human responses (e.g., his personal perceptions and experiences)
c. The babysitter's learning needs

SCENARIO TWO

Imagine that you just admitted Mr. Nelson, a 41-year-old businessman who has acute abdominal pain. He's never been in the hospital and tells you he hates everything about hospitals. He's been vomiting for 2 days and is unable to keep any food down. His abdomen is distended, and he has no bowel sounds. He is scheduled to go to the operating room at 2 PM for emergency exploratory surgery. He tells you he's worried because his brother died in the hospital. Suddenly he doubles over and says, "This is really getting worse!" You take his vital signs, and they are as follows: T 101° F, P 122 beats/min, R 32 breaths per minute, BP 140/80 mm Hg. These signs are the same as those taken an hour ago, except that before, his pulse was 104 beats/min.

Cluster the information in the preceding scenario that helps you determine the following:
a. Mr. Nelson's physical status
b. Mr. Nelson's human responses (e.g., his personal perceptions and experiences).

SKILL 6.7: Distinguishing Relevant from Irrelevant

Definition

Deciding what information is *pertinent* to understanding specific health concerns and what information is *immaterial*.

Why This Skill Is Needed for Clinical Reasoning

When faced with a lot of information, narrowing it to *only the pertinent facts* prevents your brain from being cluttered with unnecessary facts. Deciding what's relevant is also an example of one of the principles of the scientific method: classifying or categorizing information into groups of related (relevant) information.

Guidelines: How to Distinguish Relevant from Irrelevant

This skill is closely related to Skill 6.6, Clustering Related Cues (Signs and Symptoms). Here, however, we're looking at this skill a little differently. In clustering related cues, you simply put related information together (e.g., you put all the respiratory data in one place, all the nutritional data in another, and so on). In this skill, you analyze the cues you put together and decide what information is related to a specific health concern. For example, if someone has constipation and you note that she has a sedentary life, poor fiber intake, and takes iron supplements, it's likely that this information is relevant to the constipation.

Distinguishing relevant from irrelevant is especially difficult for novices because being able to do this depends on having problem-specific knowledge and experience. Here are some strategies that can help you determine what's relevant, even with limited knowledge:

1. List (or map) the abnormal data you collected. Then ask yourself, "What is the connection between this (data) and that (data)?" *Example:* What is the connection between someone's shortness of breath and rapid pulse?
2. Ask the person to identify relationships among signs and symptoms. *Example:* Can you think of any relationship between your shortness of breath and something that happened today?

CLINICAL REASONING EXERCISES

Find example responses in Appendix I (page 222).
   Read the following scenarios and then answer the questions that follow them.

SCENARIO ONE

Imagine you work in community health and make a visit to Mrs. Roberts, who is 80 years old and had a cerebrovascular accident (CVA) a month ago. Today you notice she seems to be increasingly confused: she knows where she is but forgets what day it is and doesn't seem to remember her daily routine. You know that confusion in the elderly can be caused by any of the following: medications, infection, decreased oxygen to the brain, electrolyte imbalance, and brain pathological conditions.

   Suppose you had the following data (a to f) in relation to scenario one. Put an **R** in front of the things that are relevant to the confusion.

   _____a. Recently started taking buspirone hydrochloride for anxiety
   _____b. Temperature 100.8° F orally
   _____c. History of myocardial infarction 5 years ago
   _____d. Seems dehydrated
   _____e. Has no allergies
   _____f. Regular diet

SCENARIO TWO

You assess Mrs. Clark, a 32-year-old patient with diabetes, who is in for a routine visit. When you ask how the new diet is going, she breaks down into tears, saying, "I'm never going to be able to do this!"

Suppose you had the following data (a to g) in relation to scenario two. Decide its possible relevance to Mrs. Clark's problem with sticking to the diabetic diet. Put an **R** in front of the things that are relevant.

_____a. Diagnosed with diabetes 2 months ago

_____b. Vital signs within normal limits

_____c. Complains of constipation

_____d. Married with three school-age children

_____e. Loves to cook

_____f. Has always been 50 pounds overweight

_____g. Allergic to aspirin

SKILL 6.8:   Recognizing Inconsistencies

Definition

Identifying cues that contradict each other. *Example:* Imagine that you're caring for "Fred" after chest surgery and he tells you that he has no pain. However, he moves very little and barely breathes when you ask him to take a deep breath. The way he's moving is inconsistent with his statements of being pain-free.

Why This Skill Is Needed for Clinical Reasoning

Recognizing inconsistencies "sends up a red flag" that tells you to probe more deeply to get to the facts. It also helps you focus your assessment to clarify the issues/signs and symptoms. For example, with Fred in the preceding section, you might say, "It seems to me that you aren't moving very well.... I suspect you have more pain than you admit. I want you to be comfortable so that you move well and can take deep breaths to clear your lungs. Is there a particular spot that's bothering you?"

Guidelines: How to Recognize Inconsistencies

1. Compare what the patient states (subjective data) with what you observe (objective data). If what the person states isn't supported by what you observe, you have inconsistent information and need to investigate further.
2. Recognizing inconsistencies requires problem-specific knowledge. For example, suppose you have the following data:
   - **Subjective Data:** Patient states, "I must have strained my back lifting my child. My right side is killing me."
   - **Objective Data:** Fever of 102.4° F; cloudy, foul-smelling urine.

   If you know how back injuries usually manifest, you know that the subjective and objective data are *inconsistent* with a back injury and *more consistent* with a urinary tract infection.
3. To recognize inconsistencies with limited knowledge:
   a. **Determine the signs and symptoms of the problem you suspect** by looking up the problem in a reference. For example, if you suspect pneumonia—something you should report immediately—look up the signs and symptoms of pneumonia.
   b. **Compare the information in the reference with your patient's data**. If your patient's signs and symptoms are different from those listed in the reference, you have inconsistencies and must investigate further. Assess the person more closely, and consider other problems that the signs and symptoms might represent. For example, are the signs and symptoms more consistent with a cold or flu than pneumonia?

CLINICAL REASONING EXERCISES

Find example responses in Appendix I (page 222).

Answer the questions that follow scenarios one and two.

SCENARIO ONE

You interview Cathy in the prenatal clinic 2 weeks before delivery. You ask her how she feels about the baby coming. She tells you she's happy that she gets to see the baby in only 2 weeks. When you ask her if she has any questions about the delivery, she tells you she's been going to birthing classes with her boyfriend and feels like she knows what to expect. You review her records and notice that her first clinic visit was 2 weeks ago, when she came with her mother.

---

a. Identify inconsistencies in the preceding scenario.
b. Explain what you might do to clarify the inconsistencies you identified.

SCENARIO TWO

You're in the grocery store and a 20-year-old woman comes up to you and says, "Please help me! I can't breathe, and my heart is racing." She is sweating profusely and says, "I feel like I'm having a heart attack and I'm going to die!" You help her sit down, then take her pulse, and find it to be 100 beats/min, regular, and strong. Her respirations are 36 per minute. She tells you she has no pain, but wants you to call an ambulance. You offer emotional support and ask someone to call 911. As you wait for the ambulance, she tells you this has happened to her several times before and that she has had an electrocardiogram, which showed normal cardiac function.

In the preceding scenario, how consistent are the signs, symptoms, and risk factors with those of a heart problem?

SKILL 6.9: **Identifying Patterns**

Definition

Deciding what patterns of health, illness, or function are indicated by patient data. *Example:* You cluster together cues of chronic productive cough, wheezing, and exercise intolerance and decide they indicate a pattern of respiratory problems.

Why This Skill Is Needed for Clinical Reasoning

Identifying patterns helps you do two things: (1) get a beginning picture of problems and (2) recognize gaps in data collection. When you recognize gaps in data collection, you can decide how to focus your assessment to gain that missing information. Using the puzzle analogy, when you put some pieces together, you start to see what the end picture will be and more readily find missing pieces.

Here's an example of how identifying patterns helps you discover missing information. Suppose you clustered together the following data:

• No bowel movement in 3 days
• Abdominal fullness
• States he's been "constipated off and on for the past month"

You may decide that the preceding cues represent a pattern of bowel elimination problems. Having recognized this pattern, you know to focus your assessment to gain more information and decide exactly what the problem with bowel elimination is. For example, you ask, "What does *off and on* mean?" The person responds, "I get so constipated I have to take laxatives, and then I get diarrhea." This added information is likely to make you suspect that the bowel elimination problem may be caused in part by laxative abuse. You then explore his knowledge of how diet, fluids, and exercise influence bowel function. You also need to find out whether a primary care provider has evaluated the bowel issue recently (changes in bowel elimination is one of the signs of cancer).

Guidelines: How to Identify Patterns

To identify patterns:
1. Analyze the cues you put together and decide which of the following patterns they represent:
   - Normal pattern (*no signs and symptoms* of the pattern are present)
   - Risk for abnormal pattern (*risk factors* for the pattern are present)
   - Abnormal pattern (*signs and symptoms* of an abnormal pattern are present)
2. After you get a beginning idea of the patterns, look for gaps in data collection by asking, "What other information might clarify my understanding of this pattern?"

⚡ CLINICAL REASONING EXERCISES

Find example responses in Appendix I (page 222).
Match the *patterns* (a to e) with the *examples supporting evidence* (1 to 5).
Patterns:
   a. Potential (risk) for ineffective sexual reproductive pattern and infection transmission
   b. Potential (risk) for impaired bowel elimination pattern
   c. Probably normal sleep–rest pattern
   d. Impaired respiratory function pattern
   e. Probably normal coping pattern
Example supporting evidence:
   1. _____ Manages daily self-care; has husband cook all meals; passes the time by knitting blankets for the homeless. Eats little fiber; just started taking codeine every 4 hours; drinks about three glasses of water daily; spends most of her time in bed; normal bowel function
   2. _____ Has just been diagnosed with genital herpes; single; worried about transmitting herpes to future sex partners and future children (during delivery)
   3. _____ Bilateral rales; respirations increased to 34 per minute; coughing up white mucus
   4. _____ States, "I can cope with my illness, so long as I have help from my husband."
   5. _____ Works nights; sleeps 4 hours in the morning and 3 hours before going to work

---

SKILL 6.10:   Identifying Missing Information

Definition

Recognizing gaps in data collection and searching for information to fill in the gaps.

Why This Skill Is Needed for Clinical Reasoning

Recognizing gaps in information and filling in those gaps prevents you from making one of the most common clinical reasoning errors: developing hypotheses or making judgments based on incomplete information.

Guidelines: How to Identify Missing Information

1. Rather than relying on your own memory, the best way to identify missing information is to reflect on recorded data and ask, "What's missing here?" You may have to print out electronic information so that you can see more of it at once.

2. If you're not sure if you need more information, ask questions like, "What difference will it make?" or "How will knowing this information change the approach to treatment?" If the information won't change your approach, then you may not need to take the time to gather it.

3. Other strategies for recognizing missing information include accomplishing all of the following clinical reasoning skills: identifying assumptions, checking accuracy and reliability, clustering related cues, recognizing inconsistencies, identifying patterns, and evaluating and correcting thinking.

? CLINICAL REASONING EXERCISES

Find example responses in Appendix I (page 222).

Go back to the Clinical Reasoning Exercises for the Skill 6.9, Identifying Patterns: Consider the information given in 1 to 5 and decide what information might be missing that could add to your understanding of the pattern.

SKILL 6.11: Managing Risk Factors—Promoting Health

NOTE: This skill deals with identifying and managing risk factors in *healthy* people. The next skill—diagnosing actual and potential problems—deals with identifying risk factors in the context of *people with existing health problems.*

Definition

Maximizing well-being by detecting and managing factors that evidence shows contribute to health problems (e.g., sedentary lifestyles contribute to many health problems).

Why This Skill Is Needed for Clinical Reasoning

As addressed in Chapter 4, in the section on "Predictive Care Models," identifying risk factors is central to being proactive, promoting health, and preventing problems.

Guidelines: How to Identify and Manage Risk Factors

1. **Assess people's awareness of—and motivation for—identifying and managing risk factors.** For example, do they know what's required for adequate nutrition, rest, exercise, and spiritual and psychological well-being? Are they able and willing to do what's needed to reduce risks? Not knowing about risk factors and not wanting do something about them are risk factors in themselves.

2. **Keep growth and development in mind**. *Examples*:
   - A woman who is pregnant or planning on becoming pregnant must consider risk factors for both herself and the fetus when taking medications. Teach her that inadequate intake of folic acid increases risk for spontaneous abortion and other problems such as spina bifida in infants.
   - After menopause, women should be aware that they should be screened for osteoporosis (decreased bone density).

3. **Look for risk factors that are known to put people at risk for a variety of common problems.** *Examples:* Obesity; poor diet; high cholesterol; tobacco use; immobility; sedentary life; stressful life; poor sleeping habits; allergies; chronic illness; extremes of age (very young or old); low socioeconomic status; illiteracy; sun exposure; and excessive use of medications, alcohol, or illicit drugs.

4. **Paying attention to social determinants of care, assess the following:**
   - Genetic, cultural, or biological factors (e.g., race, family history, and personal history predisposing one to health problems)
   - Behavioral factors (e.g., problems with anger management, attention-deficit disorders)
   - Psychosocial and/or economic factors (e.g., lack of emotional support, poverty)
   - Environmental factors (e.g., air quality)
   - Age-related factors (e.g., women after menopause are at risk for osteoporosis; infants are at risk for ear infections)
   - Sexual-pattern factors (e.g., whether the person is sexually active and with whom)
   - Safety-related factors (e.g., whether seat belts are worn, whether small children ride in car seats, whether the home environment is safe)
   - Disease-related factors (e.g., someone with chronic lung disease is at risk for pneumonia; someone with diabetes is at risk for skin problems)
   - Treatment-related factors (e.g., complicated medication or treatment regimen)
5. **Teach the importance of managing risk factors to prevent costly, debilitating illnesses.**
   For more strategies on risk management, review "Predictive Care Models" starting on page 105, and go to the following web pages:
   - Harvard Center for Risk Analysis (http://www.hcra.harvard.edu)
   - The Centers for Disease Control and Prevention (http://www.cdc.gov)
   - The Agency for Healthcare Research and Quality (https://www.ahrq.gov/)
   - *Healthy People 2020* (http://www.healthypeople.gov/)
   You also can look up "risk factors" in the index of up-to-date textbooks or on Google (you can find excellent tables on common diseases and risk factors).

⚡ CLINICAL REASONING EXERCISES

Find example responses in Appendix I (page 223).
1. You assess a 25-year-old man and determine that he is healthy. What questions might you ask to identify risk factors for possible problems?
2. You assess a 72-year-old woman and find that she is healthy, but she says, "I tend to be a little clumsy—I lose my balance." Why should you be concerned about this?
3. A 50-year-old man says, "I'm getting to the age where I should be doing more to look after myself, and I want to know more about my risk factors." How do you respond?

SKILL 6.12:   Diagnosing Actual and Potential Health Problems

NOTE: This skill deals with identifying risk factors in the context of people *with existing health problems*. The preceding skill deals with risk factors in the context of *healthy* people.

Definition

Ensuring that your patient's actual and potential problems are correctly identified based on evidence from the health assessment and patient records. This skill includes (1) ensuring that signs and symptoms of health problems that are beyond your practice scope are referred to the appropriate health care professional; (2) choosing the name that best describes the problem (the definitive diagnosis); (3) determining the cause(s) and contributing factors of the problem; and (4) providing the evidence that leads you to believe the diagnosis, problem, or issue is present. It also includes *differential diagnosis*: identifying signs and symptoms, creating a list of suspected problems, and weighing the probability of one problem against that of another that's closely related). This is similar to what the National Council of State Boards of Nursing (NCSBN) calls *cue recognition and generating hypotheses.* [1]

Why This Skill Is Needed for Clinical Reasoning

This skill is important for the following reasons:

1. Making definitive diagnoses (the most specific, correct diagnoses) is key to being able to determine the *specific actions/treatments* designed to prevent, manage, or resolve them. If you miss problems, are too vague about the problems, or name them incorrectly, you have made a diagnostic error that may cause you to:
   - Initiate actions that aggravate the problems or waste time
   - Omit essential actions required to prevent and manage the problems
   - Allow problems to go untreated
   - Influence others to make the same mistake you did
2. You don't fully understand the problems—or know what to do about them—until you know what's causing or contributing to them.
3. Predicting potential problems and complications helps you:
   - Know what signs and symptoms to look for when monitoring the patient
   - Anticipate what could happen if things get worse and be prepared for complications (for example, when patients have their jaws wired, keep a wire cutter nearby in case of issues with choking or aspiration
4. Providing the supporting evidence that led you to the diagnosis helps others understand the problem better. For example, compare the two following problem statements and decide which one gives a better picture of the problem:
   - Potential for violence
   - Potential for violence related to anger management problems as evidenced by history of previous violence and refusal to attend anger management programs

The previous bullet here gives an example summary statement for a diagnosis. Alternatively, use a diagram or map as shown in Fig. 6.2.

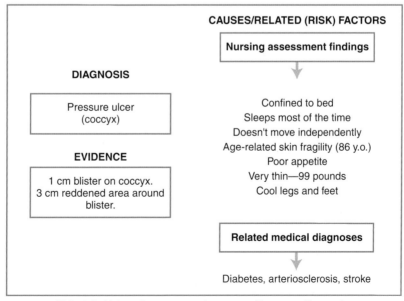

FIG. 6.2 Using diagrams and maps to illustrate diagnosis.

Guidelines: How to Diagnose Actual and Potential Problems

1. Review the "how to" guidelines listed in Skill 6.5, Making Inferences (Drawing Valid Conclusions).
2. Realize that if your knowledge and expertise are limited, you are at risk for making any one of the following diagnostic (problem identification) errors:
   - Making a diagnosis or naming the problem without considering whether the data may represent a different problem altogether (e.g., assuming indigestion signifies gastric reflux or upset stomach instead of possible coronary problems).
   - Not considering all the relevant data because of a narrow focus (e.g., not looking for other coronary symptoms because you decide that the person simply has indigestion).
   - Failing to recognize personal biases or assumptions. *Example:* Thinking that someone is faking pain because he doesn't look like he's in pain. Knowledgeable nurses know that people handle pain differently and that often outward signs of pain are not present, even though the person is experiencing significant discomfort. This is especially true for people with chronic pain.
   - Overanalyzing ("analysis paralysis") and delaying taking action.

Actual Problems

1. **Verify that your information is correct and complete.** If you're not sure what to do next, report signs and symptoms to a more qualified nurse before going on to complete problem identification.
2. **Avoid drawing conclusions or identifying problems based on only one cue or one source** ("More than one cue, more likely it's true. More than one source, more likely of course.").
3. **Cluster abnormal data** (cues/signs and symptoms).
4. **Begin the process of differential diagnosis—create a list of problems that may be suggested by the signs and symptoms.** Box 6.1 gives an example checklist to consider possible problems.
   - After you complete your list of suspected problems, compare your patient's signs and symptoms with the signs and symptoms of the problems you suspect. Some call this phase "testing hunches (hypotheses)."
   - Name the problems by using the term that most closely matches your patient's signs and symptoms. *Example:* If your patient's signs and symptoms match the signs and symptoms of *anxiety* better than *fear,* label the problem *anxiety.*
5. **Determine what's causing or contributing to the problems.**
   - Always consider whether it's possible that medications, medical problems, or allergies are causing the problems.
   - Ask the patient and significant others if they can identify factors that are contributing to the problems.
   - Consider whether there are factors related to age, disease process, treatments, medications, or life changes that could be contributing to the problems.
6. **As appropriate, use the following strategies:**
   - Draw a map to clarify relationships among problems and signs, symptoms, or risk factors.
   - Use the Systematic Problem Analysis Worksheet (Fig. 6.3) to systematically consider possible causative factors.
7. **If a summary diagnostic statement is required, use the memory jog PRE (problem, related risk factors, evidence) to describe the following:**
   P—Problem
   R—Related factors (risk and contributing factors)
   E—Evidence (patient data) that led you to conclude the problem exists
   Example: Pain related to left rib fracture as evidenced by rating of 8 on pain scale.

BOX 6.1   Checklist for Identifying Actual and Potential Problems

1. List current medications (include over-the-counter and herbal drugs). Ask yourself whether any of the patient's problems could be related to any of the medications (remember SODA).
   Side effect?
   Overdose?
   Drug interaction?
   Allergy or Adverse reaction?
2. List current and past allergies, diseases, surgeries, or trauma.
3. Consider whether any of the patient's current problems are related to questions 1 or 2.
4. Complete the following checklist:

	(Circle those that apply)			
Is there a risk for infection (self or transmission to others)?	Yes	No	AR	Pos
Is there a problem with breathing?	Yes	No	AR[1]	Pos[2]
Is there a problem with circulation?	Yes	No	AR	Pos
Is there a problem with comfort?	Yes	No	AR	Pos
Is there a problem with nutrition?	Yes	No	AR	Pos
Is there a problem with urinary or bowel elimination?	Yes	No	AR	Pos
Is there a problem with fluid or electrolyte balance?	Yes	No	AR	Pos
Is there a problem with the ability to think or perceive the environment (cognitive issue)?	Yes	No	AR	Pos
Is there a problem with communication?	Yes	No	AR	Pos
Is there a problem with safety (risk for injury or falls)?	Yes	No	AR	Pos
Is there a problem with sleeping or exercising?	Yes	No	AR	Pos
Is there a risk for impaired skin integrity?	Yes	No	AR	Pos
Is there a problem with coping or stress?	Yes	No	AR	Pos
Is there a psychological, developmental, or self-esteem problem?	Yes	No	AR	Pos
Is there a sociocultural problem?	Yes	No	AR	Pos
Is there a problem with roles, relationships, or sexuality?	Yes	No	AR	Pos
Does the person have a problem with taking medications?	Yes	No	AR	Pos
Does the patient require teaching?	Yes	No	AR	Pos
Is there a problem with health maintenance at home?	Yes	No	AR	Pos
Is this admission going to cause difficulties at home?	Yes	No	AR	Pos
Is there a problem with personal or religious beliefs?	Yes	No	AR	Pos
Is there a problem with coping or managing stress?	Yes	No	AR	Pos
Could this person be pregnant?	Yes	No	AR	Pos

[1]AR = At risk for problem (no signs and symptoms present, but risk factors are evident).
[2]Pos = Possible problem (insufficient data, but you suspect a problem).
Source: © 2018 R. Alfaro-LeFevre. www.AlfaroTeachSmart.com.

SYSTEMATIC PROBLEM ANALYSIS WORKSHEET

Instructions:

1. List the focus problem, diagnosis, issue, or in box below.
2. Put a check mark in all boxes on the right that correspond to factors that contribute to the problem, diagnosis, or issue you identified.
3. Decide what factors must be managed and who will manage them.
4. Use back of page or figure of man as needed.

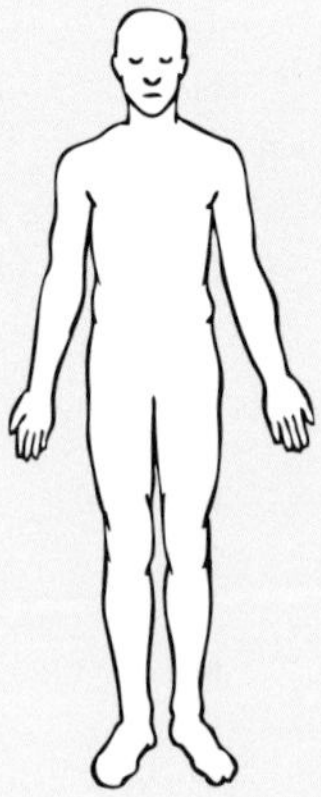

CONTRIBUTING OR RELATED (RISK) FACTORS

Actual / potential diagnosis, problem, or issue

1. Main reason for admission or contact?

2. Vulnerability—constitutional or age-related factors?
☐ Age ____ Weight ____ Height ____ Mental Status? ____
☐ Communication ability? ☐ Smoker? ☐ Drinker (alcohol)?
☐ Skin status? ☐ Nutrition-hydration status?
☐ Mobility or self-care problems?
☐ Bowel elimination or urine elimination problems?
☐ Immune system status? ☐ Overall health status/resilience?
☐ Other?

3. Allergy, medication, or treatment-related factors?
☐ Allergies?   ☐ Considered all meds (Rx, OTC, herbal)?
☐ Treatments?

4. Co-existing medical problems, injuries, or pathophysiology?
☐ Neuro?   ☐ Resp?   ☐ Cardiac-circulatory?   ☐ GI?   ☐ GU?
☐ Diabetes? ☐ Hypertension?   ☐ Depression?   ☐ Other?

5. Environmental factors? Patient identified factors?
☐ Current environment (include work)?   ☐ Role-related?
☐ Other factors?

6. Comfort factors? Mobility problems? Self-care problems?
☐ Pain level? ☐ Pain management? ☐ Self-mobile? ☐ Other?

7. Socioeconomic, spiritual, cultural factors?
☐ Family issues? ☐ Coping problems? ☐ Support systems limited?
☐ Other?

FIG. 6.3 Systematic Problem Analysis Worksheet.

GUIDING PRINCIPLE

Diagnosis is incomplete until you identify not only the problems but also the underlying causes and contributing factors of the problems. Clearly and specifically identifying both the problem and its cause(s) is key to determining specific interventions to resolve it.

Predicting Potential Problems and Complications

1. Find out the patient's allergies, medications, treatments, and current and past medical and nursing problems.
2. Look up problems and complications often associated with those things noted in step 1.

  Examples: If the person has diabetes, there is a risk for foot ulcers and poor healing. If your patient just had a myocardial infarction (MI) and has an arterial line in place, determine common potential complications of MI (e.g., congestive heart failure, arrhythmias, pericarditis, MI extension, and cardiac arrest) and of the arterial line (e.g., thrombus or emboli).

3. Name the potential problems/complications. For example, if someone is taking an anticoagulant, the person has a potential for bleeding.

⏼ CLINICAL REASONING EXERCISES

Find example responses in Appendix I (page 223).

Read the following scenarios and then complete the instructions that follow them.

SCENARIO ONE
You just admitted Nigel to the psychiatric unit. He is agitated but won't talk to anyone. You check previous records and note that he has a history of striking caregivers.

Write a summary statement that best describes the potential problem in the previous scenario. Alternatively, draw a map or diagram.

SCENARIO TWO
Elaine is in the recovery room after having an emergency appendectomy under general anesthesia. She's very groggy and extremely nauseated.

Predict Elaine's potential complications.

SCENARIO THREE
Susan is a single working mother of three children. She tells you that she has never been a very organized person and is having trouble coping with the many demands on her time. Her children look healthy and happy, but her house is cluttered and she appears disheveled.

Write a summary statement that best describes the problem, using the PRE (problem, related [risk] factors, evidence) format.

SCENARIO FOUR
Imagine that you're caring for a 41-year-old man with four fractured ribs.

What other information do you need to determine whether he is at high risk for respiratory problems?

SKILL 6.13:   Setting Priorities

Definition

In this section, setting priorities is defined in two ways: (1) differentiating between problems needing immediate attention and those requiring subsequent action, and (2) deciding what problems must be addressed in the patient record.

Why This Skill Is Needed for Clinical Reasoning

This skill is important for the following reasons:

- **If you don't know how to set priorities, you may cause life-threatening treatment delays.** For example, if you don't assign high priority to dealing with symptoms of congestive heart failure (CHF), it can rapidly progress to pulmonary edema and death.

- **If you give equal attention to major and minor problems, you may not have the time you need to manage the most important ones.** Not only will your patients suffer, but you will constantly feel disorganized and overwhelmed.
- **All problems that must be managed to achieve the overall outcomes must be recorded in the patient record.**

Guidelines: How to Set Priorities

NOTE: "Managing Your Time" (Skill 7.6 in Chapter 7) gives more strategies for setting priorities inside and outside of the clinical setting. Chapter 4 details how to set priorities to delegate safely and effectively (page 109).

1. Ask patients to name two main problems they are experiencing right now.
2. Apply the *20/80 Rule* (you have 100% of things you need to do; determine the 20% that *must* be done now and the 80% that can wait).
3. Apply the principles and strategies described in the following shaded section.

Setting Priorities: Principles and Strategies

Principles of Setting Priorities

- **Setting priorities is a fluid, changing process.** The order of priority changes, depending on the seriousness and relationship of the problems. *Example:* If abnormal lab values are at life-threatening levels, they are likely to be highest priority; if your patient is having trouble breathing because of acute rib pain, managing the pain may be a higher priority than dealing with a rapid pulse, because the pain is causing the rapid pulse.
- **Setting priorities requires:**
  - **Understanding the "the big picture" of all the patient's problems** (e.g., having a multi-disciplinary list of current nursing problems, medical problems, and treatment regimens; knowing the *overall* expected outcomes of care).
  - **Determining the relationships among the problems:** If problem Y causes problem Z, problem Y takes priority over problem Z. *Example:* If pain is causing immobility, pain management is a high priority.
  - **Choosing an appropriate method of assigning priorities.** For example, for identifying initial urgent priorities, some nurses use the ABC method (make sure the patient has no threats to *Airway, Breathing, or Circulation*); emergency department health teams focus on prioritizing care to save *life, limbs, and vision*.
- **Maslow's Hierarchy of Needs**, as follows, is a helpful model for setting priorities, especially when answering question on the NCLEX.[2]

  Priority 1. Physiological needs—Life-threatening problems (or risk factors) posing a threat to physiological needs (e.g., problems with breathing, circulation, nutrition, hydration, elimination, temperature regulation, physical comfort)

  Priority 2. Safety and security—Problems (or risk factors) posing a threat to safety and security (e.g., environmental hazards, fear)

  Priority 3. Love and belonging—Problems (or risk factors) posing a threat to feeling loved and a part of something (e.g., isolation or loss of a loved one)

  Priority 4. Self-esteem—Problems (or risk factors) posing a threat to self-esteem (e.g., inability to perform normal activities)

  Priority 5. Personal goals—Problems (or risk factors) posing a threat to the ability to achieve personal goals

Steps for Setting Priorities

1. **Ensure patient and caregiver safety and prevention of infection transmission.**
2. **Assign high priority to first-level priority problems (immediate priorities): Remember "ABCs plus V and L" as listed next.** *Exception:* With cardiopulmonary resuscitation (CPR) for cardiac arrest, start chest compressions before giving breaths of air (for up-to-date CPR guidelines, see http://www.americanheart.org).

   Airway problems

   Breathing problems

   Cardiac and **c**irculation problems

   +

   Vital signs concerns (e.g., fever, hypertension, hypotension)

   Lab values that are life threatening (e.g., low blood sugar)
3. **Attend to second-level priority problems:**
   - Mental status change (e.g., confusion, decreased alertness)
   - Medical problems requiring immediate attention (e.g., a diabetic who hasn't had insulin)
   - Pain
   - Urinary elimination problems
4. **Address third-level priority problems (later priorities):**
   - Health problems that don't fit into the earlier categories (e.g., problems with lack of knowledge, activity, rest, family coping)

❓ CLINICAL REASONING EXERCISES

Find example responses in Appendix I (page 223).

1. If the expected outcome is *will be discharged home in 5 days and able to manage colostomy care,* which of the following problems must be addressed in the patient record?
   a. Anxiety related to inability to return to work for 6 weeks
   b. Patient education: Colostomy care
   c. Pressure ulcer related to colostomy drainage
2. What is the most immediate priority in the following scenario?

SCENARIO

Mr. Potter, a 64-year-old construction worker, is admitted with right calf thrombophlebitis. He is a smoker and has a cold, which is causing frequent sneezing and a productive cough. The doctor has ordered bed rest, warm soaks, and anticoagulants, with bathroom privileges for bowel movements only. Mr. Potter tells you he needs to use the bathroom. Then he mentions that he has been having chest discomfort.

SKILL 6.14: Determining Patient-Centered (Client-Centered) Outcomes

Definition

Describing exactly what results will be observed in the patient to show the expected benefits of care at a certain point in time. *Example:* Twenty-four hours after endotracheal intubation for open-heart surgery, the patient will be able to breathe independently without the tube.

Why This Skill Is Needed for Clinical Reasoning

On a daily basis, outcomes (results) are often implied—if you're doing something to fix a problem, you obviously expect to see an improvement in the problem. However, in complex situations, outcomes are stated according to very specific rules, Identifying individualized patient-centered outcomes promotes efficiency because it helps you:

- Explain why the treatment plan is worthwhile (they outline the expected benefits of care).
- Pay attention to *individual* patient responses.
- Motivate key players—knowing the benefits and time frame for outcome achievement prompts patients and caregivers to initiate actions in a timely fashion.
- Determine priorities (you need to know the *overall expected outcomes* of care before you can decide what's most important and what must be done first).
- Determine specific interventions designed to achieve the outcomes.

Guidelines: How to Determine Patient-Centered (Client-Centered) Outcomes

1. **Partner with the patient and caregivers to develop outcomes together.** Be realistic, considering:
   - Physical health state; overall prognosis
   - Growth and development; psychological/mental status
   - Spiritual, cultural, and economic needs
   - Expected length of stay
   - Available human, material, and financial resources
   - Other planned therapies for the client
2. **Realize that expected outcomes may be identified** from a **problem** or **intervention** perspective, as follows:
   - **Outcomes identified for problems** describe exactly what will be observed in the patient to show that the problems are resolved (or managed). For example, what will be observed when a patient no longer has trouble feeding himself or herself?
   - **Outcomes identified for interventions** describe the desired response to the intervention. For example, what will be observed in the patient after you irrigate the nasogastric tube?

GUIDING PRINCIPLE

There are dynamic relationships among problems, interventions, and outcomes. If you aren't achieving desired outcomes, ask questions like, "Are we sure that we identified the problems correctly?" "Have we tailored these outcomes to this patient's individual circumstances?" and "Are the outcomes realistic and has the patient been included determining them?"

---

3. **To determine expected outcomes for problems. Reverse the problem—describe what will** be observed in the patient when the problem no longer exists or is managed at an acceptable level (see the following diagram).

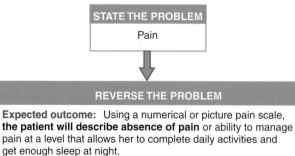

STATE THE PROBLEM
Pain

REVERSE THE PROBLEM
Expected outcome: Using a numerical or picture pain scale, **the patient will describe absence of pain** or ability to manage pain at a level that allows her to complete daily activities and get enough sleep at night.

4. **To determine expected outcomes for interventions.** Describe what will be observed in the patient to demonstrate that the desired response to the intervention has been achieved (see the following diagram).

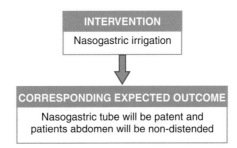

5. **To ensure that outcomes are specific,** they should have the following components:
   - **Subject:** Who is expected to achieve the outcome? Or what part of the patient will be observed to demonstrate the expected benefit?
   - **Verb:** What will the person do (or what will be observed) to demonstrate outcome achievement?
   - **Condition:** Under what circumstances will the person do it?
   - **Performance Criteria:** How well will the person do it?
   - **Target Time:** By when will the person be able to do it?

   Examples: "By Friday, Jim will walk with a walker to the end of the hall." Or, "By Friday, the skin on the bottom of the heel will be intact and free from signs of irritation."

6. **Use observable, measurable verbs** (verbs that describe things you can clearly see, hear, feel, or smell).
   - **Use verbs like these:** Explain, describe, state, list, demonstrate, show, communicate, express, walk, gain, and lose.
   - **Don't use verbs like these:** Know, understand, appreciate, feel (these aren't measurable because no one can read someone else's mind to find out if they know, understand, appreciate, and so on).

7. **In complex cases, develop both short- and long-term outcomes. Use short-term outcomes as stepping stones to long-term outcomes.** *Examples:* (Short term) "After 1 week, Fred will be able to bathe and dress himself with assistance." (Long term) "After 4 weeks, Fred will be totally independent in performing his morning care."

Use SMART to remember key features of expected outcomes:
   Specific
   Measurable
   Agreed upon by all parties
   Realistic
   Time-bound

---

8. **To give a summary statement that guides evaluation, use "as evidenced by" to describe exactly what behaviors will indicate that the outcome has been met.** *Example:* "The patient will demonstrate diabetes management as evidenced by the ability to state how insulin works, perform glucose monitoring, adjust insulin dose according to blood sugar level, and use sterile injection technique."

❓ CLINICAL REASONING EXERCISES

Find example responses in Appendix I (page 223).

Determine a specific, client-centered outcome for each of the following:

1. Pressure ulcer related to age, obesity, and prolonged bed rest
2. Suction patient PRN (as needed)
3. Irrigate Foley catheter every 4 hours
4. Endotracheal intubation
5. Leg muscle weakness related to prolonged bed rest as evidenced by inability to walk the length of the hall without assistance

---

SKILL 6.15:   Determining Individualized Interventions

Definition

Identifying specific nursing actions that are tailored to the patient's needs and desires and are designed to (1) prevent, manage, and eliminate problems and risk factors; (2) reduce the likelihood of undesired outcomes and increase the likelihood of desired outcomes; and (3) promote health and independence.

Why This Skill Is Needed for Clinical Reasoning

To prevent and resolve health problems, you must know how to develop safe, individualized interventions that are specific to each patient's particular situation. Focusing on individual patient needs and desires gives the patient a sense of autonomy and helps you design a plan that's more likely to be followed. Knowing how to tailor the interventions to increase the likelihood of success and decrease the likelihood of harm is the key to safety, efficiency, and patient satisfaction.

Guidelines: How to Determine Individualized Interventions

1. **Involve patients, families, and caregivers in decision-making early.** They are the ones who can help you tailor interventions in ways that are likely to succeed. Tell patients that your role is not only to take care of them but also to help them know how to take care of themselves when you're not there.
2. **Identify interventions that aim to monitor and manage both the problems and their underlying contributing factors.**

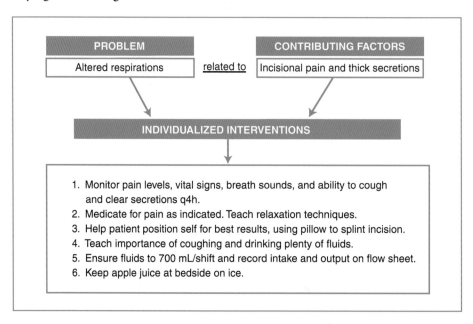

3. **Give high priority to designing interventions aimed at managing the factors that are contributing to the problems.** For example, if your patient does not move or cough well after surgery because of incisional pain, a high-priority intervention will be to manage the pain.

GUIDING PRINCIPLE

Be sure that your independent interventions aren't attempting to treat a problem that needs medical management by a more qualified professional. *Example:* Unrelieved pain may indicate there's a life-threatening problem that needs immediate medical attention; continuing to treat the pain may mask critical symptoms and put the patient at significant risk.

---

4. **Identify the problems and risk factors that must be monitored and managed to achieve the overall outcomes, and then ask the following:**
   - "How will we monitor the status of the problems and risk factors?" ("What will we assess?" "Who will assess it?" "How often will we assess it?" "How will assessments be recorded?")
   - "What must be done to (1) manage or eliminate the risk (contributing) factors?" (2) "Manage or eliminate the problems?" (3) "Promote safety and reduce risk for harm?" (4) "Teach the person what he or she needs to know to be independent?"
5. **Consider the interventions you identified, and ask the following:**
   - "Have I predicted the *expected benefits* for this particular patient?"
   - "Have I predicted *undesired responses* and identified ways to minimize them?"
   - "Do I know the level of evidence that supports getting the desired results to my interventions in this situation?" *Example:* "Are your interventions recommended by textbooks? By policies, procedures, or standard plans? By clinical practice guidelines?"
   - "Have I weighed the risks of the intervention against the benefits?"
   - "What can we do to increase the likelihood of getting desired results and reduce the risk for doing harm (getting undesirable results) in this specific patient's situation?"
6. **Remember the PPMP (predict, prevent, manage, promote) approach:**
   - **Predict potential complications, and be ready to manage them.** Sometimes you can't do much about the cause of the problems, but you can prevent and manage the symptoms and potential complications of the problems. *Example:* If someone has just had his jaws wired shut, you can't do much about it, but you must be prepared to handle the potential complication of aspiration by having suction equipment and wire cutters nearby.
   - **Identify interventions that not only treat problems and risk factors but also promote optimum function, independence, and well-being.** *Example:* Stress the benefits of walking at least 20 minutes a day. Be sure that patients have a paper and pen to write down things they need to remember. Ask patients what you can do to make things more convenient for them.
7. **Keep in mind both direct-care interventions (things you do directly for or with the patient, such as helping him or her get out of bed) and indirect-care interventions** (things you do away from the patient, such as monitoring lab results).

GUIDING PRINCIPLE

When determining interventions, remember, SEE, DO, TEACH, RECORD: Consider what you need to see (assess), what you or the patient needs to do, what you need to teach, and what you must record. Example:
- **See:** Assess ability to walk with walker in the room before allowing the patient to go out in the hall alone.
- **Do:** Have him or her walk the length of the hall three times per day.
- **Teach:** Reinforce that research shows that walking will increase muscle strength and reduce fatigue.
- **Record:** Record pulse and blood pressure before and after walking at least once per day.

❓ CLINICAL REASONING EXERCISES

Find example responses in Appendix I (page 224).

1. Determine specific interventions for each of the following problems and corresponding outcomes.

Problem	Corresponding Expected Outcome
a. Risk for dehydration related to diarrhea and insufficient fluid intake	Will maintain adequate hydration as evidenced by drinking 4 quarts of clear liquids per 24-hour period
b. Risk for anxiety related to insufficient knowledge of hospital procedures	By the end of today, will relate knowledge of hospital procedures and express ways of managing anxiety
c. Pain related to arthritic joints as evidenced by statements of pain with range of motion for the past 20 years	After application of heat and assistance with range of motion, will rate pain on a scale of 0 to 10 and express that joint pain doesn't prohibit movement or sleep

2. Imagine you're doing a home visit with an 86-year-old woman who is asthmatic and is on chemotherapy for ovarian cancer. She is independent but likes to spend much of her day reading in bed. She is 5 feet tall and weighs 93 pounds. Determine all the factors she has that may contribute to a risk for pressure ulcer. Then decide what, if anything, will be done to manage each contributing factor.

3. Answer the questions after the following scenario.

SCENARIO

You make a home visit to a Russian family with three children, ages 5, 7, and 10. Their home is next to a forest full of deer ticks. The mother is upset because she keeps finding ticks on the children, and she knows Lyme disease comes from tick bites. She's told the children not to go into the forest, but she suspects they disregard her instructions. Now the mother is considering punishing the children when she finds a tick on them, hoping this will make them more careful.

You look up Lyme disease and learn that the best treatment is prevention of tick bites. You then identify the following problem and expected outcome:

Problem: Infection risk related to tick bites.

Expected outcome: The children will have a decreased risk for tick bites and infection as evidenced by their wearing insect repellent when outside, avoiding tall grassy areas, and monitoring themselves and each other for ticks.

a. What might happen if the children are punished when a tick is found on them?
b. What might happen if you reward the children for finding ticks?
c. What interventions might safely motivate the children to participate in spotting ticks and avoiding bites?
d. What specific interventions could you use to achieve the expected outcome listed for this situation?

SKILL 6.16:   Evaluating and Correcting Thinking (Self-Regulating)

Definition

Reflecting on your thinking for the purpose of ensuring accuracy, safety, and improvement—for example, looking for flaws, deciding whether your thinking is focused, clear, and in enough depth—and then making adjustments as needed.

Why This Skill Is Needed for Clinical Reasoning

Developing sound clinical reasoning skills requires you to self-regulate, which means reflecting on your thinking and asking yourself questions like, "How clear am I about what's going on here?" "What could I be missing?" "How can I be sure that my reasoning is correct?" "Am I holding myself to high standards?" "Do I know what I'll do if things go wrong?" "What creative approaches might work here?" "What peers or experts can I get to dialogue with me so that I better understand the thinking that should go into a situation like this?"

Guidelines: How to Evaluate and Correct Thinking (Self-Regulating)

Evaluating and correcting thinking is an ongoing process. Because the nursing process is a major tool for clinical reasoning, the following shaded section gives example questions you should be asking at various phases of ADPIE.

Questions to Ask to Reflect on Reasoning

Assessment and Diagnosis
- To what degree were the patient and key stakeholders involved in the process?
- How well do I understand my patient's perceptions, wants, and needs?
- What assumptions could I have made?
- How complete is data collection?
- How accurate and reliable is my information?
- How sure am I of the conclusions I've drawn?
- Should I be reporting some signs and symptoms immediately—could this be a medical problem that requires more qualified management?
- How well does the patient's data support that the problems I identified are correct?
- Have I missed any other problems that could be indicated by the patient's data? What alternate problems/hypotheses should I consider?
- How well have I identified underlying causes, contributing factors, and risk factors?
- Have I identified both nursing problems and problems requiring a multidisciplinary approach?
- Were patient strengths and resources identified?
- Have I made sure that safety issues and patient education needs were identified?

Planning
- To what degree did I involve the patient and key stakeholders in setting priorities and developing the plan?
- Have I missed any problems that must be addressed in the plan of care?
- How well do the outcomes reflect the expected benefits of care?
- Are the expected outcomes realistic, clear, and client-centered?
- Have I considered the undesired responses to interventions and identified interventions to reduce the likelihood of them happening?
- Did I consider both the problems and the outcomes when identifying interventions?
- Did I consider client preferences when developing the plan?
- Have I anticipated patient responses and individualized interventions to this specific patient and situation?

Implementation
- How well did I involve the patient in daily decision-making?
- How well am I monitoring patient responses?
- What is the status of the problems identified during assessment and diagnosis?
- Am I missing any new problems?

Continued

Questions to Ask to Reflect On Reasoning—cont'd

- Should I be doing anything differently? Are the interventions still appropriate?
- Do I need to address any safety issues?
- Have I identified and recorded changes we need to make?

Evaluation
- Where does the patient stand in relation to achieving major desired outcomes?
- How accurately and completely have I completed each of the previous phases?
- What suggestions do the patient and key stakeholders have for improvement?

There are no Clinical Reasoning Exercises for this skill, because opportunities for evaluating and correcting thinking have been provided throughout the other skills sections.

SKILL 6.17: Determining a Comprehensive Plan/Evaluating and Updating the Plan

Definition

Ensuring that the priority problems and corresponding outcomes and interventions are recorded on the patient record; keeping the plan up to date.

Why This Skill Is Needed for Clinical Reasoning

Developing a comprehensive plan and ensuring that the major care plan components are recorded (1) forces you to think about the most important aspects of giving care; (2) promotes communication between caregivers; and (3) provides data for evaluation, research, legal, and insurance purposes.

Guidelines: How to Develop a Comprehensive Plan/Update the Plan

1. Recognize that determining a comprehensive plan requires all of the previous skills listed here, as well as understanding the purpose and components of the recorded plan.

Purpose and Components of Plan of Care

Purpose
1. Promotes communication between caregivers
2. Directs care, interventions, and documentation
3. Creates a record that later can be used for evaluation, research, legal, and insurance purposes

Care Plan Components (use the memory jog EASE)
   Expected outcomes
   Actual and potential problems that must be addressed to reach overall outcomes
   Specific interventions designed to achieve the outcomes
   Evaluation statements (progress notes)

2. Identify the major problems and interventions yourself. Then:
   - Check the patient record to see whether your patient's problems and interventions are addressed by pre-established plans, policies, or doctor's orders.
   - Compare your patient's situation with the interventions on pre-established plans.
   - Modify or add interventions if needed (e.g., your patient may have mobility issues that need to be added to the pre-established plan).
   - Update the patient records to ensure that any new problems, risk factors, or interventions are communicated in the appropriate place.

🔍 CLINICAL REASONING EXERCISES

Find example responses in Appendix I (page 224).

1. Consider each of the following expected outcomes and corresponding patient data and decide whether the outcome has been achieved, partially achieved, or not achieved.

   a. **Expected outcome:** Will manage own wound care by day 3 after surgery as evidenced by ability to demonstrate how to manage wound packing. **Data:** Patient says that managing wound packing shouldn't be his concern and feels he's incapable of doing so.

   b. **Expected outcome:** Will drink at least 4 quarts of fluid as evidenced by keeping a written record of fluid intake. **Data:** Patient's record indicates 5 quarts of fluid intake daily.

   c. **Expected outcome:** The baby will be discharged home with parents able to perform CPR. **Data:** Father demonstrates CPR well. Mother has trouble establishing airway.

2. Identify two priority problems in following scenario; then develop a comprehensive plan to resolve the problems. Include an overall expected discharge outcome, outcomes for each problem, and specific interventions.

SCENARIO

It's Monday, June 29. You admit Mrs. Ankiel, who has just suffered anaphylactic shock after a bee sting. She is expected to be discharged by Tuesday, June 30. The doctor gives Mrs. Ankiel an emergency epinephrine injection kit and tells her, "The nurse will teach you how to use it." Mrs. Ankiel still has hives all over her body and says her itching feet are driving her crazy. You find that placing her feet in cool water every so often helps her discomfort. She is still slightly wheezy from the bee sting reaction.

When you ask her about using the injection kit, she replies, "No way!" Her husband, who is retired, says, "I'll be glad to learn." It's decided that it's satisfactory to discharge Mrs. Ankiel on June 30, with her husband able to demonstrate how to give epinephrine in an emergency.

---

3. Suppose a protocol on the EHR states that on the first day after surgery, your patient should have the Foley catheter out and be voiding normally. It's now the second day after surgery, and when you check the intake and output record, you see that she is voiding 30 mL every hour. What should you do, and why?

4. Suppose you're reviewing someone's chart to determine whether a satisfactory plan of care is present. What four care plan components will you look for?

REFERENCES

1. NCSBN. Measuring the right things. In: *Focus (Winter)*. 2018:12.

2. Maslow A. *Motivation in personality*. New York: Harper & Row; 1970.

Interprofessional Practice Skills: Communication, Teamwork, and Self-Management

LEARNING OUTCOMES

After completing this chapter, you should be able to:

1. Explain why communication, teamwork, and self-management skills are central to interprofessional practice.
2. Demonstrate achievement of the outcomes listed at the beginning of each skill in this chapter.

3. Use specific strategies that help you succeed as a team member or leader.

KEY CONCEPTS

Change; conflict; constructive feedback; customer service; empowered partnerships; patient satisfaction; teamwork; time management. *See also previous chapters.*

HOW TO USE THIS CHAPTER

This chapter helps you develop interpersonal, teamwork, and self-management skills—for example, managing your time and learning how to get past "the sting" of criticism so that it helps you grow. When you know how to communicate effectively and build positive relationships with patients and team members, you spend less time getting sidetracked by interpersonal and "human nature" problems and more time fully engaged in progress.

HOW THE SKILLS ARE ORGANIZED

Listed in alphabetical order, each skill is presented in the following format: (1) name of the skill, (2) definition of the skill, (3) learning outcomes, (4) thinking critically about the skill, (5) how to accomplish the skill, and (6) critical thinking exercises. To promote in-depth discussion and learning, content is presented in a way that can help you plan a seminar for each skill. In addition to reviewing the recommended resources at the end of each skill, seminar participants should search the Internet, especially YouTube, for related resources and videos. **There are no example responses for this chapter** because all of the exercises are Think, Pair, Share exercises.

SKILL 7.1: Communicating Bad News

Definition

Knowing how to convey honesty, empathy, and responsibility when giving information that may have a negative impact on someone.

Learning Outcomes

After completing this section, you should be able to:
1. Explain what happens when you avoid giving bad news.
2. Identify strategies to help people deal with the impact of getting bad news.
3. Determine how you can reduce your stress when faced with giving bad news.
4. Improve your ability to give bad news.

Thinking Critically About Giving Bad News

No one likes to give bad news because no one likes to get it. Too often, we avoid this unpleasant task altogether (and run the risk of making things worse). You may not be the one who actually gives the bad news—for example, cancer diagnoses are given by physicians only; organ donation is requested by organ transplant team members—but you're likely to be the one who needs to be there to help patients *deal with the impact* of the bad news.

Getting bad news may be better than getting *no* news. Researchers report that uncertainty about a diagnosis causes more anxiety and can be more stressful than actually knowing that you have a serious illness. Once people have a diagnosis, they usually gain some understanding and control. Whether you're dealing with life-threatening or patient satisfaction issues, knowing how to give bad news can make the difference between making a difficult situation worse and giving patients and families the information and support they need.

How to Give Bad News

The following gives guidelines for giving bad news in two different situations: (1) giving bad news related to health status (Table 7.1) and (2) giving bad news related to patient satisfaction issues (Table 7.2).

TABLE 7.1 Giving Bad News Related to Health Status	
Steps	**Rationale**
1. **Determine who has the authority and qualifications to give the bad news.** Usually, this is the primary care provider, such as the doctor or nurse practitioner.	**Most organizations have policies related to who can give patients certain information.** Depending on the impact of the news (e.g., if the news is about biopsy results, severe illness, or death), the patient and family are likely to have questions that must be answered by the most qualified professional. Always check your facility's policies regarding patient confidentiality and Health Insurance Portability and Accountability Act (HIPAA) privacy laws.

Continued

TABLE 7.1   Giving Bad News Related to Health Status—cont'd

Steps	Rationale
2. **Have the professional who is best qualified (or who has developed the best relationship with the person) give the news.**	**The messenger matters.** Bad news is often met with powerful emotions of disappointment and anger. Receiving bad news in a caring, straightforward way from trusted professionals softens the blow. It's easy to feel that a provider who is too busy to give the bad news has betrayed you. It takes a strong, logical mind not to want to "shoot the messenger." Making sure that those who know the patient best—for example, a trusted nurse or a chaplain—are present helps reduce feelings of being abandoned or helpless.
3. **Choose the setting—ensure privacy, and avoid using the phone.**	**How and where the person gets bad news matters.** Using the phone doesn't allow for appropriate assessment and support.
4. **Find out what the person already knows or suspects.**	**This simplifies the process** and helps clarify what you need to say.
5. **Give a warning shot.**	**Saying things like, "I have bad news" or "I'm sorry to have to tell you this"** prepares people for the emotional blow they are about to receive.
6. **Be direct, tell the news, and give time for it to sink in.** (Silence is golden.)	**Being direct helps people get the main information first, in a logical way.** Bad news takes time to digest—patients often need to get through shock and anger before they can move on to dealing with the impact of the news. Sometimes, all that is needed is someone to remain present, listening quietly as feelings are sorted out. You have to name the feelings before you can tame them.
7. **Respond to emotions with empathy.** Continue to use silence as a strategy. Use nonverbal gestures, as appropriate (e.g., put a hand on the person's shoulder). Help the person deal with feelings of blame.	**Each person is unique, with a range of emotional responses.** Letting people know that their emotions are understood helps them deal with strong feelings. Think about this analogy: Aspirin reduces fever and physical discomfort. Being allowed to express thoughts and feelings reduces anxiety and psychological discomfort. Bad news often brings feelings of blame. *Examples of statements that convey empathy and reduce blame:* "I'm sorry this is happening." "There's nothing that could have been done." "This is no one's fault." "It's not worth blaming … it will only make things worse … we need to deal with the problem." "We'll help you through this." *Examples of statements that don't help:* "I know how you feel." "It's God's will." "God only gives you what you can bear."
8. **Ask whether there are any questions or special requests**, especially related to spiritual and cultural needs.	**Hearing their questions and special requests helps you identify their most important needs.** Nurses are accountable for paying attention to spiritual and cultural needs. *Examples:* "Tell me what we can do right now for you." "Is there someone we can call?" "Do you have a specific religion?" "Can I get the hospital chaplain?" "What can I do?"
9. **Keep a positive tone, be realistic, and give hope.** End with a plan, and be sure the person has a printed list of resources.	**Having hope and hearing a realistic, positive attitude sets the tone for dealing with the bad news.** Hope is the "tonic" that sustains people through difficult times. *Examples:* "This is tough news … but having a positive attitude is important." "Don't jump to conclusions or let yourself be driven by worst-case scenarios." "Don't give up hope … we'll use all our resources." Having a plan mobilizes the patient and team toward dealing with the problem. A printed list of resources is essential for later, when the patient goes home, the information sinks in, and the patient starts thinking independently about how to handle the problem.
10. **Follow up** to see how things are going.	Some people may need more direction and support than others. Don't assume. Find out how they're doing.

Source: © 2018 R. Alfaro-LeFevre. http://www.AlfaroTeachSmart.com

TABLE 7.2 Giving Bad News Related to Consumer and Patient Satisfaction Issues	
Steps	**Example**
1. **Give bad news in a timely way.** Offer an apology, and don't try to hide the situation.	**"I'm sorry to tell you** we won't be able to do your x-ray today."
2. **Showing accountability, explain what happened and why.**	**"Your appointment card says today, but** somehow we have you scheduled in our book for next week. I'm not sure how this happened, but you can be sure that I'll find out."
3. **Pause to give the person a chance to express thoughts and feelings.** Listen attentively.	Silence of 3–5 seconds encourages the person to gather his or her thoughts and speak his or her mind and tell you what's most important.
4. **Present alternative solutions, and give pros and cons of each.** Get the patient's point of view.	**"I could schedule the x-ray for later today, but** we get better pictures if you fast for 12 hours before the x-ray. I realize you'd have to go home and come back and that you'd like to get it over with. I think it's worth waiting to be sure we get a good-quality x-ray. Would that be okay for you?"
5. **Recommend a course of action.** Include (a) how the plan addresses the problem and (b) how the plan addresses hardships resulting from what happened.	**"I think the best solution is** to schedule the x-ray as soon as possible. Because you've already had enough problems, I'll do my best to schedule you whenever it's convenient for you. I'll also find out who made this mistake and see what we can do to prevent this from happening again."
6. **Reaffirm your goals and vision for the future.** Include (a) key points that give confidence to those involved and (b) the time frame for expected results.	**"We're here to serve you the best way we can.** Soon we'll have a system that allows you to confirm appointments over the phone. We hope to have the system in place by May. Everyone will be encouraged to call and confirm their appointments when they get home."
7. **Follow up** to see if results were satisfactory.	**"I'm notifying our community relations department.** They'll call you to see if everything was resolved to your satisfaction. Please feel free to call and discuss anything you'd like with them too. We want you to feel satisfied with your experience with us. Please let me know if you still have problems."

Source: © 2018 R. Alfaro-LeFevre http://www.AlfaroTeachSmart.com.

CRITICAL THINKING EXERCISES

 Think, Pair, Share

With a partner, in a group, or in a journal entry:
1. Watch some of the videos on YouTube for giving bad news. Then discuss the following:
   - Your best and worst experiences with how someone gave you bad news
   - The emotions you feel when giving bad news
   - Your experiences with how people have responded to getting bad news
   - The similarities and differences between giving bad news related to patient satisfaction and giving bad news related to health status
2. Imagine that you have to tell someone that his mother has been admitted to the intensive care unit after a car accident. Using the steps for giving bad news related to health status in Table 7.1, develop a plan for how you will do this.
3. Imagine you have to tell someone that she has to wait 2 hours to see the doctor because the doctor has other urgent problems. Using the steps for giving bad news related to patient satisfaction issues in Table 7.2, develop a plan for how you'll do this.
4. Discuss where you stand in relation to achieving the learning outcomes listed at the beginning of this skill.

Recommended

Bumb M, Keefe J, Miller L, Overcash J. Breaking bad news: an evidence-based review of communication models for oncology nurses. *CJON* 2017;21(5):573–580. doi: 10.1188/17.CJON.573-580

Meyer E. *On being present, not perfect.* 2015. Retrieved from https://ceagent.com/tag/ted-talk/

Raymond R. Breaking bad news to patients: experts offer best practices. 2017. Retrieved from https://thedo.osteopathic.org/2017/02/how-to-break-bad-news-to-patients-experts-offer-best-practices/

See also Recommended in the next skill.

SKILL 7.2:   Dealing With Complaints Constructively

Definition

Using complaints as an opportunity to identify system issues and improve or restore patient/consumer satisfaction.

Learning Outcomes

After completing this section, you should be able to:
1. Explain the value of complaints.
2. Identify strategies for dealing with difficult patients and consumers.
3. Express more confidence about dealing with complaints.

Thinking Critically About Complaints

Dealing with complaints makes most of us uncomfortable—and often defensive. But complaints are actually an opportunity to improve both patient satisfaction and system problems.

Complaints help you:
1. Correct problems before they become worse or happen to someone else.
2. Identify trends in unmet needs of patients and consumers.
3. Respond in ways that let consumers know their experience matters to you and your organization.
4. Find out about complaints before people start complaining to others.

Whether you're dealing with mildly frustrated individuals or aggressive people who seem to be looking for a reason to be mad, keeping your emotions in check, using specific strategies, and staying focused on common goals help you improve satisfaction and reduce your stress.

How to Deal With Complaints Constructively

1. **You often can soothe angry people with just a little affirmation of their problem and a commitment to solve it.** For example, "I understand this is upsetting. Let me see what I can do."
2. **Don't take things personally.** Pay attention to what is being said and rein in the natural tendency to be defensive; assume there's a good reason for the complaints (these reasons may be unclear at first).
3. **Use the following approach to recover trust and satisfaction.**

> **Managing complaints: LAST (Listen, Apologize, Solve, and Thank)**[1]
> **Listen.** Encourage patients/consumers to clarify what happened (e.g., "Help me understand what happened"). Listen attentively and avoid placing blame, becoming defensive, or thinking of excuses.

Apologize. Be sincere about being sorry for the person's experience. You may not be admitting guilt; you're apologizing on behalf of the organization.

Solve. Make sure you understand the problem from the patient/consumer's perspective; then do something to solve it or find someone who can. Ask the person what you can do to make it right; tell him or her what you're going to do, and report back once you've done it.

Thank. Thank the person for bringing the issue to your attention and for his or her patience and understanding.

4. If you come in late to the situation, stay quiet, listen, and ask to verify your understanding of the problem.
5. Try to learn from the patient/consumer's experience; treat them as though they were your favorite celebrity, hero, friend, neighbor, or your grandmother.

CRITICAL THINKING EXERCISES

Think, Pair, Share

With a partner, in a group, or in a journal entry:

1. Discuss the strategies in the following video: *How to give great customer service: The LAST method.* (Website). Retrieved from https://www.engvid.com/how-to-give-great-customer-service-the-last-method/.
2. Imagine this: Someone tells you one of your patients has numerous complaints. You go to the room, introduce yourself, and ask about the problem. The patient's wife immediately becomes hostile and tells you to "just get out." What do you do and why?
3. Share how you feel when you have made complaints (e.g., angry, guilty, frustrated).
4. Give an example of a time when you thought about complaining but decided it wasn't worth it. How did this make you feel? Who lost the most in this situation?
5. Describe your best and worst experiences with making a complaint.
6. Decide where you stand in relation to achieving the learning outcomes listed at the beginning of this skill.

Recommended

Doyles A. *Nurse interview questions about patient complaints.* 2018. Retrieved from https://www.thebalancecareers.com/nurse-interview-questions-about-patient-complaints-2062663

Texas Medical Association. *How to handle patient complaints.* 2017. Retrieved from http://www.texmed.org/Template.aspx?id=4110

How to deal with patient complaints. 2015. Retrieved from https://blog.jobmedic.co.uk/how-to-deal-with-patient-complaints

See also Recommended in Skill 7.1 ("Communicating Bad News") and Skill 7.5 ("Managing Conflict Constructively").

SKILL 7.3:   Developing Empowered Partnerships

Definition

Building mutually beneficial relationships based on the belief that people have the right and the responsibility to make their own choices.[2]

Learning Outcomes

After completing this section, you should be able to:
1. Compare and contrast a parental model and an empowered partnership model.
2. Explain the benefits of empowered partnerships.
3. Identify ways to deal with barriers to developing empowered partnerships.
4. Build empowered partnerships with patients, families, colleagues, and peers.

Thinking Critically About Building Empowered Partnerships

Developing empowered partnerships with peers, colleagues, and patients requires a shift in thinking from a parental model ("I'll take care of you") to an empowered partnership model ("It's your life, and you have rights and responsibilities as well as I do; we both should grow and learn from our experience together"). Table 7.3 lists phrases that illustrate these two models.

Because partnering with patients and families is the key to getting the results you need, it's also central to critical thinking. From getting mutual agreement on desired outcomes to identifying care approaches, apply the saying, "Nothing about me without me." Keep patients involved in all decision-making.

How to Develop Empowered Partnerships

1. **Be sure you can explain the concept of an empowered partnership as described in this section.** While you can't balance power in all relationships—for example, in adult–child partnerships, adults have more power—the goal is to balance the power *as much as possible*. The following are examples of empowered partnerships:
   - Nurse–patient (or client)/Nurse–family
   - Educator–learner/Preceptor–new nurse
   - Nurse–nurse/Nurse manager–staff nurse/Nurse–unlicensed worker
   - Nurse–physician/Nurse–dietitian
2. **As much as possible, get agreement from partners on the following statements:**
   - "We're both clear about our joint purpose, and we're both responsible."
   - "I can be trusted; I promise to be honest."
   - "We should make decisions together as much as possible."
   - "We'll both agree to rules for resolving conflict between us."
   - "We both should expect to grow and learn from our experience together."
   - "We're each responsible for our own emotional well-being (if I feel bad about something, it's my responsibility to do something about it)."
   - "We both have the right to say no, so long as no harm is done."
   - "I choose to be here, so nobody's to blame."
   - "If one of us sees the other engage in unsafe or unethical conduct, we have the responsibility to address it appropriately."
   - "We're both responsible for the outcomes (consequences) of our actions."

TABLE 7.3 **Parental Versus Empowered Partnership Model**	
Parental Model	**Empowered Partnership**
I want to look after you.	How can I empower you to be able to be independent?
I know what's best for you.	You know yourself best. Tell me what you'd like to see happen, what's most important to you.
You should do as I say.	I want you to be able to make informed choices.
I'm responsible for you.	We share a common purpose, and we're both responsible for what happens.

NOTE: With nurse–patient relationships, the statements on the preceding page may not be so because nurses are often held more accountable than patients. For example, nurses don't have the right to say no if it jeopardizes patient care. Patients often have few choices about where they are.

3. **Make the choice to:**
   - Rise to the challenge of *taking charge* over the comfort of *remaining dependent*
   - Give up some of the power; take calculated, thoughtful risks; and be willing to do the work needed to be independent
4. **Aim to provide the following:**[2]
   - Nonjudgmental acceptance; space for self-expression
   - Respect for each other's boundaries; structure for conflict resolution
   - Encouragement for growth in the areas where one is limited (expect both partners to grow)
   - Coaching skills that transform (coaching that truly affects the learner's attitudes and skills)
5. **Recognize that people may be uncomfortable in an empowered partnership because they may be:**
   - Used to being taken care of and not accustomed to taking responsibility
   - Unwilling to accept the responsibility that comes with power
   - Unwilling to give up some of the power they're accustomed to having
   - Having difficulty making the required shift in thinking (they don't truly believe in the benefits of partnership)
6. **Coach those who aren't accustomed to the roles and responsibilities of being in a partnership** (this change takes time).
7. **Keep the focus on mutually agreed-upon outcomes**—these are what inspire you both to work together (e.g. we agreed you should be independent).

❓ CRITICAL THINKING EXERCISES

Think, Pair, Share

With a partner, in a group, or in a journal entry:
1. Discuss how establishing partnerships with peers is different from establishing partnerships with patients.
2. Address how establishing an empowered partnership is affected by the following:
   - How long you have contact with the patient (e.g., 1 day versus 1 week)
   - The patient's health state (e.g., critically ill versus independent)
   - Growth and development (e.g., How do you partner with a child or an elderly person?)
3. Explain what's meant by the following statement: Partnership is an attitude as much as a model for relationships.
4. Think of a time that you had to complete a complex task with someone. How did it go? What were the dynamics? Would you say that the experience was one of an empowered partnership? What went well, and what would you do differently if you did it again?
5. Decide where you stand in relation to achieving the learning outcomes listed at the beginning of this skill.

Recommended

Jethwani K, Sperber J. *Who gives us the right to "empower."* 2017. Retrieved from https://catalyst.nejm.org/gives-right-patient-empowerment/
The Empowered Patient Coalition (Website). Retrieved from http://empoweredpatientcoalition.org/
Greene J. *How to empower others in the workplace: a guide for support teams.* 2018. Retrieved from https://www.askspoke.com/blog/support/empower-others-workplace/

SKILL 7.4:   Giving and Taking Constructive Feedback

Definition

Being able to give (and respond to) comments about performance in ways that promote growth and improvement.

Learning Outcomes

After completing this section, you should be able to:

1. Discuss the effect of emotional responses to negative feedback.
2. Determine how you can turn feedback you receive into opportunities to grow.
3. Explain why being uncomfortable with giving constructive feedback can lead to unsafe patient care and stunted growth.
4. Identify strategies for giving constructive feedback.

Thinking Critically About Giving and Taking Constructive Feedback

Giving constructive feedback is not easy. Receiving feedback that feels like you're being criticized can be devastating. Offering constructive feedback not only helps you avoid letting little issues become big ones; it's crucial to safe, effective care and performance improvement.

Consider the possible consequences related to safety and performance in the following examples of staff who avoid giving constructive feedback (taken from actual focus groups discussing factors that contribute to errors):[3]

- **Nurses focus group:** "A group of nurses describe a peer as careless and inattentive. Instead of confronting her, they double-check her work—sometimes running into patient rooms to re-take blood pressures or redo safety checks. They've 'worked around' this nurse's weakness for over a year. The nurses resent her but never talk to her about their concerns. Nor do any of the doctors who also avoid her and compensate for her."
- **Physicians focus group:** "A group of eight anesthesiologists agree a peer is dangerously incompetent, but they don't confront him. Instead, they go to great efforts to schedule surgeries for the sickest babies at times when he is not on duty. This problem has persisted for over 5 years."

Nothing makes people bristle more quickly than unfair, unskillful, or unsolicited criticism. Knowing how to give constructive feedback in a supportive way can make the difference between alienating others and helping them learn. Knowing how to respond to criticism—to be objective and work through the negative aspects of feedback—reduces your stress and helps you understand exactly what you need to work on.

GUIDING PRINCIPLE

Whether or not feedback is useful depends on the relationship you have with the person giving or receiving the feedback. Without mutual trust, feedback is unlikely to be viewed constructively.

How to Give and Take Constructive Feedback

The following gives strategies for giving and taking constructive feedback.

Giving Constructive Feedback

- **Before giving feedback,** think about how you can give it in a supportive way that focuses on the goal of improvement and success. Aim to give the feedback in the way a mentor or coach would give it, rather than a critic.

- State the *results* of the behavior you observe (what you see or hear). *Example:* "I don't mean to be critical, but when I care for the same patients you do, there's a lot of clutter at the bedside. I get overwhelmed because I need to feel organized when giving patient care."
- **Be sensitive to personality differences** (personalities of both the giver and the receiver of feedback greatly affect whether the feedback is viewed as constructive).
- **Give feedback frequently** and in a timely way (this way it's viewed as being more sincere); "catch" people being effective and reward them with positive feedback.
- **Start with what's being done right** (e.g., "Here are the things I see you do right"). Next, focus on what could be *improved* (rather than on what's *wrong*).
- **Stay fully engaged in the communication;** listen actively to avoid misunderstandings or make assumptions.
- **Be aware that constant negative feedback can hinder progress** by making people fear failure.
- **Replace the word *criticism*** with *feedback, advice, recommendation, suggestion, observation,* or *opinion* (e.g., "May I give you some advice?").
- **Change the word *constructive*** to *practical, helpful,* or *useful* (e.g., "May I give you some practical advice?").
- **Ask for permission or clarification** ("May I tell you what I see?" or "Help me understand what you're trying to do.").
- **Remember that compliments are energizing and "feed the soul"**; as Mark Twain said, "I can live for two months on a good compliment."

Taking Constructive Feedback

- **Keep in mind that receiving constructive feedback is a complex issue** that's closely linked to self-esteem. Being told that you could improve or do things differently often brings up feelings of being wrong or not good enough. These gut reactions cloud key issues and hinder your ability to be objective.
- **If you find yourself getting the intense negative feelings** that come with receiving negative feedback, say to yourself, "I'm getting upset. I'd better take a deep breath, calm down, and listen. If I work to be objective and not take things personally, I might learn something when I think about this later when I'm less stressed."
- **Learn to befriend negative feedback,** evaluating it objectively. Someone wants you to succeed, or she or he would not have bothered to share her of his thoughts. Not all feedback is given constructively, but try to focus on what you can learn.
- **Ask yourself, "Have I heard this same feedback** from other people?"
- **If you agree with the negative feedback**, acknowledge that the feedback is useful and think about what you can do about it.
- **Don't make excuses,** don't be defensive, and try to see the benefits of the feedback.
- **Practice personal feedback** by monitoring your own behavior and paying attention to how others respond to you.
- **Don't let false pride, rationalization, or other negative feelings get in the way** of your growth.
- **Remember that no one's perfect,** but we can all improve. Be prepared to expend some physical and emotional energy to change.
- **Don't dwell on negative feedback when you're tired**—wait until a day or two later when you're refreshed and more likely to be objective. *Example:* Suppose you give a group presentation and get some negative comments. If you revisit the evaluations a week after the presentation—when you're rested—you'll probably see what was valid criticism from the *group as a whole* and what was simply *one or two attendees' points of view.*

CRITICAL THINKING EXERCISES

Think, Pair, Share

With a partner, in a group, or in a journal entry:

1. Think about a time when someone gave you negative feedback. What happened, and how did you feel? What made things better or worse? What did you learn in the long run?
2. Recall a time when you tried to give constructive feedback to someone for the sake of improvement. What happened and how did you feel? Would you do it differently if you had to do it again?
3. One of my workshop participants told me that one of her students told her, "I saw a nurse who must have stuck the patient at least five times with the same needle." Discuss what you could you do to address this behavior if you saw this happen or if a peer told you the same thing.
4. Decide where you stand in relation to achieving the learning outcomes listed at the beginning of this skill.

Recommended

Sherman R. 3 steps to give more effective difficult feedback. 2017. Retrieved from http://www.emergingrnleader.com/3-steps-to-give-more-effective-difficult-feedback/

McKay D. How to get the most from your performance review. 2018. Retrieved from https://www.thebalancecareers.com/how-to-get-the-most-from-your-performance-review-526101

Receiving Criticism. (Website). Retrieved from http://www.youmeworks.com/receivingcriticism.html

Henman P. How to deal with criticism in the workplace. 2018. Retrieved from https://woman.thenest.com/deal-criticism-workplace-7127.html

See also Recommended in the next skill.

SKILL 7.5:   Managing Conflict Constructively

Definition

Being able to make conflict work in positive ways (learning, growth, and improvement).

Learning Outcomes

After completing this section, you should be able to:

1. Compare and contrast your usual approach to dealing with conflict with that of other people you know.
2. Describe common physiological and emotional responses to conflict.
3. Use conflict resolution strategies to make conflict work in positive ways.

Thinking Critically About Conflict

Conflict comes from human instinct. From the beginning of mankind, when survival of the fittest reigned, humans instinctively protected their territory and reacted with suspicion to people different from themselves. Today, many of us subconsciously protect our territory and react negatively toward others when things aren't going the way we expect.

Conflict can be mild (e.g., quietly opposing an idea or action) or it can be severe (e.g., showing sharp disagreement and anger). For many, the word *conflict* has negative connotations, bringing feelings of discomfort and dread. Most of us want to live in a world where everyone gets along and everything goes smoothly. Critical thinking requires being able to understand and exchange

TABLE 7.4   Positive and Negative Outcomes of Conflict

Negative Outcomes	Positive Outcomes of Managing Conflict Constructively
Increased stress	Reduced stress
Decreased productivity	Increased productivity; performance improvement
Poor relationships and feelings of isolation	Better relationships and interactions; increased harmony
Wasted time and energy	More time and energy for real progress
Frustration, anger, and hopelessness	Improved ability to clarify main issues and find creative solutions
Lack of growth	Opportunity to improve bothersome things
Poor self-esteem	Improved self-esteem

different viewpoints, wants, and needs and to come to a sincere agreement about what's most important. When you know how to manage conflict constructively, you're more likely to have positive outcomes and spend less time dealing with the negative outcomes of conflict (Table 7.4).

How to Manage Conflict Constructively

1. Gain insight into your natural style of dealing with conflict (Box 7.1). Make a commitment to use your strengths and work on weaknesses in an objective, purposeful way.
2. Learn to recognize patterns and appearances of conflict early. Be aware of verbal and nonverbal behaviors that signal that conflict may be developing (e.g., withdrawal, frequent verbalization of problems).
3. Practice using conflict management strategies (Box 7.2).
4. Use a comprehensive approach to assessing and managing conflict:
   - **Recognize that it takes courage to confront.** People who confront usually have given a lot of thought to what's happening and have been struggling with how things are going for a while).

BOX 7.1   Managing Conflict: What's Your Style?

AVOIDERS pull away. They ignore issues or withdraw from people they feel are causing conflict. Avoiders often get along well with others because they focus on promoting peace and harmony. However, they tend to allow problems to persist and place little importance on their own needs. As a result, they miss opportunities to make improvements and tend to "explode" when things finally get to be too much, even though the trigger issue may be minor.

ACCOMMODATORS (SMOOTHERS) give up their own needs and try to make others feel better. Members of this group often struggle with inner conflicts because they secretly wish to speak their minds. They, too, can explode, damaging relationships because of failure to honestly confront issues that are important to them.

FORCERS try to get their way even if it means others have to give up what they want or need. They're minimally interested in or aware of what others need and don't really care if they are liked.

COMPROMISERS give up part of their wants and needs and persuade others to give up part of their wants and needs. They think they get win-win solutions but may be settling for minimally acceptable solutions that continue the conflict (because they assume everyone has to lose something in negotiations rather than persisting to find answers that fully satisfy everyone involved).

COLLABORATIVE PROBLEM SOLVERS make it a rule to fairly face issues together. This group has equal concern for both the issues and the relationship. They see conflict as a means of improving relationships by gaining understanding and reducing tension. They look for solutions that allow everyone to win by identifying areas of agreement and differences. They evaluate alternatives and choose solutions that have the full support of the key parties involved.

BOX 7.2 Mad About You: Managing Conflict

1. Listen with the intent to understand the other person's point of view before presenting your own.
2. Take a deep breath, and keep a lid on your emotions. It's hard to think clearly when your adrenaline is flowing.
3. Using "I" messages and a nonthreatening tone of voice, explain how the problem is affecting you and what you'd like to happen. *Examples:*
   - "I feel [name the feeling]."
   - "When I see or hear [state the problem]."
   - "I would like [state the change you want to happen]."
4. Ask yourself: "What can I find in this situation that I'm doing to contribute to the problem?" You have more control over things that you're doing to contribute to the problem than over things that others are doing to contribute to the problem.
5. Get rid of old baggage (feelings and preconceptions you have because of things that have happened in the past); for example, thinking, "I'm just not the type of person who can handle conflict, so she knows she can get her way."
6. Look for deep issues. For example, say, "Tell me what's really bothering you." (Keep repeating this if the answer is "I don't know.")
7. Be willing to hear things you don't like to hear. You need honest feedback to work through the issues.
8. Ask for help from those involved. For example, "Can we agree to not be so hard on one another?"
9. Change your approach to managing conflict depending on the situation (one size doesn't fit all). For example, many nurses use avoidance as their main approach to resolving conflicts.
   - Use collaborative problem-solving as the overall, optimum way to manage conflict. Because this approach takes more time than you may have at the moment, initially you may need to use one of the following approaches. You also may need to use all the following methods as stepping-stones to collaborative problem-solving.
   - Use avoidance only when trying to delay confrontation until a more appropriate time, when a time-out is required, or when issues are of minor importance in relation to the overall goal.
   - Use accommodation or smoothing when the goal is to preserve relationships or encourage others to express themselves.
   - Use compromise when time is too limited for a full collaborative approach and there are two equally empowered sides that must reach agreement yet maintain a positive relationship. Find a common ground to achieve temporary settlement that at least satisfies each side's main objectives.
   - Use forcing only when there isn't time for discussion (e.g., in an emergency), when you must implement unpopular changes, or when all other strategies have failed and the change is required.

- **Don't jump to conclusions:** Hold your opinions until you're sure of all the facts. Check your strong feelings and assume the person has good intentions (it may not seem like it, but most people don't intend to offend or do wrong).
- **Remember that there are three ways to view the situation:** (1) the way you see it, (2) the way the other person sees it, and (3) the way it really is.
- **Stay focused on the relationship and common values and goals (e.g., "We're both committed to good patient care.").** Don't nitpick on small issues—look at the big picture, and address the impact that the major behaviors have on achieving goals.
- **Choose an appropriate time and place to open discussion** (ensure privacy and find a convenient time for those involved).
- **Foster an atmosphere of trust and sincere desire to face issues fairly together;** encourage free exchange of ideas, feelings, and attitudes.
- **Be willing to persevere** until you clearly understand the issues, values, and goals of the key players involved.

BOX 7.3   Being Assertive Without Being Aggressive

- Try to understand completely before responding. To be sure you understand correctly, paraphrase what you heard (e.g., "I understand you're completely frustrated.").
- State your own feelings, thoughts, and needs clearly, in a nonthreatening way.
- Stand up for your own rights while showing respect for the rights of others.
- Pay attention to cultural and personality differences.
- Convey needs and wants by using "I" messages to address how you feel about the specific behavior that disturbs you (e.g., "I was embarrassed and hurt when I saw you walk away from our conversation" rather than, "You made me feel like such a jerk when …").
- Value yourself and act with confidence—don't feel guilty when you say "no" ("I'm sorry, but I can't do that.").
- Own responsibility and speak with authority—use eye contact, a direct body posture, and a controlled voice volume and tone (you may need to adapt this if cultural differences are involved).

BOX 7.4   How to Negotiate

1. Clarify the results you want to achieve (e.g., "I'd like to have a schedule that works for everyone").
2. Explore the needs and wants of all parties; determine common and conflicting needs; work to find mutually agreeable solutions.
3. Build and maintain a communication climate that supports problem-solving under stress.
4. Think about various proposals; decide whether to reject, reframe, or accept them.
5. Decide the worst-case scenario (what you're willing to accept even if it's not exactly what you want). Don't accept anything that's below your worst-case scenario. Discuss any offer that's less than you'd like but better than your worst-case scenario.

- **Look for win-win solutions** (you may have to compromise a little bit). Try to find several solutions to the problems, evaluating each solution with the key players involved.
- **Make a conscious effort to stay calm,** help others stay calm, and keep the focus on the positive outcomes of resolving the conflict and building the relationship.
- **Take a break,** ask for a truce, or get help from outside sources as needed. Allow for time out, but keep interacting until all parties agree to the solution.
- **Set up a time to revisit issues** to see if the solutions are actually being carried out and helping to reduce the problem.
5. Use the strategies in Box 7.3 to be assertive without being aggressive.
6. Apply principles of negotiation (Box 7.4).

CRITICAL THINKING EXERCISES

Think, Pair, Share

With a partner, in a group, or in a journal entry:

1. In relation to Box 7.1, **identify your usual way of dealing with conflict.** After considering your own style, think about what styles you've encountered and how they affect you and the conflict resolution process.
2. **Recall a time when you had a difficult conflict.** What could you have done to handle the situation better? What style(s) may have achieved a better outcome?
3. **Share your stories about conflict with others,** asking for a different viewpoint on what was going on in and what styles and strategies might help.

4. **Practice using "I" messages.** Change the following statements to ones that send "I" messages.
   - "You never listen to me."
   - "I wish you wouldn't be so sloppy all the time."
   - "You make me feel like I'm the one who causes all the problems."
   - "You make me feel insignificant when you ignore me like that."
   - "Why are you always attacking me?"
5. **Use role-playing to practice assertive communication and conflict resolution.** Get a partner. Have one of you be the manager in the following situation and the other be the staff nurse. **Here's the situation:** A staff nurse is angry because he didn't get a specific day off, even though he had put in a written request well ahead of time. He needs the weekend off for his daughter's birthday. The manager spent hours trying to find proper coverage but couldn't honor his request because two other nurses also needed to be off and were turned down for their requests the previous month.
6. Decide where you stand in relation to achieving the learning outcomes listed at the beginning of this skill.

Recommended

Deschene L. *Twenty things to do when you're feeling angry with someone.* Retrieved from http://tinybuddha.com/blog/20-things-to-do-when-youre-feeling-angry-with-someone/

Mind Tools. *Conflict resolution: resolving conflict rationally and effectively.* Retrieved from http://www.mindtools.com/pages/article/newLDR_81.htm

Conflict Resolution Skills (Website). Retrieved from https://www.helpguide.org/articles/relationships-communication/conflict-resolution-skills.htm

See also Recommended in Skill 7.4, Giving and Taking Constructive Feedback.

SKILL 7.6: Managing Your Time

Definition

Making the most of the time you have by getting organized and staying focused on major priorities (working smarter, not harder).

Learning Outcomes

After completing this section, you should be able to:
1. Explain how an activity diary (or log) helps you manage your time.
2. Describe how to set priorities based on your personal and professional goals.
3. Identify ways to organize your life to make the most of your time.
4. Determine ways to improve your ability to manage your time in the clinical setting.

Thinking Critically About Managing Your Time

Do you sometimes feel like you're in a race against time from sunup to sundown? It's hard to think critically when you're constantly bombarded by things you should do (or didn't get done). Your performance suffers and you feel stressed because you never complete what you started out to do. Gaining control over the time you have by setting priorities and applying the insights and strategies in this section reduces your stress and improves your performance.

How to Manage Your Time

This section is organized into the following headings:(1) Determining What Must Be Done, (2) Ranking Priorities, (3) Organizing Your Schedule and Work, and (4) Streamlining Work in the Clinical Setting.

Determining What Must Be Done

1. **Determine and record your personal, professional, and work goals.** Keep them in a readily accessible place. These goals serve as a guide to help you prioritize and organize.
2. **Start an activity diary (or log).** For several consecutive days, write down everything you do. Include what you do, the amount of time you spend doing it, and the time of day you do it. It should look something like this:

Activity Log	
Time	**Activities and Tasks**
8:00 to 8:30 AM	Drive to health club
8:30 to 9:00 AM	Work out
9:00 to 9:45 AM	Drive to class
10:00 to 11:15 AM	Class
11:15 AM to 1:00 PM	Have lunch, hang out with friends
1:00 to 2:15 PM	Class
2:15 to 5:00 PM	Miscellaneous unscheduled tasks

3. **After a few days, analyze your log and arrange each of the activities and tasks** according to the following categories:
   - Must do (essential) activities and tasks
   - Should or could do (or can be delegated to someone else) activities and tasks
   - Nice to do (if you had more time) activities
   - Not necessary (time waster) activities and tasks
4. **Be sure that things under your "must do" category reflect your personal and professional or work goals.** If they don't, decide whether you truly must do them.
5. **Determine whether there are things missing on your "must do" list.** Add these to the list.
6. **Find ways to spend most of your time each day on the "must do" list.** Figure out how to get rid of time wasters. *Example:* In the preceding activity log, you could get rid of an hour's driving by working out at home instead of at the health club.
7. **Review the list of "nice to do" activities.** Ask, "Are there things on this list that I could be delegating to someone else?" If so, who is the best person(s) to do the tasks? What would be the results in the long run?
8. **Consider whether you could combine some activities.** For example, if you have specific educational goals, you might listen to educational tapes while driving.

Ranking Priorities

1. **Determine first-, second-, and third-order priorities** and clarify the rationale for your choices:
   - First-order priority: Must do—important and urgent
   - Second-order priority: Must do—important but not urgent
   - Third-order priority: Nice to do—not important and not urgent
2. **For each priority, consider the following:**
   - How much time you have
   - Whether you (and only you) can do what needs to be done, or whether you can delegate the task(s) or parts of the task(s) to others
   - Whether technology can help you be more efficient (e.g., mastering computer skills)
   - Whether paying someone to get things done better or more quickly will improve your results or give you more time to spend on tasks related to major goals
   - Whether there is a cheaper way of accomplishing the task

Organizing Your Schedule and Work

1. **Review your personal, professional, and work goals.** Organize your time to get the tasks related to your *most important goals* done *first*.
2. **Work on major priorities when you perform best** (e.g., some people work better in the morning; others do better at night).
3. **Plan break time, eat healthily, drink lots of water, and sleep regular hours.** Include time for exercise and stress reduction (this helps you be more productive by avoiding low energy levels).
4. **Organize your environment for optimum productivity.**
5. **Make a "to do" list for each day, and estimate the time each activity on your list will require.** Be sure that your list includes only those activities that you must or should do.
6. **Reserve time in your daily schedule for unexpected events.** Life is unpredictable.
7. **For long-term (or large) projects, keep a master list to refer to periodically.** For each project, map out interim target dates that ensure you will complete the project in a timely way or by the designated deadline.
8. **Avoid the human tendency to put off large projects** or find excuses to avoid things you don't enjoy. Procrastination is a major time waster.
9. **Don't expect or demand perfection.** Letting go of a task once it's done is crucial for managing time. Perfectionism can also be a time waster!
10. **Look for ways to streamline work,** as in the following section.

GUIDING PRINCIPLE

To avoid oversights, keep all scheduled activities within the same organizing system (e.g., an electronic calendar), rather than keeping multiple or duplicate systems. For example, don't keep separate work and social calendars.

Streamlining Work in the Clinical Setting

1. **Be sure you're familiar with principles of delegating and setting priorities in the clinical setting** (see "Delegating Safely and Effectively," Chapter 4, and Skill 6.13, "Setting Priorities," Chapter 6).
2. **Arrive at least 15 to 20 minutes early** to gather your thoughts, get the big picture of what's happening on the unit, and get focused and plan your day.
3. **Use an electronic or print tool** to organize your day and keep information handy (don't rely on memory; you'll have too many interruptions).
4. **Cluster activities before entering a room**—think ahead and anticipate needs (e.g., a need for pain medication).
   - Label all supply shelves and cabinets clearly for easy access.
   - Organize supply and medication carts so that the commonly used items are easily found.
5. **Set limits on what you agree to do.** If you think you need more staff, say so.
6. **Ask for "no interruptions"** when you need to stay focused.
7. **Stay hydrated and make time for meals and breaks** to maintain energy level.

❓ CRITICAL THINKING EXERCISES

Think, Pair, Share

With a partner, in a group, or in a journal entry:

1. Identify three personal or professional goals that you want to accomplish within the next year.

2. Keep an activity diary for 3 consecutive days during the week. Be sure to include all activities for work, school, and home. In relation to the goals you identified in number 1, analyze the diary and:
   - Determine the "must do" activities that will help you achieve your goals for the next year.
   - Identify time wasters, and decide how you might eliminate them.
   - Rank the "must do" activities by assigning priorities (first-order, second-order, or third-order priorities).
   - Ask yourself whether there are some things you should be doing to achieve your personal and professional goals. Add these to the list.
   - Share what you learned from doing the earlier items.
   - Share time management strategies that work in your personal life.
3. Describe strategies that help you manage your time in the clinical setting.
4. Decide where you stand in relation to achieving the learning outcomes listed at the beginning of this skill.

Recommended

The Power of Full Engagement: The Four Energy Management Principles That Drive Performance. (Website). 2015. Retrieved from https://fs.blog/2015/06/the-power-of-full-engagement/

Ohama R. *Time management for right brained diverse thinkers*. 2006. Retrieved from https://prezi .com/clffljwnsywa/time-management-for-right-brained-diverse-thinkers/

MindTools. *Time management*. Retrieved from http://www.mindtools.com/pages/main/newMN_ HTE.htm

SKILL 7.7: Navigating and Facilitating Change

Definition

Knowing how to chart a course to successfully adapt to change (and help others do the same).

Learning Outcomes

After completing this section, you should be able to:
1. Recognize your usual response to change.
2. Identify strategies to help you navigate change.
3. Determine how to facilitate change in others.

Thinking Critically About Change

As Will Rogers said, "Even if you're on the right track, you'll get run over if you just sit there." Change is a part of life, and as many have said, "Sometimes in the winds of change, we find our true direction." Knowing how to plot a course through the many changes we face—and how to help others do the same—helps you move from feeling disrupted and frustrated to feeling a sense of progress and accomplishment.

How to Navigate and Facilitate Change

This section first gives strategies to help you navigate change, and then it gives strategies to help you help others deal with change.

Strategies to Navigate Change

1. Curb the tendency to keep the status quo just because it's easy and comfortable.
2. When first faced with change, suspend judgment and explore reasons for the required change. Navigating change doesn't mean embracing change uncritically—it means clarifying the pros and cons and making reasoned decisions about whether the change is worthwhile.

3. Make sure you understand why the change is being made and how you feel about it. If you can get something out of the change, it helps you accept it. If you have strong feelings against making the change, you need to explore and work through them.

4. Identify barriers to making the change and find ways to deal with them. *Example:* Make yourself a "cheat sheet" when learning new technology.

5. Ask for help. If you express the problems you have, others may be able to help. You also may identify concerns that are bothering everyone.

6. Expect the natural sequence of events often associated with adapting to change, seen in Box 7.5.

Strategies to Facilitate Change in Others

1. Include key stakeholders to determine how the change will affect those involved. Be clear about the positives and negatives from their perspectives (e.g., "This will require effort and time on your part, but when we're done we'll all have it easier.").

2. Clearly describe both the required changes and the expected benefits.

3. Clarify changes in roles and responsibilities.

4. Get support from formal and informal group leaders (they can make or break progress).

5. Allow people to explore how the change will affect their daily lives (e.g., when one group moved to electronic health records, several nurses said, "You know how we love our paper!").

6. Encourage involvement in finding ways to make the change easier.

7. Convey an understanding of negative feelings and extra work associated with having to make changes. Provide necessary resources and support until the change has been fully implemented.

8. Involving key stakeholders, identify barriers to making the change and find ways to deal with them. For example, if workers are expected to take time to practice using a new computer system, provide extra personnel to do ordinary chores.

9. Be clear about timelines. Key players must know exactly what change is expected to occur and by when.

10. Ask for ownership of responsibility for change (both leaders and subordinates own some of the work). Be patient. Adapting to change takes time.

BOX 7.5   Adapting to Change: Four Stages

1. **LOSING FOCUS.** Expect some confusion, disorientation, and forgetfulness at first. You may be unsure about boundaries and responsibilities. Ask for clarification, keep notes, and use to-do lists.

2. **DENIAL.** You may want to minimize or deny the effect the change has on you. However, connecting with and dealing with feelings helps you move forward. Acknowledge how you feel about what you lose and gain by making the change.

3. **ANGER OR DEPRESSION.** If you feel angry, discouraged, or frustrated:
   - Vent your anger in a safe place. Be careful with whom, how, and where you ventilate. Your words can come back to haunt you. Find someone who'll listen without being affected by your feelings (e.g., someone who has gone through the change you're experiencing, not someone who also is struggling and who may be pulled down by your negativity).
   - Use stress management strategies (e.g., exercise helps diffuse anger and frustration).
   - Keep away from negative people, or soon you'll feel the same way.
   - Stay focused on what you'll gain from making the change. Be patient with yourself, let go of the past, and take it one step at a time. Make a conscious effort to think critically and not emotionally.

4. **MOVING FORWARD.** Seek opportunities to use the new skills and procedures you've learned. Celebrate small successes, recognizing how far you've come and what you learned along the way.
   - Share your experience with those who may not have come as far as you have.
   - Remember to represent your organization positively in public, even if you don't feel that way at the moment.

CRITICAL THINKING EXERCISES

Think, Pair, Share

With a partner, in a group, or in a journal entry:

1. Share your best and worst experiences with navigating and facilitating change. Discuss what made them your best and worst experiences.
2. Describe a personal or work change that you experienced that wasn't your choice (e.g., moving to a new home, a change in job description). Think about how you felt at the time and the effect it had on your ability to make the change. Identify some things you could have done to make the change easier.
3. Share a time you tried to help someone else change.
   - How successful were you?
   - What, if anything, would you do differently?
4. Study Box 7.6 on transformational change. Discuss the difference between change that transforms and change that conforms.
5. Decide where you stand in relation to achieving the learning outcomes listed at the beginning of this skill.

Recommended

McGraw P. *4 stages of readiness for change*. 2018. Retrieved from https://www.drphil.com/advice/the-4-stages-of-readiness-for-change/

Sherman R. *The speed of change*. 2018. Retrieved from http://www.emergingrnleader.com/the-speed-of-change/

Hopkin M. *How leaders navigate change*. 2018. Retrieved from https://leadonpurposeblog.com/2017/04/17/how-leaders-navigate-change/

Acuff J. *How to navigate the 4 types of work-life change*. 2015. Retrieved from https://www.youtube.com/watch?v=RRwHjnz0LTc

---

BOX 7.6   Transformation Change: Four Ways We Change

1. **Pendulum change:** I was wrong before, but now I'm right.
2. **Change by exception:** I'm right, except for …
3. **Incremental change:** I was almost right before, but now I'm right.
4. **Paradigm change:** What I knew before was partially right. What I know now is more right but still only part of what I'll know tomorrow.

Paradigm Change Is Transformational

Paradigm change combines what's useful about old ways with what's useful about new ways and keeps us open to looking for even better ways. We realize:

- Our previous views were only part of the picture.
- What we now know is only part of what we'll know later.
- Change is no longer threatening: it enlarges and enriches.
- The unknown can then be friendly and interesting.
- Each insight smooths the road, making the change process easier.

Paradigm Shift

A paradigm shift occurs when there's a change from one way of thinking to another. It's a transformation, almost a metamorphosis. It doesn't just happen—it's driven by agents of change (leaders and staff who support the change).

Modified from Ferguson M. *Aquarian conspiracy: personal and social transformation in our time*. West Minster, MD: Penguin Random House; 2009.

SKILL 7.8:   **Preventing and Dealing With Mistakes Constructively**

Definition

Knowing how to prevent, detect, correct, and learn from errors.

Learning Outcomes

After completing this section, you should be able to:

1. Define the terms *error, sentinel event, near miss, hazardous condition,* and *safety culture.*
2. Explain how to determine the seriousness of a mistake.
3. Describe the relationship between communication and errors.
4. Identify circumstances that lead you and others to make mistakes.
5. Identify strategies that help you create safety nets for your patients and team members.
6. Decide what to do when you make (or witness someone else make) a mistake.
7. Explain the importance of creating a culture in which error reporting is encouraged more than punished.

Thinking Critically About Preventing and Dealing With Mistakes

To quote a nursing professional development specialist, "Mistakes affect people and families for a lifetime! No one wants to make a mistake that hurts someone. Learning about a safety culture and how to prevent, learn from, and deal with mistakes is critical."[4]

Errors can be your worst nightmare, or they can be stepping-stones to learning and improvement. And sometimes they can be both. Dealing with mistakes is a complex issue that includes considering legal consequences (in some states, it's the law that patients be informed of errors; mistakes sometimes end up in malpractice litigation). This section addresses what errors are considered to be serious; why errors happen; and how to prevent, detect, correct, and learn from them.

There are two major types of errors:
1. **Commission**—doing the wrong thing (e.g., giving the wrong medication)
2. **Omission**—failing to do the right thing (e.g., not ensuring safety)

There are three common reasons for mistakes:
1. **Execution errors**—doing the right thing incorrectly
2. **Rule violation**—going against current rules or policies
3. **Wrong plan**—when actions proceed as planned but fail to achieve the intended outcome because the planned action or original intention was wrong

Too many people have a one-size-fits-all mindset when it comes to dealing with mistakes. Deep down, they believe that all errors are bad, that all errors happen because of lack of knowledge or laziness, and that the best way to deal with people who make mistakes is to punish them. However, this approach shames those involved, doesn't examine the real causes of errors, and does little to reduce the incidence of mistakes—it only reduces the *reporting* of mistakes (if people expect punishment, they'll *hide* errors). When errors aren't reported, opportunities to fix related problems are missed and mistakes are likely to be repeated.

Most mistakes happen for many reasons and in spite of good intentions. To promote a safety culture, we must change the mindset from "mistakes shouldn't happen" to "when dealing with humans, mistakes will happen for various reasons." We must share our mistakes freely so that we can work together to find ways to prevent future mistakes. Box 7.7 shows common causes of patient care errors.

BOX 7.7 Common Causes of Patient Care Errors

1. **Miscommunication and communication failures:** Eighty percent of serious medical errors involve interpersonal miscommunications, especially between caregivers during the transfer of patients.* Other communication failures include transcription errors, use of abbreviations, illegible handwriting, incorrect interpretation of physician's orders, use of verbal orders, failure to record medications given or omitted, and unclear medication administration records.
2. **Errors or omissions in medication reconciliation** when patients are admitted or transferred from one unit to another (medication reconciliation is a formal process for creating a complete and accurate list of a patient's current medications and comparing the list to those in the patient record or medication orders).
3. **Failure to ensure the "11 Rights of Medication Administration"**

Right patient	Right assessment	Right to refuse
Right drug	Right route	Right evaluation (follow-up)
Right dosage	Right time	Right documentation
Right reason	Right patient education	

4. **Not following policies and procedures:** Lack of attention to safeguards in medication administration procedures intended to prevent errors.
5. **Interruptions and distractions:** Just as pilots maintain a sterile cockpit—no socializing on landings and take-offs—nurses must avoid interrupting one another and create quiet "no interruptions zones."
6. **Human and system problems:** These include things like nurses with little experience being assigned patients with complex conditions; nurse fatigue (sleep deprivation, consecutive hours worked without breaks or little time off); rotating shifts; poor staffing; distractions and interruptions; the practice of floating nurses to unfamiliar units; hospital and pharmacy design features; and drug manufacturing problems (e.g., look-alike and sound-alike drug names, look-alike packaging, confusing and unclear labeling, failure to specify drug concentrations on dose calculation charts).

*Dingley C, Daugherty K, Derieg M et al. Improving patient safety through provider communication strategy enhancements. Retrieved from https://www.ahrq.gov/

Key Terms Related to Examining Mistakes

The following terms are important to understand to develop and maintain in-depth error prevention strategies:

- **SENTINEL EVENT:** A patient safety event (not primarily related to the natural course of the patient's illness or underlying condition) that reaches a patient and results in death, permanent harm, or severe temporary harm. The following are also considered sentinel events: (1) suicide of any patient receiving care, treatment, and services in a staffed around-the clock care setting or within 72 hours of discharge, including from the hospital's emergency department (ED); (2) unanticipated death of a full-term infant; (3) discharge of an infant to the wrong family; and (4) abduction of any patient receiving care, treatment, and services.[5] The term *sentinel* is used because of its relationship to a sentinel guard—a soldier who stands guard to keep people safe. Sentinel events are so serious that they signal the need for immediate investigation to ensure they don't happen again.
- **CLOSE CALL, NEAR MISS, OR "GOOD CATCH":** A safety event that did not reach the patient but poses a significant chance of a serious adverse outcome if it happens again.[5] *Example:* If a physician almost operates on the wrong site but this is caught just in time, it's a near miss. Near misses may be considered sentinel events, but they may not be reviewed by The Joint Commission under its sentinel event policy.

- **HAZARDOUS CONDITION:** Any set of circumstances (other than the patient's own disease or condition) that significantly increases the probability of a serious adverse event.[5] *Example:* Nurses who have too many acutely ill patients to give appropriate care.
- **NO HARM EVENT:** A safety event that reaches the patient but does not cause harm.[5] *Example:* A patient who has been prescribed a regular diet receives an 1800-calorie diabetic lunch tray.
- **ROOT CAUSE ANALYSIS (RCA):** The process for identifying *deep underlying cause(s)* of a mistake—the "root(s)" of errors. Requires examining in detail what happened, why it happened, who was involved, all factors that contributed to the mistake, and what can be done to prevent it. *Example:* Thoroughly examining what happened with a medication error in order to identify the major contributing factors (e.g., a nurse may have had inadequate knowledge to give a new medication, but the *root cause* of the lack of knowledge may be that there's no policy in place to ensure that new drugs aren't introduced unless all nurses have the required knowledge—this is considered a *system* problem).
- **FAILURE MODE EFFECT ANALYSIS (FMEA):** FMEA is a systematic, proactive approach to error prevention that aims to build systems that promote safety and prevent accidents. FMEA assumes (1) that errors are not only possible but likely, despite knowledgeable and careful health care professionals; and (2) that it's too much to ask individuals alone to be responsible for errors. Instead, the responsibility is placed on the interprofessional group that engages in a never-ending process of quality improvement to assess and correct areas in which errors are likely. FMEA aims to design a system in which critical or catastrophic errors can't happen. *Example:* Wrong-site surgeries that are prevented by a strict policy that includes several "checkpoints" to ensure that the correct surgery in the correct person in the correct body part is done.

How to Prevent and Deal With Mistakes Constructively

1. **Make patient and caregiver safety a part of the health team code of conduct** (Box 7.8).
2. **Make it a point to look for errors and flaws in thinking.** In important or emergency situations, check, check, and check again—the more you check, the more you find.
3. **Remember that all mistakes aren't created equal**—in addition to knowing the difference among a sentinel event, near miss, or hazardous condition, you should know the following different types of mistakes, what things cause them, and how you can prevent them.
   - **MENTAL SLIPS:** These mistakes happen when there's a lapse in your attention to what you're doing or when there's a lapse in short-term memory. *Example:* You're on the way to check an IV, but you're interrupted to help lift someone up in bed. You then forget that you were on the way to check the IV and go on to another task. *Prevention:* Use electronic or print tools that prompt you to do important tasks (e.g., check IV every hour). Get your charting done as soon as possible to help you notice when you've forgotten to do something.

BOX 7.8   Safety and Error Prevention: Code of Conduct

As a member of this group/team, I agree to keep patient and caregiver safety and welfare as the primary concern in all interactions, including:

- Following policies and procedures and using evidence-based practices.
- Being vigilant and monitoring for care practices that increase risks for errors.
- Remembering that no one is perfect and all humans are vulnerable to making mistakes.
- Taking responsibility for being "a safety net" when helping co-workers, anticipating what they may need, and pitching in to prevent mistakes (e.g., "I think that glove is contaminated, let me get you a new one." "Here's a new needle.").
- Making it a team principle that "If we witness unethical or unsafe practices, it's our responsibility to address it (first directly with the person, then through policies and procedures if warranted)."

Checklists, protocols, and computerized decision aids all help reduce mental slips because they relieve you from relying on short-term memory, the aspect of memory that becomes most imperfect under stress or fatigue.

- **COMMUNICATION ERRORS:** These mistakes happen when people misunderstand each other. *Example:* You're working in the emergency department and just spoke to Dr. French about one of your patients, Mrs. Moran. A few minutes later, Dr. French comes to you and says, "Would you send her to x-ray?" nodding in the direction of another patient. You don't see him nod in the other direction and assume Dr. French is referring to Mrs. Moran. *Prevention:* Repeat what you hear to clarify verbal interactions ("You want me to send Mrs. Moran to x-ray?"). Check written orders to clarify verbal orders.

- **KNOWLEDGE ERRORS:** These mistakes are due to insufficient knowledge. *Example:* You cause unnecessary side effects by giving an IV drug too quickly because you didn't know it should be given slowly. *Prevention:* Be sure you find out the answers to who, what, why, when, and how in the context of each individual patient situation before you give any drug or perform any intervention.

- **LEARNING ERRORS:** Although these mistakes often include knowledge errors, learning errors usually are related to several different factors associated with being in a learning situation (e.g., doing something for the first time or being stressed). *Example:* You change sterile dressings for the first time. You contaminate your glove by slightly touching an unsterile field. You don't notice it because you're focused on assessing the wound. *Prevention:* A surefire way to avoid learning errors is not to try anything new, which makes no sense. Many students hide from new experiences because they're afraid of making mistakes. This just postpones the inevitable. The best way to avoid learning errors is to be prepared and to practice, practice, practice in as safe an environment as possible (e.g., in a skills lab). In risky situations, it's best to have a more experienced nurse guide performance, give advice, or actually handle the task at hand.

- **RELYING TOO MUCH ON TECHNOLOGY:** These mistakes happen when you allow technology to think for you, without wondering if there's a flaw in the system. *Example:* Someone complains that a heating pad is too hot. You check the setting and see that it's in the "low" position. Instead of carefully feeling the pad yourself, you explain that it's probably okay because it's set on low. *Prevention:* Read all instruction manuals carefully. Don't trust machines more than your own knowledge and perceptions. Don't allow technology to think for you: think with it.

- **SYSTEM ERRORS:** These mistakes are related to something wrong with the way things are accomplished within the facility as a whole. *Examples:* Drugs that aren't given because the pharmacist is overloaded and unable to dispense the drug in a timely manner, errors that happen because a policy or procedure is unclear, or errors that happen because a facility uses a lot of per-diem personnel who are more at risk for making mistakes. *Prevention:* Report possible system problems to the risk management or performance improvement department. Create a multidisciplinary panel to examine possible and actual system problems.

4. **Always determine how serious the error is.** Serious errors need to be examined more closely, prevented more meticulously, and detected and corrected more quickly than less serious errors.

GUIDING PRINCIPLE

To determine the seriousness of a mistake, answer two questions:
1. **What harm could this mistake cause** (consider harm in terms of human morbidity, mortality, and suffering first; then in terms of inconvenience, cost, and lost time)? If you're unable to predict harm, get help.
2. **Is this mistake a sentinel event, near miss, or hazardous condition?**

5. **Follow policies and procedures,** and be sure you understand the rationale behind them. These are designed by experts to prevent, detect, and correct errors early.
6. **When using checklists, think about each item carefully.** Checklists are supposed to jog your brain, not replace it.
7. **Involve patients and families.** Educate them and encourage them to become participants in preventing errors by verifying that they're getting the right treatments and medications and by speaking up when they have questions.
8. **Never give a medication or perform an intervention without knowing why it's indicated for each particular person.** Be careful about multitasking.
9. **Involve experts** (e.g., if you're unsure about the best way to give medication, ask a pharmacist).
10. **Look after yourself.** If you're rested and use stress management strategies, you're less likely to make mistakes.

What to Do When Mistakes Happen

1. **Determine the seriousness of the error** as soon as it's recognized, and take immediate steps to prevent or reduce harm (get help if needed).
2. **Follow policy and procedures for dealing with mistakes,** including how to report and record the mistake. Standards and some state laws mandate that patients be informed when mistakes happen.
3. **Chart actions taken to address the error** (e.g., increasing the frequency of monitoring or a transfer to another unit).
4. **Curb the tendency to focus too much on guilt** and not enough on what can be learned from the mistake.
5. **Explore the specifics of the incident objectively, examining the procedures and circumstances leading to the errors.** Consider the value of sharing the mistake with others to alert them of the possibility of its happening again.

NOTE: For more information on error prevention, check the index for the following topics: Quality and Safety Education for Nurses; competencies; safety culture; standard tools; miscommunication; read-back rules; repeat-back rules; time-outs; nursing surveillance; dangerous situations; failure to rescue; and strategies to identify, interrupt, and correct errors. Box 7.9 shows key organizations involved in preventing errors and promoting safety.

BOX 7.9 Key Patient Safety Websites

- Patient Safety Network: http://www.psnet.ahrq.gov
- Patient Safety Organization Program: pso.ahrq.gov/with_PSO
- Hospitals in Pursuit of Excellence: http://www.hpoe.org/
- National Patient Safety Foundation: http://www.npsf.org
- Partnerships for Patients: http://partnershipforpatients.cms.gov/
- The Joint Commission (TJC): http://www.jointcommission.org
- TJC Center for Transforming Healthcare: http://www.centerfortransforminghealthcare.org/
- The National Academy of Medicine: http://www.nationalacademies.org/hmd/
- Quality & Safety for Nursing Education (QSEN): http://www.qsen.org/
- Canadian Patient Safety Institute: http://www.patientsafetyinstitute.ca
- Canadian Institute for Health Information: http://www.cihi.ca
- Accreditation Canada: http://www.accreditation.ca

CRITICAL THINKING EXERCISES

Think, Pair, Share

With a partner, in a group, or in a journal entry:
1. Address the implications of the following statements:
   a. Being ignorant doesn't merely mean not knowing; it means not knowing what you don't know. Being educated means knowing precisely what you don't know.
   b. As a nurse it's your responsibility to be alert not only to situations that might cause you to make mistakes but also to situations that may cause others to make mistakes.
2. Respond to the following:
   a. How do you feel when you make a mistake?
   b. What can you do to help someone else who has made a mistake?
   c. How can you help correct error-prone systems and increase checks to prevent medication errors?
3. Share examples of a sentinel event, near miss, hazardous condition, mental slip, knowledge error, learning error, and system error.
4. Share your personal (or a family's or friend's) experiences with errors.
5. Watch a baseball game and notice how the players back one another up and provide "safety nets" in case of overthrown balls. Notice that the crowd yells at players who don't back up other players. How does this apply to what you see in the health care setting?
6. Discuss the following PowerPoint presentation (single slide): *The ABCs of Patient Safety*. Retrieved from www.mspatientsafety.com/ABCsofpatientsafety.ppt
7. Decide where you stand in relation to achieving the learning outcomes listed at the beginning of this skill.

Recommended

Patient Safety Network primers. Retrieved from: https://psnet.ahrq.gov/primers

AHRQ. Surveys on patient safety features.™ Retrieved from https://www.ahrq/sops/index.html

Darrah J. *Charting the course to fewer medical errors*. 2018. Retrieved from http://nursing.advanceweb.com/charting-the-course-to-fewer-medical-errors

McDonald S. *Medical errors*. 2017. Retrieved from https://ceufast.com/course/medical-errors

Rosenberg K. Missed nursing care increases risk of death after surgery. AJN 2018;118(1):56–57. doi: 10.1097/01.NAJ.0000529718.83040.20

Khan A, Coffey M, Litterer K, et al. Patient and family centered I-PASS study group. *JAMA Pediatr* 2017;171:372–381. Retrieved from https://psnet.ahrq.gov/resources/resource/30900?utm_source=ahrq&utm_medium=en-3&utm_term=&utm_content=3&utm_campaign=ahrq_en3_14_2017

SKILL 7.9: Transforming a Group Into a Team

Definition

Knowing how to create a group in which the members work together to achieve shared outcomes within a specific time frame.

Learning Outcomes

After completing this section, you should be able to:
1. Describe the common stages of team building.
2. Describe strategies that transform groups into teams.
3. Participate more effectively as part of a team.
4. Ensure that patients are key members of the health care team.

Thinking Critically About Teamwork

How well a team works together makes the difference between having unhappy patients and staff and great patient outcomes and job satisfaction. Yet building a team isn't easy. Team members need to be nurtured as the team evolves from being a group of diverse strangers to a group that values common goals and brings together diverse talents and strengths.

True teamwork occurs when all team members are:

1. Committed to common goals and a high level of productivity
2. Energized by their ability to work together
3. Concerned about how team members feel during the work process
4. Committed to including patients and their caregivers as key team members

Consider the differences in what's happening in the two groups in the following scenarios.

SCENARIO TWO GROUPS: NO TEAMWORK VERSUS TEAMWORK

Group 1 consists of several nurses who have worked together for the past 6 months. They don't feel like they're working as a team and want this to change. Their manager, Jane, is a busy person who has a demanding boss. Under pressure, Jane barks orders and personally takes over some tasks. The staff responds by doing what they are told or lying low until things calm down. There is minimal group participation in problem-solving and decision-making. The nurses want to execute their responsibilities in a satisfactory way. But no one has given thought to the need for group goals or concerted group action. Morale is low, and everyone talks about how unhappy they are.

Group 2 consists of several nurses who also have worked together for 6 months. By contrast, these nurses are energized and proud of their successes. Like Group 1, their manager, Terri, also is a busy person with a demanding boss. However, when the pressure is on, Terri stops the action and convenes a problem-solving discussion, focusing on common goals and getting input from team members. Better solutions are found because the pressure is channeled into a spirit of "let's fix this together." These nurses enjoy a sense of growing and improving together—work is more than just a job.

How to Transform a Group Into a Team

Knowing how to communicate and build trust are the cornerstones of teamwork. Respect personality and cultural differences and get agreement on a code of conduct. Be aware of messages sent by behavior. For example, if you consistently show up late for work, shirk responsibility, give excuses, or are arrogant or defensive, you need to be aware of the messages these behaviors send to the rest of the team. On the other hand, if you use behaviors like always being on time, being willing to help, accepting responsibility, and being open to suggestions, you send altogether different messages.

Teamwork requires empowerment, a willingness and commitment to "let go" of "having it your way" for the benefit of the group. There are five stages of empowerment: (1) letting go of self-promotion; (2) believing that others are capable and competent; (3) trusting others; (4) being willing to forgo your own processes, plans, or strategies to give others a chance; and (5) sharing the outcomes and celebrating success.[6]

GUIDING PRINCIPLE

Being an effective health care team member requires building relationships with co-workers and ensuring that patients and their caregivers are viewed as key team members.

Box 7.10 shows the common stages of team building. Box 7.11 gives team-building strategies for team leaders and members.

BOX 7.10 Team-Building Stages

1. **FORMING:** Group members start to get to know one another, testing each other's values, beliefs, and attitudes. Basic goals and tasks are defined, roles assigned, and ideas shared.
2. **STORMING:** Conflict begins, often because of misunderstandings or disagreements about what realistically can get done and how exactly things will get done. More testing goes on in this phase, with some people asking themselves questions like, "How much am I willing to do?" This is a time to maintain high standards, provide emotional support, and aim to get consensus (agreement from everyone). Beware of false consensus during this phase; some people will say they agree when they really don't (just to avoid further conflict). Because this is a stressful stage, you may need to take more breaks.
3. **NORMING:** The group becomes more cohesive and really wants to work together in a positive way. Group members agree on rules—for example, when meetings will be held, who should attend, what the proper lines of communication are, and how problems and disagreements will be handled. At this point the leader needs to be sensitive to group values, asking for votes to determine common needs and desires.
4. **PERFORMING:** Team members begin to bond to one another and function well together with a good understanding of roles, responsibilities, and relationships.

BOX 7.11 Team-Building Strategies

1. **Team leaders should:**
   - Create a shared vision of the team's mission or purpose: Everyone must be committed to reaching clearly defined outcomes.
   - Stress that everyone is responsible for preventing errors and improving outcomes by analyzing current practices and pointing out improvements that could be made.
   - Turn diversity to the team's advantage (e.g., assign tasks based on individual strengths and preferences as much as possible).
   - Ask for consensus in decisions (everyone agrees to agree), rather than settling for a majority vote.
   - Keep team members well informed so that everyone understands the big picture; help them recognize common stages of team building.
   - Use team huddles (brief meetings to share goals and priority tasks) at the beginning of each day and as needed.
   - Recognize team members for their contributions.
2. **Team members should:**
   - Come to agreement on roles, responsibilities, and proper lines of communication.
   - Work hard to meet responsibilities and deliver what they promise.
   - Get involved and contribute to the good of the group.
   - Stay focused on the big picture of what the team is trying to accomplish.
   - Make a conscious effort to overcome the human tendency to focus narrowly on self; too often, team members have difficulty seeing other members' struggles because they themselves are working so hard.
   - Actively participate in team huddles.
3. **Leaders and team members should:**
   - Use behaviors that promote trust and create a caring and energized environment.
   - Follow the "Platinum Rule" (treat others as they want to be treated instead of assuming they want to be treated the same as you do).[7]
   - Show enthusiasm—it's contagious and it energizes others.
   - Address and resolve conflicts early—push for high-quality communication.
   - Pay attention to group process and where the team is in relation to the stages of team building.
   - Recognize individual and team efforts; be a good sport and help new teammates make entry.
   - Support creativity and new ways of doing things.
   - Broaden skills; offer to try new tasks or to cross-train.
   - Promote group learning by collecting, sharing, and analyzing information.
   - Spend fun time together (here's where relationships grow).

CRITICAL THINKING EXERCISES

Think, Pair, Share

With a partner, in a group, or in a journal entry:

1. Discuss some of the TeamSTEPPS strategies and tools available at http://teamstepps.ahrq.gov/. TeamSTEPPS was developed by the Department of Defense's Patient Safety Program together with the Agency for Healthcare Research and Quality to improve communication and teamwork skills among health care professionals. TeamSTEPPS is scientifically rooted in more than 20 years of research and lessons from the application of teamwork principles.

2. Share your story about a group you currently belong to. In what team-building stage is the group (see Box 7.10)?

3. Share your best and worst experiences with being part of a team. Consider what went right and why you think it went right, and what went wrong and why you think it went wrong.

4. Discuss what humans can learn from the geese in *Pulling Together Simple Truths* (3-minute inspirational video at https://www.youtube.com/watch?v=7ZqNpDNDKAc).

5. Practice brainstorming as a group. Get in a group of four to eight persons. Have one person be the recorder, writing on a flip chart or blackboard. Identify a problem you'd like to resolve or a situation that could be improved (e.g., how you could get teenagers to come to a meeting on sex education). For 30 minutes, without interruptions, have group members share ideas to be recorded for all to see. Choose the three best suggestions. After you finish, spend 10 minutes discussing the group dynamics during the brainstorming session.

6. Decide where you stand in relation to achieving the learning outcomes listed at the beginning of this skill.

Recommended

Agency for Healthcare Research and Quality. *TeamSTEPPS*. Retrieved from http://teamstepps.ahrq.gov/

Moore J, Everly M, Bauer R. Multigenerational challenges: team-building for positive clinical workforce outcomes. *OJIN* 2016;21(2):Manuscript 3. DOI: 10.3912/OJIN.Vol21No02Man03

DiVincenzo P. Team huddles: a winning strategy for safety. *Nursing* 2017;47(7):59–60 doi: 10.1097/01.NURSE.0000520522.84449.0e

Huddles tip sheet. 2016. Retrieved from https://www.pioneernetwork.net/wp-content/uploads/2016/10/Huddles-Tip-Sheet.pdf

See also Recommended in Skills 7.3 to 7.5, "Developing Empowered Partnerships," "Giving and Taking Constructive Feedback," and "Managing Conflict Constructively."

REFERENCES

1. How to give great customer service: The L.A.S.T method. (Website). Retrieved from https://www.engvid.com/how-to-give-great-customer-service-the-last-method/.

2. Block P. *Stewardship: Choosing service over self-interest, 2nd Ed*. San Francisco: Berrett-Koehler; 2013.

3. Vitalsmarts. *Silence kills: The study overview*. Retrieved from https://www.vitalsmarts.com/resource/silence-kills/; 2011.

4. Konzelmann, N. Personal communication.

5. The Joint Commission. *Sentinel Events*. Retrieved from https://www.jointcommission.org/assets/1/6/CAMH_24_SE_all_CURRENT.pdf; 2017.

6. Whiting, S. Personal communication.

7. Alessandra, T. The platinum rule. Retrieved from www.alessandra.com/abouttony/aboutpr.asp

Concept Mapping: Getting in the "Right" State of Mind

WHAT IS CONCEPT MAPPING?

Concept mapping is a learning strategy that uses the right brain (creative hemisphere) to enhance your ability to see relationships, identify major ideas, and understand information. With concept mapping, you simply draw your personal view of key concepts and how they relate to one another. Unlike outlining, which uses the left brain (logical hemisphere), mapping is flexible, has few rules, and is easy to learn (left brain–dominant people may struggle at first). Mapping boosts your ability to grasp and remember complex relationships because there are few words (less clutter) on the page, and you can focus *on the concepts and relationships* (without worrying about writing or outlining rules). Study Fig. 1, which shows key points of this paragraph; compare how your brain handles this paragraph versus how it handles the map.

Fig. 2 shows a map of how the brain works.

WHEN DO YOU USE MAPPING?

You can use mapping for various purposes, including the following:
- Taking notes or learning new content
- Mapping the care planning process or how symptoms relate to one another
- Writing papers or preparing presentations
- Preparing for exams
- Brainstorming
- Facilitating group problem-solving

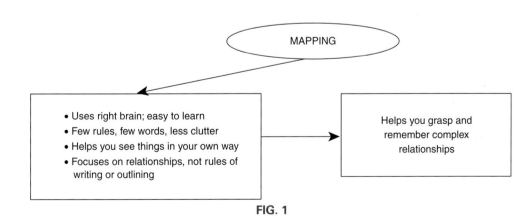

FIG. 1

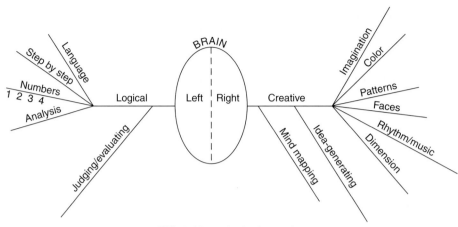

FIG. 2 How the brain works.

WHAT ARE THE BENEFITS?

Consider the benefits of mapping.

General Benefits

- Faster than regular note-taking
- Highlights key ideas and gets rid of the irrelevant information
- Helps you quickly gather, review, and recall large amounts of information
- Increases brainpower available for learning and problem-solving by reducing energy used on concerns about structure and documentation
- Gives you a "visual" that helps you clarify relationships
- Helps you retain what you learn because you "play with the information" in your own way as you make your map

Group Benefits

- Promotes communication (keeps everyone focused on the main issues)
- Facilitates problem-solving (generates more ideas, helps group suspend judgment)
- Makes ideas and relationships clear

HOW MAPPING PROMOTES CRITICAL THINKING

Concept mapping facilitates the "productive and analytical phases" of critical thinking—the phase when you gather information, identify relationships, and produce new ideas. After you complete this productive phase, you can get in touch with your left brain talents and move to the "judgment phase"—you evaluate your map and form opinions or judgments: Is it accurate? Is it useful? Can you refine your map to make it more accurate and useful?

STEPS FOR MAPPING TO PROMOTE CRITICAL THINKING

1. **Put the central theme or concept** in the center, at the bottom, or at the top of the page, and draw a circle around it (e.g., see the first map in this section).
2. **Place the main ideas relating to the concept** on lines (or in circles) around the central theme.

3. **Add details** by putting them on lines (or in circles) connecting them to the main ideas.
4. **Use key words or simple pictures** only; keep it legible.
5. **Make sure no idea stands alone.** If you can't connect an idea with something on the page, it's irrelevant to the central theme.
6. **Don't allow yourself to slow down** over concerns about where to place words (this is your left brain habit trying to dominate). Instead, let your ideas flow and use lines to show connections.
7. **Use colors** to highlight the most important ideas.
8. **Evaluate your map and revise as needed.**

Nursing Process Summary

NOTE: The following phases are iterative (interrelated, dynamic, and repetitive), not linear. All phases begin with **assessment** to ensure the most up-to-date data.

Assessment

Purpose: Collect and record data to provide the information needed to:
- Predict, prevent, detect, manage, and resolve problems, issues, and risks.
- Clarify expected outcomes.
- Identify individualized interventions to achieve outcomes and to promote optimum health, function, and independence.

Diagnosis/Outcome Identification

Purpose: Analyze patient data to (1) clarify realistic expected outcomes (benefits of care) and (2) identify the problems, risks, or issues that must be managed to achieve the outcomes. During this phase, in addition to clarifying outcomes, you:
- Identify signs and symptoms that may indicate the need for referral to a more qualified professional (report these immediately).
- Confirm or rule out suspected problems.
- Determine the patient's resources, strengths, and use of healthy behaviors.
- Reflect on thinking to determine whether (1) patient participation in the process has been at an optimum level; (2) data are accurate and complete; (3) assumptions have been identified and reasoning tailored to the individual patient and circumstances; (4) conclusions are based on facts (evidence) rather than guesswork; and (5) alternative conclusions, ideas, and solutions were considered. **Reflecting on thinking applies to all the phases, but is placed here because it requires analysis, which is the focus of this phase.**

Planning

Purpose: Ensure that there's a complete, recorded, outcome-focused plan that's tailored to the individual patient and circumstances. The plan should be designed to do the following:
- Include the most qualified members of the interprofessional team to manage the problems (e.g., RN? PCP? nutritionist?).
- Specify short-term and long-term outcomes, if indicated.
- Monitor and manage priority problems, issues, and risks.
- Promote optimum comfort, function, independence, and health.
- Coordinate care and include patients as partners in decision-making.
- Achieve the desired outcomes safely, efficiently, and cost-effectively.
- Include teaching to help patients make informed decisions and become independent.
- Provide a record that can be used to monitor progress and communicate care.

Implementation

Purpose: Put the plan into action.

- Assess the patient to determine whether interventions are still appropriate and the patient is ready.
- Prioritize, delegate, and coordinate care as indicated, including patients and other caregivers as partners in decision-making and care.
- Prepare the environment and equipment for safety, comfort, and convenience.
- Perform interventions, and then reassess to determine patient responses.
- Make immediate changes as needed; update the recorded plan if required.
- Record patient data and responses to monitor progress and communicate care.

Evaluation

Purpose: Determine where the patient stands in relation to desired outcomes; consider how the process can be improved.

- Assess the patient status to determine whether expected outcomes have been met and what factors promoted or inhibited the success of the plan.
- Report progress (or lack of progress) to key members of the interprofessional team.
- Plan for ongoing assessment, improvement, and patient independence.
- Discharge the patient or update the plan as indicated.

Source: © 2019 R. Alfaro-LeFevre. No use without permission.

Examples of CTIs Within the 4-Circle Model

EXAMPLES OF CTIs WITHIN THE 4-CIRCLE MODEL

INSTRUCTIONS: Going clockwise, matching boxes circles. CTIs are abbreviated.

CIRCLE #1
- Self-aware; authentic
- Effective communicator
- Curious / inquisitive
- Self-disciplined
- Confident / resilient
- Analytical / insightful
- Autonomous / responsible
- Honest / upright
- Alert to context
- Proactive
- Patient / persistent
- Logical and intuitive
- Creative
- Realistic / practical
- Open and fair-minded
- Sensitive to diversity
- Reflective / self-corrective
- Improvement-oriented

CIRCLE #2
- Ensures safety and infection control
- Applies standards, ethics codes, and nursing process principles
- Teaches patients, self, and others
- Assesses comprehensively
- Checks accuracy/reliability
- Distinguishes normal from abnormal and relevant from irrelevant
- Recognizes missing information
- Considers alternative explanations and solutions
- Determines individualized outcomes
- Weighs risks and benefits; individualizes interventions
- Manages risks, predicts complications, promotes optimum well-being
- Sets priorities
- Applies evidence/research
- Identifies ethical issues
- Delegates appropriately

CIRCLE #4
- Manages IVs, N/Gs, injections
- Suctions airways
- Manages drains & suction equipment
- Inserts / manages catheters
- Changes sterile dressings
- Uses health information technology

(1) Critical Thinking Characteristics

(2) Intellectual Skills (Theoretical & Experiential Knowledge)

CRITICAL THINKING ABILITY

(4) Technical Skills

(3) Interpersonal, Communication, & Self-management Skills

CIRCLE #3
- Uses skilled communication
- Upholds healthy workplace standards
- Promotes teamwork
- Gives and takes constructive feedback
- Addresses conflicts fairly
- Facilitates learning and safety cultures
- Leads and motivates others
- Facilitates and navigates change
- Manages stress, energy, and time

Source: © 2019 R. Alfaro-LeFevre. *Evidence-based critical thinking indicators.* No use without permission

Example of Patients' Rights and Responsibilities*

Dear Health Care Consumer:

State law requires that your health care provider or facility recognize **your rights** while receiving medical care and that you respect *their right* to expect certain behavior on your part as a patient. You have the right to (1) be treated with courtesy, respect, and protection of your privacy and (2) to receive prompt and reasonable responses to questions and requests.

You have the right to be informed of the following:

- Who is providing medical services and who is responsible for your care
- Your diagnosis, planned course of treatment, alternatives, risks, and prognosis
- What patient support services are available (e.g., interpreters, community services)
- Whether treatment is experimental or for research purposes (and to give or refuse your consent to participate)

You also have the following rights:

- To refuse treatment, except as otherwise provided by law
- To have impartial access to medical treatment or accommodations, regardless of race, national origin, sexual orientation, religion, physical handicap, or payment source
- To be given treatment for any emergency condition that will deteriorate on failure to receive treatment
- To express any grievances about any violation of your rights as stated by state law through the grievance procedure of your health care provider or facility and appropriate state licensing agency
- To file complaints against a health care professional, hospital, or ambulatory surgical center with the Agency for Health Care Administration (**Note:** Appropriate information for how to reach each state's agency must be listed here.)
- To receive the following (upon request):
  1. Full information and necessary counseling on the availability of financial recourses for your care
  2. A reasonable estimate of the charges for medical care before treatment
  3. Information about whether your health care provider or facility accepts the Medicare assignment rate before treatment
  4. A copy of an itemized bill that is reasonably clear and understandable and, on request, to have charges explained

You have the following responsibilities:

- Provide your health care provider with accurate and complete information about your complaints, past illnesses, hospitalizations, medications, and other matters relating to your health
- Follow treatment plans recommended by your providers

---

* Adapted from various documents on patients' rights.

- Report unexpected changes in your condition to the health care providers
- Keep appointments and, if you're unable to do so for any reason, notify your provider or facility
- Ensure that the financial obligations of your health care are fulfilled as soon as possible
- Comply with health care provider and facility rules and regulations affecting patient conduct

Source: Alfaro-LeFevre R. Handouts © 2020 http://www.AlfaroTeachSmart.com

DEAD ON!!—A Game to Promote Critical Thinking

The point of this game is to be sure that you give key parts of thinking the time and attention they require, therefore promoting thinking that's more likely to be "dead on." **Instructions:** Get six balls and put the letters D, E, A, D, O, N on each one. Start with **the "D" ball,** and toss it to someone in the group. Ask the group to focus on answering the questions listed under **"D"** provided next. Once you have exhausted thoughts on **the "D" ball,** do the same for each of the remaining balls. Be sure to <u>stay focused</u> on the <u>current</u> ball. For example, if someone expresses <u>feelings</u> rather than <u>facts</u> with the first ball, point out that the rules are that emotions are addressed when the **"E"** ball is up for discussion.

D = Data
- What <u>data</u> (facts) do you have?
- What <u>other data</u> do you need?
- What <u>assumptions</u> have you made, and what data might validate or negate them?

E = Emotions
- What emotions (gut reactions) are there (your own, others')?
- What's your intuition telling you, and what data might validate or negate it?
- How are values affecting thinking (yours, other people's)?

A = Advantages
- What's the vision and specific advantages (benefits/outcomes) for the <u>patient or client</u>?
- What are the specific advantages (benefits/outcomes) <u>for the key stakeholders</u>?
- What are the specific advantages (benefits/outcomes) for <u>you</u>?

D = Disadvantages
- What could go wrong (what are the risks)?
- What are the specific inconveniences/risks for the <u>patient, client and others</u>?
- What are the specific inconveniences/risks for <u>you</u>?
- What problems or issues <u>must</u> be addressed to get results (achieve outcomes)?
- How much work will it take, and do you have the necessary resources?

O = Out of the box
- Go out of the box—think of creative approaches!
- What can we do to decrease the disadvantages?
- What can we do to increase the likelihood of seeing the benefits?
- How can technology help?
- What research is there that might apply?
- What human resources are willing to help?

N = Now what?
- What problems, risks, or issues <u>must</u> be addressed in the plan?
- Does the plan include patient/client and key stakeholder requests?
- What professional, community, and informal resources can help?
- What interventions are needed to get results and avoid risks?
- What does all this imply?
- What did we miss when addressing the other balls? (Go through each of the balls again.)

Source: Retrieved from www.AlfaroTeachSmart.com

Key Brain Parts Involved in Thinking

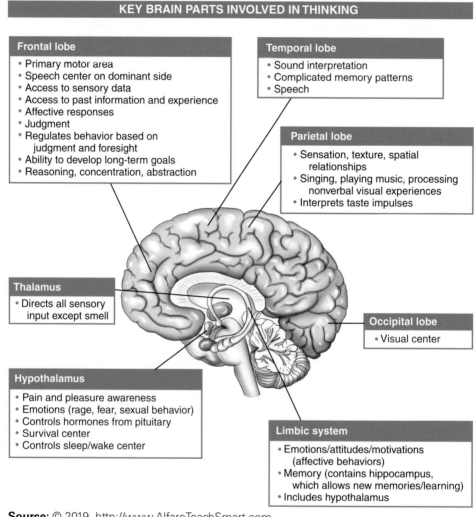

KEY BRAIN PARTS INVOLVED IN THINKING

Frontal lobe
- Primary motor area
- Speech center on dominant side
- Access to sensory data
- Access to past information and experience
- Affective responses
- Judgment
- Regulates behavior based on judgment and foresight
- Ability to develop long-term goals
- Reasoning, concentration, abstraction

Temporal lobe
- Sound interpretation
- Complicated memory patterns
- Speech

Parietal lobe
- Sensation, texture, spatial relationships
- Singing, playing music, processing nonverbal visual experiences
- Interprets taste impulses

Thalamus
- Directs all sensory input except smell

Occipital lobe
- Visual center

Hypothalamus
- Pain and pleasure awareness
- Emotions (rage, fear, sexual behavior)
- Controls hormones from pituitary
- Survival center
- Controls sleep/wake center

Limbic system
- Emotions/attitudes/motivations (affective behaviors)
- Memory (contains hippocampus, which allows new memories/learning)
- Includes hypothalamus

Source: © 2019. http://www.AlfaroTeachSmart.com

Example SBAR Communication Tool

SBAR is pronounced *S-BAR* and stands for *situation, background, assessment, recommendation*. SBAR forms vary, depending on the purpose and setting. **Have patient records handy, and be sure you can readily communicate all of the following information.**

S   SITUATION: Briefly state the issue or problem: What it is, when it happened (or how it started), and how severe it is. Give the signs and symptoms that make you concerned.

B   BACKGROUND: Give the date of admission and current medical diagnoses. Determine the pertinent medical history, and give a brief synopsis of the treatment to date (e.g., medications, oxygen use, nasogastric tube, IV lines, code status).

A   ASSESSMENT: Give the most recent vital signs and any changes in the following:

- Mental status, neurological signs
- Respirations
- Pulse, skin color
- Comfort, pain
- GI status (nausea, vomiting, diarrhea, distention)
- Urine output
- Bleeding, drainage
- Other: _____

R   RECOMMENDATION: State what you think should be done. For example:

- Come see the patient now.
- Get a consultation.
- Get additional studies (e.g., CXR, ABG, EKG, CBC, other).
- Transfer the patient to ICU.
- How frequently do you want vital signs?
- If there's no improvement, by when do you want us to call you?

Abbreviations in box explained: *ABG*, Arterial blood gases; *CBC*, complete blood count; *CXR*, chest x-ray; *EKG*, electrocardiogram; *GI*, gastrointestinal; *ICU*, intensive care unit.
Source: Summarized from many online SBAR resources.

Results of Two Studies Describing Critical Thinking Skills

SCHEFFER AND RUBENFELD[1]

- **Analyzing:** Separating or breaking down a whole into parts to discover their nature, function, and relationships
- **Applying standards:** Judging according to established personal, professional, or social rules or criteria
- **Discriminating:** Recognizing differences and similarities among things or situations and distinguishing carefully as to category or rank
- **Information seeking:** Searching for evidence, facts, or knowledge by identifying relevant sources and gathering objective, subjective, historical, and current data from those sources
- **Logical reasoning:** Drawing inferences or conclusions that are supported in or justified by evidence
- **Predicting:** Envisioning a plan and its consequences
- **Transforming knowledge:** Changing or converting the condition, nature, form, or function of concepts and contexts

THE AMERICAN PHILOSOPHICAL ASSOCIATION DELPHI REPORT[2]

- **Interpretation:** Categorizing, decoding sentences, and clarifying meaning
- **Analysis:** Examining ideas, identifying arguments, and analyzing arguments
- **Evaluation:** Assessing claims and assessing arguments
- **Inference:** Querying evidence, conjecturing alternatives, and drawing conclusions
- **Explanation:** Stating results, justifying procedures, and presenting arguments
- **Self-regulation:** Self-examination and self-correction

REFERENCES

1. Scheffer B, Rubenfeld M. A consensus statement on critical thinking in nursing. *Journal of Nursing Education.* 2000;39:353.
2. Facione P. *Critical thinking: What it is and why it counts.* Retrieved from, https://www.insightassessment.com/Resources/Importance-of-Critical-Thinking/(language)/eng-US; 2018.

Response Key for Exercises in Chapters 1 to 6

Note: Remember that these are *example* responses, not the *only* responses. You may have a response that is different but equally as good as the example. The main point is to learn by evaluating the thinking you put into completing the exercises. If you have a question, ask your teacher. There are no responses listed for *Think, Pair, Share* questions.

CHAPTER 1 EXERCISES

1. **A.** (a) safety, (b) welfare (c) priority **B.** critical **C.** (a) process (b) clinical judgment **D.** context **E.** CTIs **F.** ADPIE **G.** (a) cycle (b) dynamic **H.** (a) ethics codes (b) laws
2. **A.** Facts are clearly observable and easily validated as true. Opinions may vary depending on personal perspectives. They may or may not be valid. **B.** The best way to determine whether an opinion is valid is to ask for the *facts* (evidence) that support the opinion. Then determine the strength of the evidence and decide whether the opinion makes logical sense.
3. CTIs are observable behaviors that are usually seen in critical thinkers. For this reason, CTI and critical thinking behaviors may be viewed as being the same thing.
4. You must clearly identify the priority problems, issues, and risks that must be managed to achieve the desired results (outcomes).
5. Your ability to demonstrate CTIs is likely to diminish (because more of your brain power is going toward learning new things and gaining a comfortable state).
6. *Context* refers to the importance of paying attention to how thinking changes depending on circumstances (one size doesn't fit all). *Confident, courage, curious,* and *committed* are important characteristics needed for critical thinking.
7. Considering thinking ahead, thinking-in-action, and thinking back helps you examine thinking in a holistic way. If you look only at one phase, you miss important parts of thinking because the circumstances of each one are different.

CHAPTER 2 EXERCISES

1. **A.** (a) personality (b) affect **B.** (a) developing (b) changing **C.** communication **D.** assumptions **E.** starting **F.** (a) hypothesis (b) conclusions **G.** self-efficacy **H.** (a) intent (b) results
2. Feelings have a great impact on what and how we think. Those of us who are driven by feelings are likely to have more problems thinking critically, especially when situations are emotionally charged. Thinking critically requires that you recognize feelings and their impact on thinking and then use your head to apply logical and ethical reasoning principles. All too often we aren't even aware of deep, strong feelings involved in certain situations. Those of us who are able to connect with emotions and give them the attention they deserve—to make them explicit, to accept them, and to recognize their influence over thinking—can facilitate more logical, objective thinking.

3. The *Golden Rule* and the *Platinum Rule* both aim at treating others well. The *Platinum Rule* stresses that we are all different and that others may not want to be treated the same way we do. For example, don't assume that just because you like to be "touchy-feely," others do too.

4. c.

5. Jack and Jill are goldfish. A cat knocked the fish tank on the floor, shattering it. You probably assumed they were people.

6. Sometimes the terms *goals* and *outcomes* are used interchangeably. However, it's more correct to use *goals* when stating *general intent* (what you aim to do) and to use *outcomes* to clearly describe what you expect *others to observe* when the goal is met. Goals are more general and may focus on what the nurse aims to do. Outcomes are very specific and focused on what the *patient* will be able to do. *Example goal:* My goal is to teach Juan about diabetes. *Example outcome:* After 3 weeks, Juan will be able to give his own insulin and state how he will manage his dosage based on his diet, activity level, and glucose monitor readings.

7. You have to apply *knowledge* CTIs to accomplish *intellectual skill* CTIs.

CHAPTER 3 EXERCISES

1. **A.** (a) know (b) ready **B.** various **C.** (a) practice (b) same **D.** (a) big (b) details **E.** debriefing **F.** formative **G.** (a) preparing (b) calm

2. You're accountable for determining the limits of your own knowledge. You're also accountable for ensuring that patients, families, and other caregivers have the knowledge they need to proceed with care safely and effectively.

3. By teaching people how to manage their health, we empower them to achieve the important outcomes of being independent and achieving optimum health. In today's fast-paced clinical setting, you must be a self-starter and be able to teach yourself how to give competent care.

4. Two common skills that are easy to lose are mathematics and second language skills. To maintain math skills, drill yourself by calculating the information yourself then double-checking it with a calculator. If you have lost some of your math skills, you need to keep a calculator handy and keep calculation formulas available for quick reference. To be safe, you need to have someone else check your math. With second languages, find opportunities to practice, listen to your second language radio or TV, and keep translation tools handy (usually electronic).

5. The purpose of remediation is to help learners gain vital skills that are either lost or never learned.

6. Using a structured tool helps learners and their preceptors or educators be "on the same page" and organized and complete during debriefing and evaluation.

7. If you study only by looking at your notes, you may be misled about how much you know. Recognizing information in your notes is not the same as having the information "in your head."

CHAPTER 4 EXERCISES

Exercises 4.1. Clinical Reasoning Principles, Thinking Like a Nurse, Decision-Making, and Thinking With HIT

1. **A.** about **B.** (a) whole person (b) responses **C.** (a) pivotal (b) flawed **D.** scope **E.** (a) broad (b) analyze **F.** (a) your (b) interpret

2. Interoperability—the ability of two or more systems to exchange and use the same information—promotes safe effective use of HIT.

3. Surveillance—monitoring to detect signs and symptoms (cues) that indicate deviations from expected patterns of health, illness, or recovery—is a key nursing responsibility.

4. Any of the following are correct: caring, compassionate care; ADL management; health promotion; complication prevention; surveillance; patient and family education; medication and treatment regimen management; mobility promotion; physical comfort; emotional comfort; care coordination; delegation; documentation; population-based care.

5. Critical thinking is guided by standards, policies, ethics codes, and laws (individual state practice acts and state boards of nursing).

6. Ruling out "the bad things" (worst-case scenarios) first prioritizes your reasoning and ensures timely treatment of major issues.

Exercise 4.2 Care Planning, Hand-offs, Predictive Care Models, Delegating Effectively, and Outcome-Focused Care

1. **A.** created **B.** (a) concepts or principles (b) concepts or principles **C.** EASE **D.** assessment and planning **E.** (a) logic or intuition (b) logic or intuition **F.** PPMP **G.** (a) falls (b) care omissions **H.** (a) decisions (b) outcomes

2. Systems-based practice—recognizing all the processes in health care systems that interact to give quality, cost-effective care—is crucial for critical thinking. Recognizing missing links within systems is central to achieving outcomes. For example, many nurses have recognized delays in care related to system issues (e.g., problems with physicians being unavailable to perform certain services). As a result, these nurses have successfully sought to increase their scope of practice to deal with issues that normally required physician attendance (e.g., postoperative intubation; lumbar punctures).

3. According to social determinants of health (the conditions in which people are born, grow, work, live, and age, as well as the wider set of forces and systems that shape the conditions of daily life), this child is vulnerable to many health issues. For example, because he is so young, he's totally dependent on his grandmother's care and judgment. Since there is no car, there may be issues with getting medication or to health care appointments. Since this family is poor, he may not be getting nutritious meals. This child should be seen by a health care professional frequently. A social service consult may be indicated.

4. In the presence of known problems, you predict the most likely and most dangerous complications and take immediate action to (1) prevent them and (2) be prepared to manage them in case they can't be prevented. *Example:* If you're going to care for someone with a wired jaw and you aren't familiar with the care of someone with a wired jaw, look it up so that you know the common and dangerous complications and how to deal with them (e.g., in this case, one dangerous complication is aspiration because the person is unable to open his or her mouth, so you would have wire cutters nearby). You also look for evidence of risk and causative factors (things we know cause problems or put people at risk for problems). You then aim to manage these factors to prevent the actual problems. *Example:* In the case of the wired jaw, you assess for nausea (a risk factor for vomiting and aspiration). If nausea is present, ask for an antinausea drug, hold food, and keep suction equipment and wire cutters nearby. Finally, you promote health and function by asking the person how he or she is handling dietary and fluid intake need and make suggestions as needed.

5. It's unlikely that the off-going nurse has adequately assessed the family's needs. It's highly unlikely that the family is doing "fine," because this is a hard time for any family. It appears as though the family has had limited involvement in the child's care. You should assess the family's needs and begin to include interventions that meet these needs in the nursing plan (e.g., allow the family to spend more time with the child).

6. MMA should trigger you to consider a priority in clinical reasoning: deciding whether a patient's signs and symptoms may be related to *Medical problems, Medications, or Allergies*. EASE helps you remember the major care plan components: Expected outcomes, Actual and potential problems that must be addressed to reach the overall outcomes, Specific interventions designed to achieve the outcomes, and Evaluation statements (progress notes).

7. You can insert a nasogastric tube if the facility permits it; you've received permission from your instructor; you have the required knowledge and level of competence; the procedure is reasonable, prudent, and safe; and you're willing to assume accountability for how you perform the procedure and the patient response to the procedure.

CHAPTER 5 EXERCISES

Exercise 5.1 Moral and Ethical Reasoning, Professionalism, and Leadership

1. (a) professional; personal (b) autonomy (c) beneficence (d) justice (e) fidelity (f) veracity (g) confidentiality (h) accountability (i) virtues (j) utilitarian; good (k) deontological; consequences

2. Ask for a family meeting to make the decision. Include an ethicist, trusted friends, or clergy to help.

3. Maintaining professional conduct guards you from being accused of inappropriate conduct; it promotes trust and protects your patients' dignity, autonomy, and privacy

4. Leaders aren't necessarily tied to positions of authority as managers are. You can find them anywhere—from managerial positions, to frontline nurses, to students. Managers tend to control their staff ("you should do as I say"), while leaders build relationships with their staff and empower and engage those around them (called circle of influence).

Exercise 5.2 Research, EBP, and QI

1. (a) rigorous (b) surveys (c) transformed (d) unchanging (e) evidence (f) improve (g) domains (h) satisfaction

2. Clinical summaries and practice alerts help busy nurses use EBP to improve care practices by giving sound, simple summaries on the most up-to-date findings on a specific topic.

3. False. Because finding and critiquing research is time consuming, this is an unrealistic expectation. Rather, staff nurses are accountable for responsibilities listed under *Frequently Asked Questions on Staff Nurses' Role*.

4. (b). Developing protocols to manage postoperative complications has a major and possibly unchanging impact on improving outcomes related to healing and survival.

CHAPTER 6 EXERCISES

Skill 6.1. Identifying Assumptions Exercises

1. There's not enough evidence to indicate that the patient needs instruction. Many people are fully knowledgeable about their diet but aren't able to stick to it. It would be better to explore the main struggles with nutrition and diet.

2. You might waste your time teaching information the patient already knows. You might alienate the patient: Who likes to be taught things they already know? The patient gets the message that you don't understand the problem—that you jump to conclusions.

3. **Scenario One. (a)** She seems to have assumed that she can create a positive attitude for Jeff by talking about advances in diabetic care. **(b)** She needed to assess Jeff's human response to

learning he has diabetes. Jeff may be well aware of advances in diabetic care but is still having trouble coming to terms with having to regulate his diet and take insulin for the rest of his life. She didn't assess before acting. **(c)** Jeff probably thinks Anita is a know-it-all because she didn't take the time to find out his point of view on the situation. It's a real turn-off when someone starts trying to change your attitude before he or she finds out what your attitude is.

Scenario Two. (a) She seems to have assumed the mother can read and that the mother will let her know if she has questions. **(b)** If the mother can't read or is embarrassed to ask questions, the child may have inadequate care from his mother. If harm results from the nurse's failure to determine the mother's understanding, the nurse may be accused of negligence.

Scenario Three. (a) The assumption seems to be that he would have the desired response to the drug without any adverse reactions. **(b)** It's likely that she was concerned that Mr. Schmidt wouldn't respond to the diuretic as expected—that he might experience an adverse reaction. **(c)** She may have thought that the physician wouldn't like it if she challenged his judgment.

Skill 6.2. Assessing Systematically and Comprehensively Exercises

1. The *body systems approach* to assessment is probably the best method. Or you may choose the head-to-toe approach and cluster signs and symptoms of medical problems after you perform the assessment.
2. A nursing model approach (*Functional Health Patterns*) together with the *body systems approach.*
3. **Scenario One. (a)** Assess the extent of Pearl's voluntary movement (can she wiggle her toes?); color of toes and skin around cast edges; whether Pearl feels numbness or tingling in her foot or leg; whether there is any edema of the leg or toes; the quality of the dorsalis pedis pulse; whether Pearl perceives a needle prick as being sharp; and whether her toes are warm or cool. **(b)** Check circulation by assessing the dorsalis pedis pulse quality and capillary refill in toes; check for nerve compression by asking her to wiggle her toes and ask whether there is any numbness or tingling. If these are satisfactory, you might choose to put a warm sock over the toes; encourage her to wiggle her toes frequently to increase the circulation, and continue to closely monitor her dorsalis pedis pulse, toe temperature, and toe sensation. **(c)** Assessing each of these helps you detect early signs of circulatory problems, nerve compression, or skin irritation. If you find one area that begins to exhibit abnormal assessment findings (e.g., edema), you should increase the frequency and intensity of assessment of other areas (e.g., skin color). Each area of assessment has specific relevance: checking movement, numbness, and sensation monitors for nerve compression; checking for color, edema, pulse quality, and warmth monitors for circulation and skin condition. **(d)** Try repositioning her leg; if symptoms persist after an hour, report the problem immediately.

   Scenario Two. (a) Look up digoxin in an up-to-date reference (or consult with a pharmacist). Then assess as follows. **To assess for therapeutic effect,** check to see if Mr. Wu's serum digoxin level is within therapeutic range (0.5 to 2 ng/mL). Determine the status of cardiac symptoms compared with baseline (status of apical and/or radial pulse rate and rhythm, lung sounds, urine output, edema, activity tolerance). **To assess for allergic or adverse reactions,** check Mr. Wu for associated signs and symptoms listed in the drug reference. **To assess for contraindications,** check Mr. Wu for associated signs and symptoms listed in the drug reference. The most common contraindications for digoxin include serum potassium levels less than 3.5 mEq/L (increases the risk for toxicity), pulse rate less than 60 or below physician-prescribed parameters, and clinical signs of toxicity or overdose. **To assess for drug interactions,** get a complete list of medications (including herbal and holistic drugs) and check with the pharmacist to find out if there are any drug interactions. **To assess for toxicity or overdose,** check Mr. Wu for associated signs and symptoms. The most common signs and symptoms of digoxin toxicity include serum digoxin level above 2 ng/mL; atrioventricular block (PR interval greater than 0.24 sec); and progressive bradycardia, nausea, vomiting, and/or visual disturbances (blurring, snowflakes, yellow-green halos around images). **(b)** If no therapeutic effect is achieved by giving a drug or if the person is experiencing adverse reactions, you need to question whether a change in dosage is necessary or whether the drug should be continued at all. If you identify contraindications to giving the drug, you need to withhold the drug. If you identify signs of toxicity or overdose, it's especially important to withhold the drug because you'd be adding to the toxicity or overdose problem.

    Scenario Three. (a) *Vital signs:* Measure temperature, pulse, respirations, and blood pressure. *Eye opening:* Call Gerome's name. Tell him to open his eyes. If he makes no response, pinch him. *Best motor response:* Ask him to move each extremity. Use a pin prick or pinch him and see if he can tell you where he feels it. If he makes no response, pinch him and note whether he flexes his extremity to withdraw from pain, flexes in spasm, or extends his extremity. *Best verbal response:* Ask him what his name is, where he is, and what day it is. *Pupillary reaction:* Determine the size of each pupil in millimeters before flashing a light into it. Then flash a light into each pupil and observe whether it constricts briskly. *Purposeful limb movement:* Check each extremity by asking Gerome to move it, observing for muscle contraction (attempts to move), ability to lift extremity, and ability to lift extremity even though you try to hold it down. *Limb sensation:* Prick each limb with a sterile needle, and ask Gerome what he feels (this may be unnecessary for Gerome, since he has a head injury rather than a spinal cord injury). *Seizure activity:* Observe for muscle twitching. *Gag reflex:* Place a clean tongue blade in the back of Gerome's throat, and see if it triggers gagging. **(b)** By monitoring all of these parameters, signs and symptoms of increased intracranial pressure can be detected early. Signs and symptoms of increased intracranial pressure are decreasing level of consciousness; increasing restlessness; irritability and confusion; stronger headache; nausea and vomiting; increasing speech problems; pupil changes (dilated and nonreactive or constricted and nonreactive pupils); cranial nerve dysfunction; increasing muscle weakness, flaccidity, or coordination problems; seizures; decerebrate posturing (muscles stiff and extended, head retracted); and decorticate posturing (muscles rigid and still, with arms flexed, fists clenched, and legs extended)—the latter two are both late signs of increased intracranial pressure. **(c)** Monitor other parameters of neurological assessment closely for other signs of increased intracranial pressure. If there are no other changes and you can indeed arouse Gerome, you don't need to be immediately concerned; however, you should increase the frequency of assessment of all parameters until you're comfortable that the increased somnolence is merely a sign of the combined effects of fatigue and existing brain swelling (rather than increasing brain swelling). If you have any questions about how to proceed, report the increased somnolence to your supervisor. **(d)** Check other neurological parameters closely, and report and record findings immediately; increase the frequency of assessment. **(e)** If the baseline pulse was rapid, this may be a normal finding. However, you should closely assess all the other assessment parameters to check for other reportable signs and symptoms. If the pulse is dropping to 60 beats/min, closely monitor all other assessment parameters and report the findings immediately (may be a sign of life-threatening increase in intracranial pressure).

Skill 6.3 Checking Accuracy and Reliability (Validating Data) Exercises

1. Talk with Mrs. Molina and explore her feelings and concerns.
2. You may be able to turn on Mr. Nola's blood glucose monitor and check it (some monitors automatically show the previous blood glucose level). If not, ask him to take it again now (quietly observe his technique). If he is proficient at performing a check for blood glucose, it's likely his previous result was correct. If the second reading is significantly different from the previous

reading, consider whether there is a relationship between the change in blood sugar reading and recent food intake or peak insulin levels. I would consider the blood sugar reading the patient took with you observing as being most valid.

3. Take it in the right arm. Take it again in 15 minutes.

4. Using "teach back" principles, explore with Mr. McGwire why he thinks he has foot ulcers. Ask him to tell you what he does to avoid getting foot ulcers. He may be very knowledgeable about diabetic care and foot ulcers and still be getting these ulcers. Review his diagnostic tests to see if the A1c (glycohemoglobin, HbA1c) is within normal range. This test indicates blood glucose levels over the long term.

Skill 6.4. Distinguishing Normal from Abnormal–Detecting Signs and Symptoms (Cues) Exercises

1. **(a)** If you assumed this was an oral temperature, you should have placed an *S* here. You may have placed a question mark here, which is actually a more correct response. You need to ask, *"How was this temperature taken?"* (orally? rectally? tympanic?) **(b)** If you assumed the patient never has rales, you should have placed an *S* here. You may have placed a question mark here, which is actually a more correct response. You need to ask questions like, *"What do the patient's lungs sound like when he's in his usual state of health? What is the respiratory rate? How far up the back can you hear the rales? Are there just a few rales, or are there copious rales? When the patient coughs, do the rales clear?"* **(c)** You may have placed an *S* here, but you really need to *ask if this is a normal pattern for the person and why the person only sleeps 3 hours at a time* (e.g., it's not unusual for mothers of newborns to sleep only 3 hours at a time because of feeding schedules). **(d)** *S.* **(e)** *O* or question mark. This is usually a normal finding, but you may have placed a question mark because you wanted to know such things as *whether there's any drainage, whether the area is hot to touch,* and *whether the patient is afebrile.* **(f)** *O.* This is normal for a 2-year-old. **(g)** *S.* **(h)** You may have placed an *S* here, but a question mark is a more correct response. Ask, *"What are the bathing practices of a person of this culture?"* **(i)** *S.* This is likely to be a normal finding, since the dialysis takes over the work of the kidney. **(j)** *S* or question mark. The pulse is somewhat slow but might be normal for someone who is young and athletic or older and on cardiac medication. You may have wanted to ask, *"What is this person's normal pulse?"* or *"Is the person taking any cardiac medications that slow the heart rate?"*

2. The italicized words in the responses to number 1 earlier are examples of what else you might want to know.

Skill 6.5. Making Inferences (Drawing Valid Conclusions) Exercises

1. I suspect this information indicates infection of some sort.
2. I suspect this information indicates financial problems.
3. I suspect this information indicates that the patient has trouble sticking to his diet.
4. I suspect this information indicates that the child wants to be sure his mother approves of his answer, or perhaps he is afraid.
5. I suspect this information indicates there is some medical reason for the grandmother's confusion (e.g., medications or brain issue).

Skill 6.6. Clustering Related Cues (Signs and Symptoms) Exercises

Scenario One. (a) Stung by a bee on the ear an hour ago; ear has no stinger, is red and swollen; no rash or wheezing; normal pulse and respirations. **(b)** Afraid he might die; wants to have a

Popsicle and watch TV. **(c)** Didn't make sure she had parents' phone number down (investigate whether this was lack of knowledge or oversight); doesn't know first aid for a bee sting.

Scenario Two. (a) 41 years old; acute abdominal pain; vomiting for 2 days and unable to keep any food down; abdomen distended; no bowel sounds; scheduled to go to the operating room at 2 PM; pain suddenly getting worse; vital signs unchanged, except pulse is increased by approximately 30 beats/min. **(b)** 41-year-old businessman; hates everything about hospitals; scheduled to go to the operating room at 2 PM; worried because his brother died in the hospital; suddenly experiencing severe pain.

Skill 6.7. Distinguishing Relevant From Irrelevant Exercises

Scenario One. (a) May be relevant because buspirone hydrochloride can cause confusion in the elderly. **(b)** May be relevant because it may be a sign of infection, which can cause confusion in the elderly. **(c)** May be relevant because it's indicative of previous cardiovascular disease, which is a risk factor for cerebrovascular accident (stroke), which may be the cause of the confusion. **(d)** May be relevant because dehydration in the elderly can cause electrolyte imbalance and confusion. **(e)** Not relevant. **(f)** Not relevant.

Scenario Two. (a) Probably relevant. It takes time to adjust to a diabetic regimen. **(b)** Not relevant (not abnormal). **(c)** May be relevant (may feel constipation is caused by new diet). **(d)** May be relevant because she has to prepare meals for others, increasing temptation. **(e)** Very probably relevant. Someone who likes to cook usually takes joy in eating a variety of foods. **(f)** Relevant. She needs to eat even less than she will when her weight is within normal limits. **(g)** Not relevant (has nothing to do with sticking to a diabetic diet).

Skill 6.8. Recognizing Inconsistencies Exercises

Scenario One. (a) It doesn't make sense that Cathy has only just started coming to the prenatal clinic but has been going to birthing classes. If she hasn't had prenatal care until now, you wonder whether she's really happy about the baby coming or realizes the importance of prenatal visits. You may also wonder why her mother, rather than her boyfriend, came to the clinic visit. **(b)** Check her records to see if there's any mention of receiving prenatal care somewhere else for the earlier part of her pregnancy; ask her where she's been going to birthing classes; ask how her boyfriend and mother feel about the baby coming.

Scenario Two. Her age is inconsistent with usual risk factors for a myocardial infarction (MI). While sweating and feeling of impending doom may be seen with an MI, the big picture here—her age, absence of pain, normal electrocardiogram—is inconsistent with an MI. Occasionally people don't have pain when they have an MI, but usually other risk factors and signs and symptoms are present. Her signs and symptoms are more consistent with those of a panic attack (see *Panic Attack or Heart Attack?* at http://www.womensheart.org/content/HeartDisease/panic_attack_or_heart_attack.asp).

Skill 6.9. Identifying Patterns Exercises

1. b; 2. a; 3. d; 4. e; 5. c

Skill 6.10. Identifying Missing Information Exercises

1. Why is she taking codeine? What factors are contributing to the lack of fiber in her diet and her inadequate fluid intake? What's the patient's knowledge of how to prevent altered bowel elimination? Why does the patient spend most of her time in bed?
2. What are the woman's feelings about having herpes? What does the woman know about herpes transmission? How does she feel about telling prospective partners about the herpes? How does the patient plan to prevent herpes transmission?

3. What are the person's other vital signs (pulse, blood pressure, temperature)? Is there a history of smoking? Is the person smoking now? How long has this pattern persisted? How does the person tolerate activity?

4. What type of help does the woman need? How does the husband feel about helping her? Are there any things the woman can do to be more independent (e.g., attend a support group)?

5. Does the person feel he's getting adequate rest? Is he taking sleeping aids? If so, what are they?

Skill 6.11. Managing Risk Factors—Promoting Health Exercises

1. Do you have any family history of health problems? What's your ethnic background? Do you smoke or use chewing tobacco? What do your usual meals consist of? Do you exercise regularly and get enough rest? How do you manage stress? Do you drink alcohol or take drugs that aren't prescribed? Are you sexually active (if so, do you use a condom and discuss sexual history with your partner)? Do you wear your seat belt? What do you do to stay healthy?

2. Her age puts her at risk for osteoporosis. The history of falls, together with the risk for osteoporosis, puts her at high risk for fractures. You need to look closely at why she is falling (e.g., balance problems? coordination problems? weakness or fatigue? vision problems? home hazards?). You should also assess calcium intake, which has to be adequate to prevent osteoporosis.

3. Reinforce that it's good to do things that, evidence shows, increase the likelihood of living longer and healthier. Give some examples, like the importance of staying active and eating well. Encourage him to discuss how to monitor and manage risk factors with his primary care provider. Stress that many studies support the importance of monitoring things like cholesterol, blood sugar, and prostate-specific antigen in a 50-year-old man. Suggest scheduling annual exams around specific times (e.g., birthday, Christmas) so that he remembers.

Skill 6.12. Diagnosing Actual and Potential Health Problems Exercises

Scenario One. Potential (risk) for violence related to agitation and previous history of striking caregivers.

Scenario Two. Potential complications: Hemorrhage, shock, vomiting with aspiration, pneumonia, infection, paralytic ileus.

Scenario Three. Altered coping related to poor organizational and time management skills as evidenced by cluttered home, disheveled appearance, and statements of having trouble coping.

Scenario Four. History of smoking or lung disease, whether the fractures are stable (risk for punctured lung), whether he has pain that is preventing him from coughing and clearing his lungs (risk for pneumonia).

Skill 6.13 Setting Priorities Exercises

1. (b) and (c) should be addressed on the patient record, either through colostomy care standards or nurse-generated plans. The anxiety would probably be dealt with informally.

2. Assessing and reporting the chest pain is top priority because myocardial infarction and pulmonary embolus are potential complications of thrombophlebitis.

Skill 6.14. Determining Patient-Centered (Client-Centered) Outcomes Exercises

1. The patient will maintain intact skin, free of signs of redness or irritation, and have a documented record of measures taken to prevent skin breakdown.

2. After suctioning, the mouth, the nose, and the lungs will be clear.

3. After irrigation, Foley catheter will be patent and draining clear yellow urine.

4. Endotracheal tube will be out by [date], with patient breathing independently.

5. After 3 days of practice, the patient will demonstrate increased muscle strength as evidenced by ability to walk the length of the hall and back by [date].

Skill 6.15. Determining Individualized Interventions Exercises

1. **(a)** Monitor fluid intake every shift. Keep iced tea (patient's preference) at the bedside on ice. Encourage drinking at least 3 quarts during the day and 1 quart at night. Reinforce the importance of maintaining adequate hydration. Record fluid intake. **(b)** Monitor anxiety level. Encourage her to express feelings and concerns. Fully explain all procedures. **(c)** Monitor comfort level. After applying heat for 30 minutes, assist with range-of-motion exercises three times a day.

2. **Contributing factors:** Age, low weight, chemotherapy, spends a lot of time in bed. **Interventions:** Monitor skin for pressure points, especially coccyx, elbows, and heels. Put a foam pad on bed. Use a sheepskin for coccyx and heels. Teach the importance of (1) changing positions frequently, spending more time out of bed, keeping skin moisturized, maintaining hydration and a healthy diet, and having a family member monitor her back and heels for redness, as well as (2) reporting skin problems to the advanced practice nurse (APN) or physician before each chemotherapy treatment.

3. **Scenario:** **(a)** It's quite likely that, to avoid punishment, the children won't report finding ticks, increasing the likelihood that the mother won't know about possible bites. It also increases the likelihood that the ticks won't be properly disposed. **(b)** It's possible that they may go looking for ticks, increasing the likelihood of being bitten. This approach might work, but the risks outweigh the benefits. **(c)** Determine children's understanding of the severity of the consequences of tick bites and the importance of finding ways to avoid them. Initiate teaching as indicated. Explain to the children that they can best help by asking for insect repellent to be applied before going outside, reporting ticks found on themselves and on each other, and avoiding tall grassy areas. **(d)** Start a rule that the children can't go outside without first applying insect repellent. Have the mother praise good behavior (e.g., asking for insect repellent) verbally, rather than offering rewards. Caution the mother not to offer rewards for finding ticks.

Skill 6.17 Determining a Comprehensive Plan/Evaluating and Updating the Plan Exercises

1. **(a)** Not achieved; **(b)** Achieved; **(c)** Partially achieved; focus teaching toward mother's needs.
2. Overall expected discharge outcome: Will be discharged home with lungs clear and husband able to demonstrate administration of epinephrine by June 29. Two priority problems, expected outcomes, and interventions follow:

Priority Problems	Expected Outcomes	Interventions
1. Altered respiratory function related to allergic response as evidenced by wheezing	By June 29, lungs will be clear and free of wheezing.	Monitor lungs sounds q 4 hr. Report increased wheezing or other respiratory symptoms. Record on respiratory flow sheet.
2. Patient (husband) education: *Epinephrine administration*	By June 29, husband will relate knowledge of action and side effects of epinephrine and when to give epinephrine and will demonstrate subcutaneous injection technique.	Assess husband's knowledge of indications, side effects, and administration of epinephrine. Initiate teaching as indicated, focusing on his preferred learning style. Record results on patient education form.

You may also have identified altered comfort related to itching feet. This is an important nursing concern and could be listed as a third priority.

3. According to the predicted care, she should be voiding normally. Assess the patient carefully, checking for bladder distention and asking the patient about urinary symptoms. Check vital signs, and bring the problem to the attention of the primary care provider.

4. Use the memory jog **EASE**: **E**xpected outcomes; **A**ctual and potential problems that must be addressed to reach overall outcomes; **S**pecific interventions designed to achieve the outcomes; **E**valuation statements (progress notes).

GLOSSARY

NOTE: If you can't find a term here, check the index.

accountability Being responsible or answerable for *your actions or inactions* (what you did or didn't do while carrying out your responsibilities).

advanced practice nurse (APN) A nurse who, by virtue of credentials (usually completion of a master's program and certification), has a wide scope of authority to act (may include treating medical problems and prescribing medications).

air embolism An air bubble that gets into the bloodstream; can be fatal.

analysis A mental process in which someone seeks to get a better understanding of the nature of something by carefully separating the whole into smaller parts. For example, if you want to know more about someone's physical health, each organ and system is examined separately.

analytics The practice of drawing conclusions and developing care approaches that are data driven (supported by rigorous analysis of data collected over time).

anaphylactic shock Extreme hypotension caused by an allergic reaction; requires immediate treatment or can be fatal.

artificial intelligence Computer systems that are able to perform tasks that normally require human intelligence.

assessment tool A printed or electronic form used to ensure that key information is gathered and recorded during assessment.

assignment The work that each staff member is responsible for during a given work period.

assumption Something that is taken for granted without proof. (*Compare with* hypothesis and inference.)

attitude A way of acting, feeling, or thinking that shows one's disposition, opinion, and so forth (e.g., a "can-do" attitude).

baseline data Information that describes the status of a problem before treatment begins.

benchmark A standard or point in measuring quality. In health care, benchmarks are determined by analyzing the data collected over time.

best practices Evidence-based approaches used to prevent and manage certain problems in ways that achieve optimum satisfaction with minimal cost.

care omission When necessary nursing actions have been overlooked (e.g., if a person has not been turned when the plan indicates the need to do so).

care variance When a patient has not performed activities or achieved outcomes within the expected time frame.

caring behavior Actions that show compassion and respect for another's perceptions, feelings, needs, and desires.

circumstances The conditions or facts attending an event or having some bearing on it. Used interchangeably with *context*.

classify To arrange or group together data according to categories.

competency The quality of having the necessary knowledge, skill, and attitude to perform an action under various circumstances.

context *See* circumstances.

critical Characterized by careful and exact evaluation; crucial.

cues *See* data.

data Pieces of information about health status (e.g., vital signs).

database assessment Comprehensive data collected when a client first enters the health care facility in order to gain information about all aspects of the health status.

deductive reasoning Drawing specific conclusions from general principles and rules; for example, "Because it is true that bacteria are killed by antibiotics, bacterial infection requires treatment with antibiotics." (*Compare with* inductive reasoning.)

definitive diagnosis The most specific, most correct diagnosis.

definitive interventions The most specific actions required to prevent, resolve, or control a health problem.

diagnose To identify and name health problems after careful analysis of evidence from an assessment.

diagnostic error When a health problem has been missed or incorrectly identified.

diagnostic reasoning A method of thinking that involves specific, deliberate use of ADPIE to reach conclusions about a patient's health status, risk factors, and health problems.

diaphoretic The condition of being sweaty, usually suspected to be a sign of illness (e.g., shock).

disposition One's attitude, customary frame of mind, or manner of response.

diuretic Drug given to enhance kidney function, thereby increasing fluid elimination from the body.

efficiency The quality of being able to produce a desired effect safely, with minimal risks, expense, and unnecessary effort.

emboli More than one embolus. (*See* embolus.)

embolus A clot that has moved through one vessel and lodged in another, reducing or totally blocking blood supply to tissues usually nourished by the vessels involved. (*Compare with* thrombus.)

empathy Understanding another's feelings or perceptions but not sharing the same feelings or point of view. (*Compare with* sympathy.)

empiric Relying solely on practical experience without considering science.

epidemiology The body of knowledge reflecting what is known about a specific health issue.

esthetics A sense of what is pleasing to the eye.

etiology The cause or contributing factors of a health problem.

expedite To make something happen in a quick fashion.

explicit Clearly and specifically expressed or described.

focus assessment Data collection that aims to gain specific information about a certain aspect of health status.

guidelines Documents that delineate how care is to be provided in specific situations.

habits of inquiry Habits that enhance the ability to search for the truth (e.g., verifying that data are correct and following rules of logic).

hospitalist   A medical doctor who manages hospital care.

humanistic   A way of thought or action concerned with the interests or ideals of people.

hypothesis   (1) A hunch. (2) An assertion subject to verification or proof. (*Compare with* assumption and inference.)

imply   To suggest by logical necessity.

indicator   An observable, measurable entity that serves to define a concept in a practical way.

inductive reasoning   Drawing general conclusions by observing a few specific members of a class; for example, "Since everyone I ever knew with a bacterial infection required an antibiotic and Jane has a bacterial infection, Jane requires an antibiotic." (*Compare with* deductive reasoning.)

infer   To suspect something or to attach meaning to information; for example, if someone is frowning, one may infer that he or she is worried.

inference   Something suspected to be true based on a logical conclusion after examination of the evidence. (*Compare with* assumption and hypothesis.)

informatics   The use of health information technology to facilitate the acquisition, storage, retrieval, and use of information by all health care professionals.

interventions   Actions done to prevent, cure, or manage health problems (e.g., turning someone every 2 hours to prevent skin breakdown).

intubation   The process of inserting a tube into an individual's bronchus to facilitate breathing.

intuition   Knowing something without evidence.

irrigate   To flush a tube (with normal saline solution or water) to keep it patent (open and flowing).

life processes   Events or changes that occur during one's lifetime (e.g., growing up, getting married, losing someone).

malpractice   The negligent conduct of a person acting within his or her professional capacity.

measurable   Capable of being clearly observed so that the quality and quantity of something can be readily determined.

medical domain   Actions a physician is legally qualified to perform. Some APNs are also qualified to treat issues normally in the medical domain.

mentor   A knowledgeable, insightful, and trusted person who helps someone else improve his or her thinking or performance.

myocardial infarction   Partial or complete occlusion of one or more of the coronary arteries, causing the death of coronary tissue.

nasogastric tube   A tube inserted through the nose, down the esophagus, and into the stomach.

negligence   Failure to provide the degree of care that someone of ordinary prudence would provide under the same circumstances. To claim negligence, it is necessary that there be a duty owed by one person to another, that the duty be breached, and that the breach cause harm.

nursing assistive personnel (NAP)   Individuals who are trained to assist licensed registered nurse in providing patient care, as delegated by the registered nurse. The term includes, but is not limited to, nurses' aides, medication aides, and other licensed or certified workers.

nursing domain   Actions a nurse is legally qualified to perform.

nursing intervention   An action taken by a nurse to facilitate a patient outcome.

nursing phenomena   Observable occurrences that are concerns of nursing; often considered "human experiences" (e.g., pain, anxiety).

objective data   Information that one can clearly observe or measure (e.g., a pulse of 140 beats per minute).

outcome   The result of interventions.

paradigm   A typical model or way of doing things.

patent   Open, so as to allow the flow of fluid or air.

policies   *See* guidelines.

preceptor   An experienced, qualified nurse assigned by a facility to facilitate learning for a less experienced nurse.

proactive   A way of thinking and behaving that anticipates and prevents problems before they happen.

procedures   *See* guidelines.

protocols   *See* guidelines.

pulmonary embolus   A clot that has blocked off circulation and oxygenation to lung tissue; life threatening.

qualified   Having the competence and authority to perform an action.

quality care   Health care services that increase the probability of achieving desired results with decreased probability of undesired results.

quality improvement (QI)   Ongoing studies designed to identify ways to promote achievement of desired outcomes in a timely, cost-effective manner while decreasing the risks for undesired outcomes.

rales   Abnormal breath sounds (crackles) caused by the passage of air through bronchi containing fluid. This sign is frequently associated with congestive heart failure.

related factor   *See* risk factor.

risk factor   Something known to contribute to (or be associated with) a specific problem. (*See also* etiology.)

signs   Objective data that cause one to suspect a health problem. (*Compare with* symptoms.)

social determinants of health   The conditions in which people are born, grow, work, live, and age, as well as the forces and systems that shape the conditions of daily life.

somnolent   Overly sleepy; difficult to arouse.

stakeholders   The people who will be most affected by care (e.g., patients, families) or from whom requirements will be drawn (e.g., caregivers, third-party payers, health care organizations).

standard of nursing care   The degree of skill, care, and diligence exercised by the members of the nursing profession practicing in the same or a similar locality. Many states refer to standards in their nurse practice acts.

standards   Authoritative statements that describe the responsibilities for which its practitioners are accountable.

subjective data   Information the patient states or communicates; the patient's perceptions (e.g., "My heart feels like it's racing.").

surveillance   The close observation of patients and their surroundings for the purpose of preventing complications or injury.

sympathy   Sharing the same feelings as another. (*Compare with* empathy.)

symptoms   Subjective data that cause one to suspect a health problem. (*Compare with* signs.)

synthesis   The process of putting pieces of information together to make a whole; for example, nurses put individual signs and symptoms together to identify actual and potential problems.

thrombi   More than one thrombus (clot). (*See* thrombus.)

thrombus   A clot that threatens blood supply to tissues. If the clot moves, it becomes an embolus. (*Compare with* embolus.)

tubal ligation   Surgery performed to cut and suture fallopian tubes to prevent pregnancy.

unlicensed assistive personnel (UAP)   Workers who are not licensed by the state but are trained to help with care of patients.

validity   The extent to which something can be believed to be factual and true.

variance in care   *See* care variance.

INDEX

Note: Page numbers followed by *f* indicate figures, *t* indicate tables, and *b* indicate boxes.